Sports Science: A Practical Approach

Sports Science: A Practical Approach

Editor: Jacob Meyer

Callisto Reference
www.callistoreference.com

Callisto Reference,
118-35 Queens Blvd., Suite 400,
Forest Hills, NY 11375, USA

Visit us on the World Wide Web at:
www.callistoreference.com

ISBN: 978-1-63239-958-8 (Hardback)

The publisher's policy is to use permanent paper from mills that operate a sustainable forestry policy. Furthermore, the publisher ensures that the text paper and cover boards used have met acceptable environmental accreditation standards.

Printed in China.

Cataloging-in-Publication Data

Sports science : a practical approach / edited by Jacob Meyer.
p. cm.
Includes bibliographical references and index.
ISBN 978-1-63239-958-8
1. Sports sciences. 2. Sports medicine. I. Meyer, Jacob.
GV558 .S66 2018
613.71--dc23

Table of Contents

Preface

Sports science studies the importance of exercise and the response of the human body to physical training. It incorporates areas such as anatomy, physiology and biokinetics. Sports science has four disciplines namely physiology of sports performance, biomechanics of sporting movement, sports psychology and sociology of sports. This book covers in detail some existent theories and innovative concepts revolving around sports science. It is an essential guide for both academicians and those who wish to pursue this discipline further.

This book has been the outcome of endless efforts put in by authors and researchers on various issues and topics within the field. The book is a comprehensive collection of significant researches that are addressed in a variety of chapters. It will surely enhance the knowledge of the field among readers across the globe.

It gives us an immense pleasure to thank our researchers and authors for their efforts to submit their piece of writing before the deadlines. Finally in the end, I would like to thank my family and colleagues who have been a great source of inspiration and support.

Editor

Multiple injuries in paramotoring: a case report to assess this sport's risks

Francesco Feletti

U.O.Radiologia, Presidio Ospedaliero di Ravenna, Viale Randi 5, Ravenna, Italia

Email address:
feletti@extremesportmed.net(F. Feletti)

Abstract: Paramotoring is a sport clearly distinct from paragliding in which the pilot flies using a special wing and wearing a motor on his back to take off. Generally paramotoring is not considered a high risk sport but since it is a relatively new sport, there aren't any reports in literature about injuries associated with its practice. We report the case of a 48 year old healthy professional athlete which had an accident during takeoff in one of his training flights and received diffuse axonal injury, vertebral fractures and anterior shoulder sprain with associated humeral trochiter fracture. We compared injuries to those connected to the practice of other aerial sports: paragliding in particular. Probably in paramotoring, unlike in paragliding, take-off is the more critical phase of flight and the use of the motor may aggravate the dynamics of trauma in case of accident. Although the patient was wearing a helmet at the time of the incident, he suffered a diffuse axonal injury: probably the impact location and impact speed compromised the effectiveness of helmet. So more research about the biomechanics of traumatic brain injuries in paramotoring is necessary to improve protection systems, such as helmets, to reduce injury risks in this sport. Furthermore padded back protection should be made obligatory when flying with power paragliding.

Keywords: Paramotoring, Power Paragliding, Diffuse Axonal Injury, Trauma, Extreme Sports

1. Introduction

Paramotoring or powered paragliding (PP) is a sport in which the pilot flies using a special wing and wearing a motor on his back to take off. PP was pioneered at the end of the 1980s and quickly increased in popularity so much that in the last few years many national and international championships have taken place all around the world.

The success of PP is mainly due to slow flying characteristics and the ability to land slowly and safely anywhere with no airframe to bend (Fig 1).

To the best of our knowledge there aren't any reports in literature about injuries associated with the practice of PP. Knowledge of the anatomical location and of the kind of injury is vital for sports medicine: helping to highlight which areas may be injured and to address the direction of future preventive research.

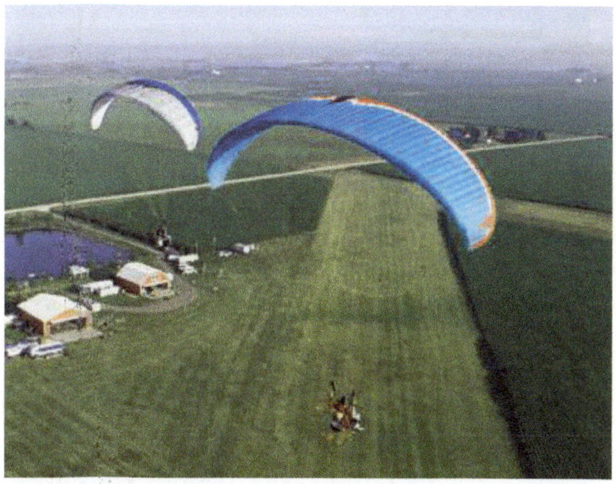

***Fig 1.** Power Paragliding. Photo courtesy of Jeff Goin, United States Powered Paragliding Association, http://www.usppa.org/.*

2. Case Report

A 48 year old healthy professional athlete had an accident during one of his training flights in good weather conditions. During takeoff, after a few meters of flight, as a consequence of a sudden and unexpected gust of wind, one side of the wing collapsed and soon after the wing collapsed: as a consequence the pilot had a hard landing. He wore a flying suit, helmet (UNI-EN 966) goggles and boots. When rescues arrived the patient was awake, apparently in touch with the environment; his cardiac function and blood circulation were stable. The paramotor frame suffered some distortion and disruption from the ground impact but there was no evidence of any pre-impact failures. The patient was immediately transported to the trauma centre.

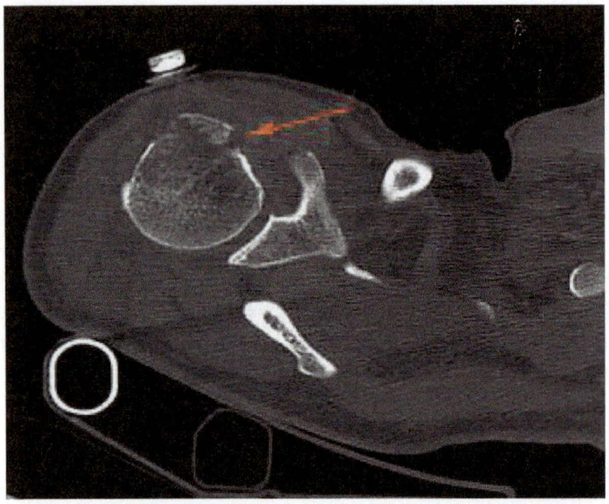

***Fig 2.** Humeral trochiter fracture: TC.*

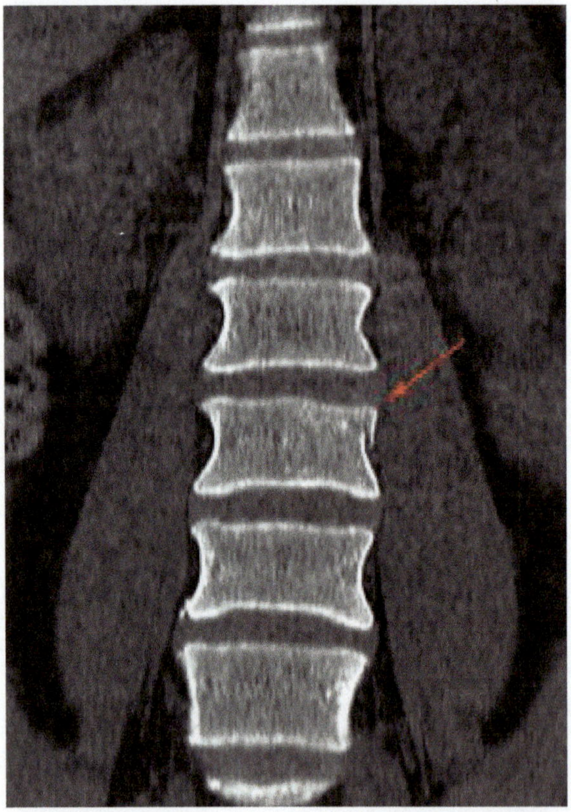

***Fig 3.** Fracture of the left superior lateral margin of L3 vertebral body.*

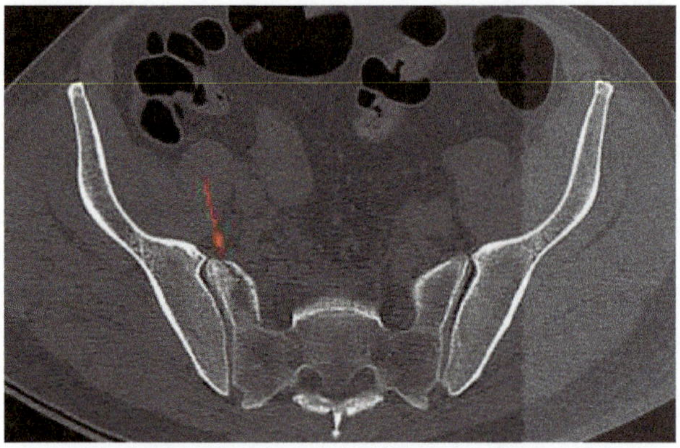

***Fig 4.** Fracture of the right wing of sacrum.*

On presentation he was able to execute simple orders but he had anarthria; his pupils were isocoric and there wasn't any ocular globe misalignment or blepharoptosis, nor evident visual field defect.

The patient had no impairment of sensitivity and muscle strength.

A plantar reflex assessment on the left showed a minimal upward response.

The patient didn't execute the commands necessary for finger-to-nose test and heel-knee test.

The Mingazzini manoeuvre was impossible because of severe hip pain especially on the right. Radiologic examinations showed anterior shoulder sprain with associated humeral trochiter fracture, the fracture of the right wing of sacrum and also fracture of the left superior lateral margin of L3 vertebral body (Fig 2, 3, 4). CT examination of the head showed a few white matter petechial hemorrhages and only minimal subarachnoid hemorrhage (Fig 5).

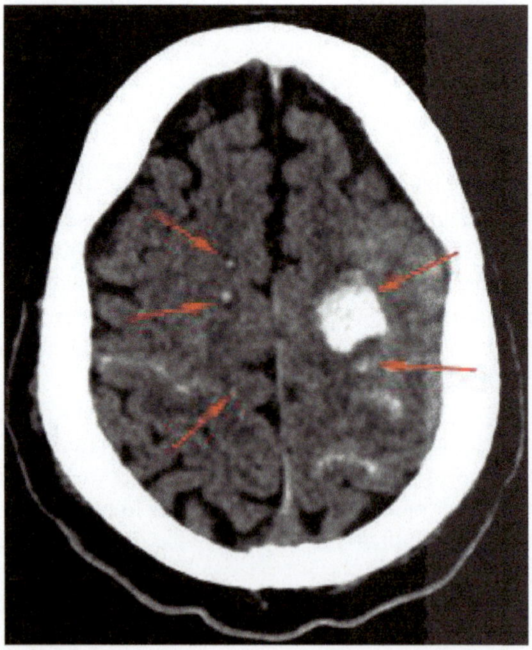

***Fig 5.** CT examination of the head: a few white matter petechial hemorrhages and only minimal subarachnoid hemorrhage.*

The patient also underwent MR imaging of the brain within 24 h: findings were consistent with the diagnosis of diffuse axonal injury (DAI) (Fig 6).

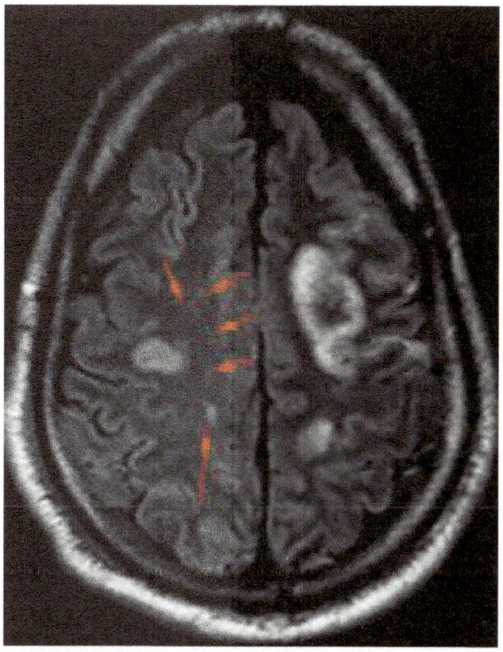

(a)

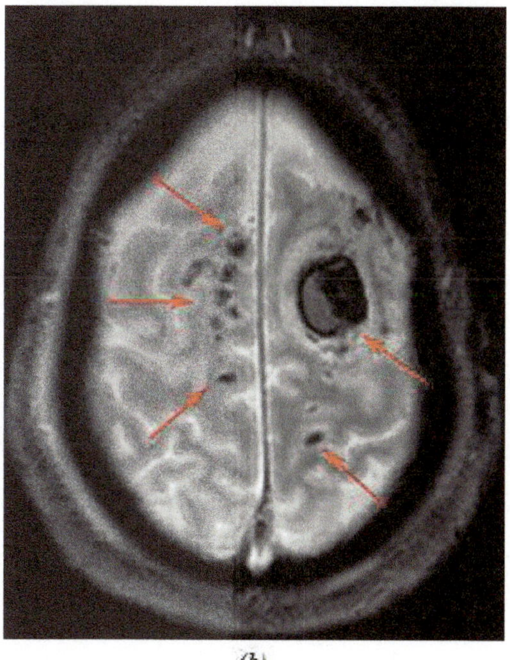

(b)

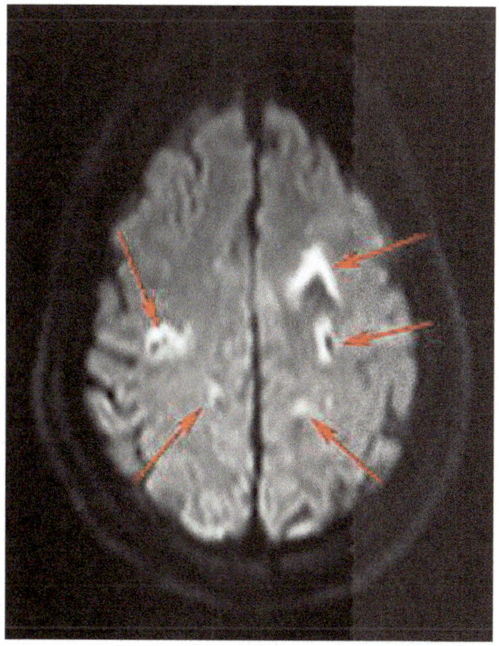

(c)

Fig 6. a,b,c. *MR of the brain shows an higher number of diffuse axonal injuries than TC a. FLAIR long TR, b. Transverse T2w FFE, c. DWI Sense.*

3. Discussion

PubMed, Embase, Cochrane, ProQuest International and Medline were searched using the terms 'paramotoring' and 'powered paragliding': we didn't find any article regarding health problems or trauma connected to the practice of this sport.

PP is a sport clearly distinct from paragliding. The way to fly the PP is greatly different from that of both paragliding and hang gliding, but also from that of light aircraft. Takeoff is the phase of flight which particularly distinguishes PP from both free flight (FF) (paragliding and hang gliding) and from other different kinds of motorized flight. In contrast to light aircrafts the motor acts on the sail, to which however is not strictly bound: in fact, the motor exerts its thrust on the crew, who is suspended from the wing by means of long cables. Unlike FF the use of a propeller allows PP to take off from flat areas without the need of a slope. Furthermore in PP crew weight contributes to the inflation of the canopy in a much less decisive way than in FF.

In spite of these differences, paragliding is the most similar to PP, compared to other aerial sports. So since the kind of injuries connected to the practice of paragliding is well known, we adopted this sport as a term of comparison. Injuries caused by FF are always sudden-onset injuries: there are no reports of overuse injuries in these sports (Rekand T, 2012).

The PP is generally considered much safer than the FF as the engine greatly simplifies both the flight and the landing, which is the most critical phase in FF. In fact the PP is generally employed in optimum atmospheric conditions, without gradients or strong wind, and in environments with few obstacles; on the contrary the optimal location and condition for FF are mountains with windy conditions.

In the case reported the cause of accident was a sudden collapse of the glide. Similarly to FF, also in PP misjudgement of wind conditions along with sudden changes of wind may cause accidents: in paragliding the collapse of the glider is the most common cause of accident in PP it could be the same (Zeller T, et al. 1992).

Whereas landing is the most dangerous phase of a flight in FF (Schulze W, et al. 2002) in the case reported, the accident happened during takeoff. It is possible that in PP takeoff is the more critical phase of flight. In fact at this stage of flight there must be balance between engine thrust, crew weight and lift of the wing and a sudden closing of the wing is very dangerous. Moreover in the PP takeoff, the displacement is mainly horizontal and the increase in altitude occurs slowly. Thus any space of fall remains long reduced, limiting emergency maneuvers. In this case the height reached was not sufficient to hazard corrective maneuvers nor to employ an emergency parachute.

In the case reported the athlete fractured the sacrum and the body of L3. In paragliding fractures between levels T11-L4 and in the sacral area are common, due to the fact that the pilot sits.In the PP it could be the same since the position of the pilot is similar.

So in PP protection systems for the back such as back protection and airbag harnesses similarly to those used in paragliding should be considered. In our case among all the injuries the head trauma was predominant. Traumatic brain injuries are common in sports accidents and may have both acute and long-lasting effects on neurocognitive function (De Beaumont L, et al. 2009. Solomon GS and Haase RF, 2008. Provenzale JM, 2010). DAI is a clinicopathological entity: widespread axonal damage is necessary for diagnosis in addition to the traumatic history (Davceva N, et al. 2012). DAI together with acute subdural haematoma are typical deceleration trauma and at the same time the two worst head injuries(Davceva N, et al. 2012). Severe brain injuries are more common among hang gliders than among paragliders because of different position of the crew during the flight (Rekand T, 2012). In paramotoring, compared to the FF the thrust of the engine and the weight of the equipment mustbe considered as elements aggravating the dynamics of trauma in case of accident; since according to Newton's law: force = mass x acceleration. Engine displacement varies between 80 cc and 250 cc and the power of the motor varies between 11 to 22,5 kw and the engine thrust is highest during takeoff. The motor is mounted on a special frame worn by the athlete: the overall weight of the equipment and the necessary plant oscillates between 20 and 40 kg. For these reasons paramotor accidents must be considered major traumas and an appropriate diagnostic protocol is mandatory.

DAI is due to angular accelerations and occurs when the head moves coronally and decelerates laterally rather than frontally (De Beaumont L, 2009. Gennarelli TA, 1983. Zwahlen RA, 2007. Wang HC, 2010. McIntosh AS 2011).

In the case reported the patient was wearing a helmet at the time of the incident but the effectiveness of helmets may be compromised due to the impact location and impact speed. It is known that the helmet decreases the linear head accelerations with limited effects in side impact conditions: similarly it has also been reported that the ability of skateboard helmets to reduce brain rotation exists but is not totally efficient (Kumar S, et al. 2012). The possibility of a fall impacting the parietal/temporal regions and of higher angular head accelerations is now considered in studies about protective headgear systems in sports and recreational accidents (Biasca N, 2010. Pellman EJ, 2003. Pellman EJ, 2003. Viano DC, 2007). In motor sports new shell and liner materials with properties optimized to minimize head and brain loads in radial, tangential and oblique impacts are always under consideration (McIntosh AS, 2011). More research about the biomechanics of traumatic brain injuries in paramotoring is necessary and in the future the same technology should be probably applied to the production of helmets for PP.

4. Conclusions

PP is a relatively new sport clearly distinct from paragliding and epidemiological studies on injuries sustained during PP are lacking. Probably in this sport, unlike in paragliding, takeoff is the more critical phase of flight and, even if PP is not considered a high risk sport, the use of the motor may aggravate the dynamics of trauma in case of accident.

Thus padded back protection should be made obligatory when flying with PP.

Finally more research about the biomechanics of traumatic brain injuries in paramotoring is necessary to adopt the best possible safety precautions and improve protection systems, such as helmets, to reduce injury risks in this sport.

Acknowledgements

The present work benefited form the input of Jeff Goin
-B.S. Aeronautical Science, Embry Riddle Aeronautical Univ.
-Capt. 737 Southwest Airlines
-Author, The Powered Paragliding Bible
-President U.S. Powered Paragliding Association

References

[1] N. Biasca, S. Wirth and Y. Tegner. "The avoid ability of head and neck injuries in ice hockey: an historical review". Br J Sports Med , 2002, vol. 36, pp. 410-427.

[2] N. Davceva, V. Janevska, B. Ilievski, G. Petrushevska and Z. Popeska. "The occurrence of acute subdural haematoma and diffuse axonal injury as two typical acceleration injuries". J

Forensic Leg Med, 2012, vol. 19(8), pp. 480-484.

[3] N. Davceva, V. Janevska, B. Ilievski, L. Spasevska and Z. Popeska. "Dilemmas concerning the diffuse axonal injury as a clinicopathological entity in forensic medical practice". Forensic Leg Med, 2012, vol.19 (7), pp. 413-418.

[4] L. De Beaumont, H. Théoret, D. Mongeon, et al. "Brain function decline in healthy retired athletes who sustained their last sports concussion in early adulthood". Brain, 2009, vol. 132, pp. 695-708.

[5] T.A. Gennarelli. "Head injury in man and experimental animals: clinical aspects". Acta Neurochir Suppl, 1983, vol. 32, pp. 1-13.

[6] V.E. Johnson, W. Stewart and D.H. Smith. "Axonal pathology in traumatic brain injury". Exp Neurol, 2012, vol. 20. [Epub ahead of print]. PMID: 22285252

[7] S. Kumar, B. Herbst and D. Strickland. "Experimental biomechanical study of head injuries in lateral falls with skateboard helmet". Biomed Sci Instrum, 2012, vol. 48, pp. 239-245.

[8] A.S. McIntosh, T.E. Andersen, R. Bahr, R. Greenwald, S. Kleiven, M.Turner, M.Varese and P.McCrory. "Sports helmets now and in the future". Br J Sports Med, 2011, vol.45: pp. 1258-1265.

[9] E.J.Pellman, D.C.Viano, A.M.Tucker and I.R. Casson. "Committee on Mild Traumatic Brain Injury, National Football League. Concussion in professional football: location and direction of helmet impacts-Part 2". Neurosurgery, 2003, pp. 53(6), vol. 1328-1340.

[10] E.J.Pellman, D.C.Viano, A.M.Tucker, I.R.Casson and J.F. Waeckerle. "Concussion in professional football: reconstruction of game impacts and injuries". Neurosurgery, 2003, vol. 53(4), pp. 799-812.

[11] J.M. Provenzale. "Imaging of Traumatic Brain Injury: A Review of the Recent Medical Literature". AJR Am J Roentgenol, 2010, vol.194 (1), pp. 16-19.

[12] T. Rekand T. "The Epidemiology of Injury in Hang Gliding and Paragliding". Med Sport Sci, 2012, vol. 58, pp. 44-56.

[13] W. Schulze, J. Richter, B, Schulze, S.A. Esenwein and K. Büttner-Janz. Injury prophylaxis in paragliding. Br J Sports Med, 2002, vol. 36: pp. 365-369.

[14] G.S. Solomon and R.F. Haase. Biopsychosocial characteristics and neurocognitive test performance in National Football League players: an initial assessment. Arch Clin Neuropsychol, 2008, vol. 23: pp. 563-577.

[15] D.C.Viano, I.R.Casson and E.J.Pellman. "Concussion in professional football: biomechanics of the struck player-part 14". Neurosurgery, 2007, vol. 61(2), pp. 313-327.

[16] H.C.Wang, Z.X. Duan, F.F. Wu, L. Xie, H. Zhang and YB Ma. "A new rat model for diffuse axonal injury using a combination of linar acceleration and angular acceleration". J Neurotrauma, 2010. vol. 27 (4), pp. 707-719.

[17] T. Zeller, A Billing and Lob G. "Injuries in paragliding". Int Orthop 1992, vol. 16, pp. 225-259.

[18] R.A. Zwahlen, L. Labler, O. Trentz , KW. Grätz and L.M. Bachmann "Lateral impact in closed head injury: A substantially increased risk for diffuse axonal injury-A preliminary study". J Craniomaxillofac Surg, 2007, vol. 35(3), pp.142-146.

2

Paroxysmal atrial fibrillation: Scuba diving or hyperbaric oxygen therapy

Raja Ben Sassi[2], Karima Taamallah[1, 3], Imen Mezoughi[2], Walid Belhaj Brahim[2], Zied Hajjej[1, 4], Hedi Gharsallah[1, 2]

[1]Université de Tunis El Manar, Faculté de Médecine de Tunis, 1007, Tunis, Tunisie
[2]Hôpital militaire de Tunis, centre d'oxygénothérapie hyperbare, 1008, Tunis, Tunisie
[3]Hôpital militaire de Tunis, service de chirurgie cardiaque, 1008, Tunis, Tunisie
[4]Hôpital militaire de Tunis, service d'anesthésie réanimation, 1008, Tunis, Tunisie

Email address:
gharsallahhedi@gmail.com (H. Gharsallah)

Abstract: Heart rhythm disorders are widely reported as complications of scuba diving but rarely after HBO therapy. We report the case of a professional diver who developed a paroxysmal atrial fibrillation after hyperbaric oxygen therapy as treatment of diving accident. It is a professional diver admitted for the treatment of a cochleovestibular desaturation accident. The initial ECG showed normal sinus rhythm. He received 10 HBO therapy sessions. We discovered a heart rhythm disorder. The ECG showed an atrial fibrillation. Heart rhythm returned to sinus after receiving FLECAIN®. Control ECG after 2 months showed a normal sinus rhythm.

Keywords: Atrial Fibrillation - HBO Therapy - Scuba Diving

1. Introduction

Scuba diving and diving in a hyperbaric chamber are two conditions that expose to the complications of overpressure. Heart rhythm disorders are widely reported as complications of scuba diving but rarely after HBO therapy.

We report the case of a professional diver who developed a paroxysmal atrial fibrillation after hyperbaric oxygen therapy as treatment of a diving accident.

2. Case Description

Our patient is a 33 years old professional diver admitted for the treatment of a cochleovestibular desaturation accident due to a 30 minutes dive at 60 meters depth. While emerging out of water he presented rotary vertigo which became disabling when he arrived to the surface. Clinical examination at the hyperbaric oxygen therapy center upon admission found a patient presenting a serious vertigo crisis with no other neurological localization signs. Eardrum examination was normal. Initial heart auscultation was normal and ECG showed normal sinus rhythm (fig 1A).

Treatment in our center consisted in a first HBO emergency recompression session at 18 m (2.8ATA) that improved partially the symptoms followed by 10 consolidation sessions. The outcome was favorable: disappearance of the vertigo at the end of treatment. Cerebro- medullary MRI showed no abnormalities. While performing a transthoracic echocardiography (in search of patent foramen ovale), we discovered a heart rhythm disorder. ECG showed an atrial fibrillation (fig 1B). The rhythm returned to normal after receiving FLECAIN®. No patent foramen ovale was found in transoesophagal echocardiography. The patient was advised not to undertake diving activities any more. Control ECG after 2 months showed a normal sinus rhythm (fig 1C).

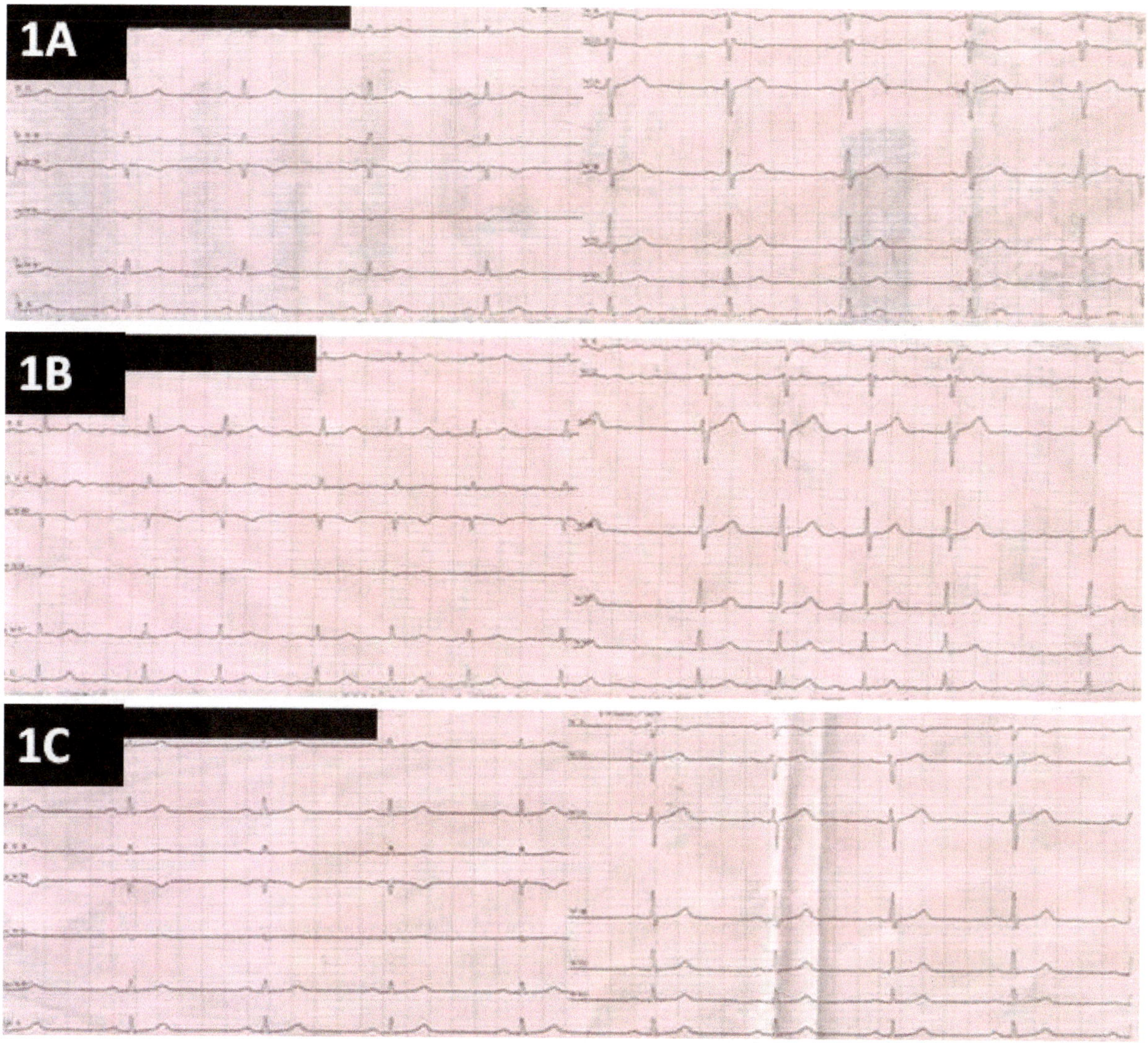

Fig 1. *Patient's electrocardiograms: 1A: Before HBO therapy, 1B: Atrial fibrillation after 10 sessions of HBO therapy, 1C: after 2months of follow up: return to sinus rythm*

3. Discussion

Paroxysmal atrial fibrillation is the most frequent supraventricular heart rhythm disorder. It is a high risk condition for thromboembolic disease. Valvular disease and myocardial injury are usually the underlying causes. In scuba diving, paroxysmal atrial fibrillation is associated to two physiopathological mechanisms. The first is mechanical related to the high pressure while emerging under water. The second is nervous via the activation of skin thermo receptors.It involves also other conditions: temperature of water, diving procedures and diving suit. In fact, conflict between the two components of the autonomic nervous system; bradycardia resulting from parasympathetic stimulation during diving on one hand and tachycardia due to sympathetic stimulation of the skin thermo receptors on the other hand, can lead to heart rhythm disorders. Some risk factors predispose to heart rhythm disorders: hereditary or acquired syndrome of long QT, hypertensive cardiomyopathy, stress and tiredness (1). Schipke et al. showed that scuba diving causes psychological stress (2).

Our patient had no cardiovascular risk factors, trans-oesophagal echocardiography showed no PFO. Nevertheless, he reported that the water was quiet cold and he was exhausted from daily diving session during the last month.

Hyperbaric oxygen therapy is a treatment procedure that consists in giving the patient oxygen at a pressure higher than the level of atmospheric pressure allowing a hyper oxygenation of the tissues. Diving accident is a type 1 recommendation *(second EUROPEAN consensus conference on the treatment of decompression illness from recreational diving. Marseille, May 9 to 11, 1996)*.The complications of HBO treatment are mostly barotraumas of the medial ear, the sinus or the lungs and toxicity due to hyperoxia. Clinical signs of hyperoxia are generally neurological. Cardiac impact is not described in literature. In fact, only one author published the occurrence of paroxysmal atrial fibrillation after a HBO session in a carbon monoxide poisoning case. He supposed that inhibition of the conduction in the atrial sinus due to hyperoxigenation led to this heart rhythm disorder (3). This case report has raised a serious controversy (4). This complication appeared after a variable period of time. Our patient was initially asymptomatic. His arrhythmia was discovered accidently after the end of the sessions. Therefore we cannot precise the exact moment of happening of this trouble. The rhythm returned to sinus after oral intake of FLECAIN®. No ECG abnormalities were detected during the follow up period.

In our case, we cannot dismiss two etiologies. The first one is scuba diving but initial ECG showed regular sinus rhythm. The second etiology is HBO treatment since it is closely related to the appearance of this arrhythmia especially as echocardiography showed no organic abnormalities. No distant recurrence was detected because there was no more exposure to scuba diving or HBO treatment.

Finally, two questions need to be answered:

1) Is ECG monitoring interesting for the patients before and after HBO sessions?
2) Can this patient take up scuba diving again?

4. Conclusion

Although Cardiac rhythm disorder due to scuba diving is a plausible hypothesis, the role played by HBO therapy in the genesis of this trouble cannot be discarded. ECG monitoring can be useful before and after HBO therapy sessions.

References

[1] M.J. Schattock, M.J. Tipton. Autonomic conflict: a different way to die during cold water immersion? J. Physiol 2012; 590(14):3219–3230.

[2] J.D. Schipke, M. Pelzer. Effect of immersion, submersion, and scuba diving on heart rate variability. Br. J. Sports Med 2001; 35:174-180.

[3] G. Celbek, B.V. BOZ. Paroxysmal atrial fibrillation after hyperbaric oxygen therapy. Am J Emerg Med 2013;31:261.e5 – 261.e7.

[4] N. Zamani. The cause of Paroxysmal atrial fibrillation: hyperbaric oxygen therapy or carbon monoxide poisoning. Am J Emerg Med. 2013;31(1):247.

Assessment of patellar alignment in different postures

Hugo Machado Sanchez[1], Eliane Gouveia de Morais Sanchez[2], Mario Antonio Baraúna[3], Roberto Sérgio de Tavares Canto[4]

[1]Master Physical Therapy, Teacher of Physical Therapy in UniRV (University of Green River), Rio Verde-GO, Brazil
[2]Master in Education (UFU), Rio Verde-GO, Brazil
[3]PhD. in Motricity Human for University of Lisboa (POR), Uberlândia-MG, Brazil
[4]Post-doctoral in Traumatology for University of Liverpool (ING), Uberlândia-MG, Brazil

Email address:
hmsfisio@yahoo.com.br (H. M. Sanchez)

Abstract: Introduction: The evaluation of Q angle is a common clinical practice however standardization regarding the best way does not exist. Objective: Compare the value of the Q angle in different static positions and rotations of lower limbs. Methods: Evaluated 56 volunteers, 30 women and 26 men, in the supine andunder static weight-bearing positions with parallel feet and with outward foot rotation. For calculate Q angle used Computerized Biophotogrammetry. Results: Have significant difference between the static weight-bearing position with parallel feet and static weight-bearing with outward foot rotation in the left side for both the sexes (p=0.00) and between the supine position with outward foot rotation and static weight-bearing with parallel feet of the left side (p=0.03), in the feminine sex. Conclusion: it is concluded that there are no differences between different positions and postures to review the Q angle, however we stress the importance of checking the relaxation of the muscles of the lower limbs.

Keywords: Q angle, Alignment, Evaluation, Computerized Biophotogrammetry

1. Introduction

The quadriceps angle, or Q angle is the angle formed by the meeting of two lines, one part of the anterior superior iliac spine (ASIS) and goes to the center of the patella, and another that goes from the tibial tuberosity to the center of patella [1-7]. It is a clinical measure used to measure knee alignment with respect to the hip, femur and tibia, as well as evaluating the alignment of the patella [5,9]. However, there is no universal acceptance of normal or abnormal Q angle due to the lack of a reliability coefficient and the different methods of measurement for this angle [7].

According to Livingston; Mandingo[8], the symmetry of the Q angle between members is also because of disagreements among different authors in their study evaluated 75 volunteers divided into three groups (no anterior knee pain , pain unilateral and bilateral pain) and verified by analysis protractor with volunteers standing upright, the values of the angles were asymmetric for the three groups, but that this asymmetry varied between groups .

Besides the Q angle assist in indicating the force vector acting on the patela[1,2,5,6,9], is also used as a criterion to identify candidates for surgery or predictor of risk of injury [5,6,9]. So that changes in the value of Q angle are associated with chondromalacia patella, lateral dislocation of the patella , patellar cartilage and erosion of the lateral condyle, femoral internal rotation, foot pronation and internal tibial torsion[3,4,7]. According Devan et al.[10], changes in Q angle in valgus knees alter the biomechanics and impairs muscle levers and therefore its functions.

The Q angle shows an inverse relationship with quadriceps strength, thus the smaller the angle the greater the force produced by the quadriceps, which assumes that individuals with above normal Q angle have lower quadriceps strength and are more subject to diseases of the joint patellofemoral [6].

The value of Q angle varies according to the sex of the patient, the state of contraction of the quadriceps and the position adopted by the patient, standing or supine [3]. The rotation of the lower limbs have direct influence on the alignment of the knees, changing them according to their placement[4,5,8,11-13]. The lack of a consensus on the normal Q angle is partly due to the absence of a standard positioning for measuring the angle [5].

The computerized biophotogrammetry uses the principle to photogrammetric images. It shows how non invasive, offering low-cost acquisition system and image interpretation, as well as the high accuracy and reproducibility. The image interpretation is the constant observation of the image to completion and issuance of a relevant report. References are marked in subjects evaluated by computerized biophotogrammetry. This demarcation is fundamental to the study and analysis of dados[11]. Other studies have already used this resource to evaluate the Q angle confirming its practicality and effectiveness [7,18].

Thus, the aim of this study was to compare the values of the Q angle in relation to supine and standing.

2. Material and Methods

To carry out this study, we randomly selected 56 volunteers - 26 men and 30 women, all undergraduates.

Included in this study university without pathological complaints in the lower limbs, and sedentary. Being excluded individuals with presence of musculoskeletal injuries in the lower limbs, lower limbs discrepancy greater than 1.5 cm, which have suffered fracture, dislocation, or previous surgery of the lower limbs, obese, with diseases of the bone, muscle or connective with neurological disorders or with sequelae of poliomyelitis and volunteers who were in the gestational period.

This study was performed after approval (opinion s/n) of the Ethics in Human Research following the existents regulations. Participants were informed about the objectives of the study and had free will to choose to participate or not the same.

The volunteers who agreed to participate in the study signed a Letter of Informed Consent and underwent an assessment where held by the same person. Then it was done filling the evaluation form that contained the personal data of volunteers, the length of the lower limbs and issues related to the exclusion criteria. Has completed filling up the identification of anatomical landmarks and placement of markers, positioning the participant to capture the image, and the photographic record.

Then, for continuation of proceedings volunteers remained barefoot and appropriate clothing (shorts or underwear), so as to be easily located and viewed the anatomical points. The identification and demarcation of anatomical points - anterior superior iliac spine and the tibial tuberosity - was through palpatory anatomy. The center point of the patella was located by using the caliper for a reliable determination of this point.

After identification of anatomical landmarks, they were marked with labels delimiting circular self -adhesive.

Demarcated the anatomical landmarks for the Q angle the process of data collection proceeded as follows.

For the standardization of the image, with the volunteer standing upright, two sites were previously demarcated on the ground, was the first demarcated following the suggestion of Livingston; Spaulding [5] , in which the feet are placed together touching medially (standing position with feet parallel - OPP), lined with an adhesive on the floor. The volunteers were instructed to keep the quadriceps muscle of both limbs relaxed, eyes to the horizon and arms along the body (Figure 1A). Then immediately proceeded to obtain the second image, in which the volunteer remained standing upright and maintained a separation of 7.5 cm heel and forefoot external rotation of 10 degrees from the midline 13 (standing position with feet abducted - OPA) , quadriceps relaxed , eyes to the horizon and arms along the body (Figure 1B). To obtain the images with the volunteers in the upright position, the camera was positioned on a tripod level and plumb to a height of 0.90 m above the ground and the distance of 2.90 m from volunteer in order to capture the image hip to foot when he was bearing.

After the collection of the second image, the volunteer was placed in the supine position, anatomical points rescheduled and instructed to maintain position without rotation of the lower limbs, ie, keeping the hip in a neutral position (lying with feet parallel - DPP), knees extended, relaxed ankle, thus keeping your feet parallel and quadriceps muscles relaxed (Figure 1C). For the acquisition of the fourth image was changed just the positioning of the feet (lying with feet abducted - DPA), which are adjusted in the same way that the second image ortostatismo[9] (Figure 1D). For this position was made a positioner that kept the legs of volunteers with external rotation desired. At this stage of acquiring images with the volunteer supine, the camera was positioned in a lateral support to the mat, parallel to the ground and at a height of 1.70m in order to capture the image of the hip to the foot of each volunteer.

The alignment of the lower limb of the volunteers was controlled by positioning / rotation of membership, without other adjustments related to the joints of the foot or hip[5].

The entire process of marking the anatomical landmarks and image acquisition was performed three times in each of four positions in said sequence, totaling 12 markings / images per volunteer so that three values was obtained for each angular position being used to statistical analysis the average of three values obtained at each position. The importance of the points between each redial picture taking in the positions analyzed was important because of the possible change of location paths adhesive when it rolled members and / or modified up posture of 9 volunteers.

Finalized the registration of these images were transported to a computer, where we proceeded to analysis using computerized biophotogrammetry through the application ALCimage 2.1 ®. Angular measurements were verified from the union of anatomical points previously marked. To calculate the Q angle was drawn a line that came from the anterior superior iliac spine to the center of the patella and thence to the tibial tuberosity by drawing an angle corresponding to the quadriceps angle.

In order to check the difference between the values of the angle Q between members postures evaluated, was used the Student t test, and the comparison between the values with and without rotation of the lower limb. To check for possible differences in Q angle cross-comparison of the four positions of each limb, was used analysis of variance (ANOVA) followed by Tukey test. The level of significance was set at p less than 5 %.

3. Results

The average age of male subjects was 21.33 ± 2.20, and female literacy of 20.81 ± 3.13 years.

In Table 1 are shown the descriptive analysis of the data for men and women bilaterally. The four positions analyzed were lying parallel feet (DPP), lying open toe (DPA) , orthostatic open toe (OPA) and standing feet parallel (OPP) .

The differences in values between right and left Q angle were calculated for males and females in all postures and positioning to assess bilateral symmetry, not finding a difference between the angular values in any of four positions evaluated for both sex (Table 2).

Table 3 shows the comparison of the angle Q between the positions of the feet, separating the lying and standing postures. When analyzed separately for each sex, found a significant difference between the values in upright positions with legs open and feet parallel on the left side in both sexes, the same as for the total group.

Comparing the positions evaluated together without cross between right and left limbs, there was statistical difference only when comparing the standing position and walk parallel orthostatic hemi body left standing open.

4. Discussion

Our evaluation of the Q angle of 56 university students of both sexes in order to assess possible variations in measurement. The evaluation was performed following a protocol previously developed based on extensive literature review. The sample was composed of students of both sexes aged 17-31 years. In this age group [2,5-7,12,13] several studies were conducted, and are present symptoms of anterior knee pain and pathologies such as patellofemoral dysfunction. Also at this age, the knees do not have bone growth, and there are degenerative diseases that could alter the angle Q.

The methodology used in the present study, we used sensitive equipment and reliable, using the caliper and computerized photogrammetry[9, 11]. The use of the caliper is suggested by France; Nester[9], as an indispensable tool for the demarcation of anatomical landmarks difficult location, minimizing errors in this item. Another important item was the demarcation and getting pictures taken at [3], allowing a more reliable the results [9]. Finally, the methodology used to select a reliable and validated tool, computerized biophotogrammetry, which allows accurate quantitation and non- invasive [11]. Studies such as Tsujimoto et al.[13] used the CT or radiography, which are reliable resources, but costly , and expose the volunteer radiation. Other tests such as Tomsich et al.[17], Kuhn et al.[4], was used a goniometer, which has questionable reliability and reproducibility.

Assessment of quadriceps angle is commonly performed unilaterally, since the members would be symmetrical. However, Livingston[18] emphasizes the need for studies with bilateral assessment of members. This study compared the Q value of the angle bilaterally resulting in a symmetry in all positions statistical analysis. Just as Herrington; Nester [7], assessing 109 volunteers in the standing position, feet parallel. This confirms the reliability of the current data, as the author mentioned herein evaluated a larger group finding similar results to this study. Already Hahn; Foldspang[11] in 339 athletes found differences between the right and left Q angles. Livingston; Spaulding[5], the reason for this difference is not yet clear, suggesting there is no explanation for this. Livingston; Mandingo[8], the difference in values between both sides, is explained by the higher tropism and muscle tone on the dominant side, which would cause a force on the patella displaces it and decreasing the value of the angle. The discrepancy between the results of the present study and Hahn; Foldspang[11], due to use of more accurate methods, is to use the average of three measurements, and the use of the caliper to locate the center of the patella.

The literature suggested the use of supine and standing postures [5,6,8,11,18], linking these to external and internal rotation of the lower limbs [5,7,19]. Another variable in the evaluation of the Q angle is contraction or relaxation of the quadriceps muscle [5,6,8,15-17,20] because the patella rises when this muscle is triggered [15,17,18,20] . That said, this study evaluated the Q angle with the quadriceps muscle relaxed ever, as well as being most used method in current studies [5,6,8,15,13,18,20] wanted to evaluate the said angle without changes imposed by the contraction muscle .

The current study evaluated 56 volunteers, asymptomatic and showed no difference between the values by changing the angular rotations of the lower limbs in the supine position. Olerud; Berg[19], assessed 34 asymptomatic individuals with internal and external rotations in the supine position, found that the amplitude of the Q angle increases in internal rotation and external rotation decreases. This difference in results is attributed to the greater number of volunteers in the current study, by using up method for localization of anatomical points more reliable, and use is the average of three values for each position, which provides greater reliability and veracity of the results presented. Comparing the values of the angle in the standing position with the leg rotated internally and externally, in both sexes, revealed no difference only on the left side. Livingston ; Spaulding[5], rated the Q angle in the standing position in 20 individuals of both sexes, through computerized analysis in three positions. They found differences in the comparison between all positions for both members. This study found similar results, since significant difference was found between the rotations in standing position, for both sexes, the left lower limb. When referring to the right side, dominant in 95 % of the population, this difference was not found. Attributed to it once more to the fact that we use is the method most thorough evaluation of this angle. As suggested by France & Nester[9], to obtain results more confident and reduce evaluation errors, material is used for precise location of the center of the patella, and takes place three measurements of the angle. In addition, this study evaluated a larger number of volunteers, giving greater credibility to our results when compared to the study of Livingston; Spaulding[5].

The right lower limb was not found difference between the placement of members with internal and external rotation bearing. Among the possible explanations is the possibility that there changes in muscle electrical activity between members of dominant and non-dominant, such a statement is quoted by Ounpuu; Winter[21], Bagesteiro; Sainburg[22] , show no difference in central motor control , keeping the muscles of the lower limbs more dominant tone. Changes in the electrical activity of muscle and torque can be present even in subjects evaluated with the request for relaxation of the muscles of the lower limb, because changes in the alignment, as tibial rotation and femoral neck antiversion generate co-contractions in the muscles of the knee and hip regardless of the wishes of the volunteer as reported by Bagesteiro; Sainburg[22]. This in turn could alter the positioning member, causing alteration of the angle Q. Another possible explanation for the difference has occurred between the dominant and non-dominant rotation is in the femur, as described by and Sanfridsson et al. [23], to report that the biomechanics of the lower limbs varies according to the position of the member may medial rotation of the femur lead to an increase of the values of the angle Q, and both, or be associated tibial rotation. However, these variables were not controlled in this study.

Livingston; Spaulding[5], after studying the Q angle in the standing position with different rotations, concluded that the ideal position is standing with feet parallel. The assessment with external rotation is not recommended because it produces discomfort to the patient and may represent an angle changed. This study agrees with the above- mentioned regarding the discomfort of maintaining external rotation once the volunteers reported more discomfort and greater difficulty maintaining quadriceps relaxed in this position. Thus Livingston; Spaulding[5] suggest that in future studies, whether used upright posture and feet parallel. Moreover, Olerud; Berg[19], report that the evaluation should be in a supine posture, and this is the best reported to evaluate the angle Q. Observing the variables, there is the conviction that an important point when evaluating the angle Q, is used for precise methodology, reducing measurement errors. How to correct posture, highlight the supine position, for not influence muscle and femoral rotations imposed by orthostatic[16]. With respect to rotation, the inner seems to be the best, being easily positioned as they do not require the positioned can be performed at any location.

This study is limited with regard to the control of the positioning of the femoral neck (femoral neck antiversion), since no radiographs were analyzed to measure this variable.

5. Conclusion

From the results obtained, it is concluded that there there is little or no difference between the analyzed positions, ie, the angle Q values do not change with the rotation member. Thus, it can be concluded that in the supine position there is asymmetry independent of the rotation angle Q of the hip, which does not occur in the standing position. From the conclusion above, it can be suggested that the Q angle can be measured in the supine position without rotation of membership, this position, easily adopted and standardized for measuring this angle clinically.

Thanks

Thanks to CAPES-PROSUP for the scholarship Master.

References

[1] Heiderscheit BC, Hamill J, Van Emmerik REA. Q-angle influences on the variability of lower extremity coordination during running. Med Sci Sports Exerc. 1999; 31(9):1313-1319.

[2] Heiderscheit BC, Hamill J, Caldwell GE. Influence of Q-angle on lower-extremity running kinematics. JOSPT 2000; 30(5):271-278.

[3] Biedert RM & Warnke, K. Correlation between the Q angle and the patella position: a clinical and axial computed tomography evaluation. Arch Orthop Trauma Surg 2001; 121:346-349.

[4] Kuhn R, Yochum TR, Cherry AR, Rodgers SS. Immediate changes in the Quadriceps Femoris angle after insertion of an orthotic device. J Maniopulative Physio Ther 2002; 25(7):465-470.

[5] Livingston LA & Spaulding SJ. Measurement of the Quadriceps Angle Using Standardized Foot Positions. J Athl Train 2002; 37(3):252-255.

[6] Herrington L & Nester C. Q-angle undervalued? The relationship between Q-angle and medio-lateral position of the patella. Clin Biomech 2004; 19(10):1070-1073.

[7] Melo de Paula GM, Molinero de Paula VR, Almeida GJM, Machado VEI, Baraúna MA, Bevilaqua-Grosso D. Correlação entre a dor anterior do joelho e a medida do ângulo Q por intermédio da fotogrametria computadorizada. Rev Bras Fis 2004; 8(1):39-43.

[8] Livingston LA & Mandingo JL. Bilateral Q angle asymmetry and anterior knee pain syndrome. Clin Biomech 1999; 14(1):7-13.

[9] France, L & Nester, C. Effect of errors in the identification of anatomical landmarks on the accuracy of Q angle values. Clin Biomech 2001; 16(8):710-713.

[10] Devan MR, Pescatello LS, Faghri JA. A Prospective Study of Overuse Knee Injuries Among Female Athletes With Muscle Imbalances and Structural Abnormalities. J Athl Train 2004; 39(3):263-267.

[11] Hahn T & Foldspang A. The Q angle and sport. Scand J Med Sci Sports. 1997; 7(1):43-8.

[12] Lathinghouse LH & Trimble MH. Effects of isometric quadriceps activation on the Q-angle in women before and after quadriceps exercise. JOSPT 2000; 30(4):211-6.

[13] Tsujimoto K, Kurosaka M, Yoshiya S, Mizuno K. Radiographic and computed tomographic analysis of the po sition of the tibial tubercle in recurrent dislocation and subluxation of the patella. Am J Knee Surg 2000; 13(2):83-8.

[14] Iunes DH, Castro FA, Salgado HS, Moura IC, Oliveira AS, Bevilaqua-Grossi D. Confiabilidade Intra e Interexaminadores e Repetibilidade da Avaliação Postural pela Fotogrametria. Rev Bras Fis 2005; 9(3):327-334.

[15] Livingston LA. The quadriceps angle: a review of the literature. JOSPT 1998; 28(2):105-9.

[16] Woodland LH & Francis RS. Parameters and comparisons of the quadriceps angle of college-aged men and women in the supine and standing positions. Am J Sports Med 1992; 20(2):208-11.

[17] Tomsich DA, Nitz AJ, Threlkeld AJ, Shapiro R. Patellofemoral alignment: reliability. JOSPT 1996; 23(3):200-8.

[18] Huberti HH & Hayes WC. Patellofemoral contact pressures: the influence of q-angle and tendofemoral contact. J Bone Joint Surg Am. 1984; 66(5):715-24.

[19] Olerud C & Berg P. The variation of the Q angle with different positions of the foot. Clin Orthop. 1984; 191:162-5.

[20] Raveendranath R, Nachiket S, Sujatha N, Priya R, Rema D. Bilateral Variability of the Quadriceps Angle (Q angle) in an Adult Indian Population. Iran J Basic Med Sci. 2011 Sep;14(5):465-71.

[21] Ounpuu S & Winter DA. Bilateral electromyographical analysis of the lower limbs during walking in normal adults. Electro Clin Neurophysiol. 1989; 72(5):429-38.

[22] Bagesteiro LB &Sainburg RL Handedness: dominant arm advantages in control of limb dynamics. J Neurophysiol. 2002; 88(5):2408-21.

[23] Sanfridsson J, Arnbjornsson A, Friden T, Ryd L, Svahn G, Jonsson K. Femorotibial rotation and the Q-angle related to the dislocating patella. Acta Radiol. 2001; 42(2):218-24.

4

Computational aerodynamics of baseball, soccer ball and volleyball

Pouya Jalilian, Patrick K. Kreun, MohammadHady M. Makhmalbaf, William W. Liou

Department of Mechanical and Aerospace Engineering, Western Michigan University, Kalamazoo, MI 49008, USA

Email address:

pouya.jalilian@wmich.edu (P. Jalilian), patrick.k.kreun@wmich.edu (P. Kreun),
m.molabaghermakhmalbaf@wmich.edu (M. Makhmalbaf), william.liou@wmich.edu (W. Liou)

Abstract: Recent advances in the computing power of modern computers have made computational fluid dynamics studies particularly interesting and feasible. We used the computational fluid dynamics method to solve the physical governing equations of the air flow around balls of popular sports in typical game conditions and investigated their aerodynamics and the flight characteristics. The work presented here describes the construction of the computational fluid dynamics models for a baseball, volleyball and two soccer balls, and the use of these models to analyze the effects of spin rate, surface pattern, and size for their respective sports. The computational results show significant correlations between ball spin rate and the aerodynamics forces, including drag and lift, for soccer ball, baseball and volleyball. For the baseball, the lift and lateral forces are shown to have also been influenced by the lace orientation.

Keywords: CFD, Baseball, Soccer Ball, Volleyball

1. Introduction

Aerodynamics in sports has attracted attention of scientists and researchers for centuries. The analysis of sporting ball aerodynamics can be traced to Newton, 1672, who studied and reviewed the flight of a tennis ball. A number of experimental and model-based techniques have been employed in studying the flight of sporting balls.

Recent advances in the field of computational fluid dynamics (CFD) have led to a dramatic rise in the pace and relative ease in which these studies can be conducted. The flexibility of CFD lends itself well to be used in investigations of a broad variety of subjects in sports. For example, CFD simulations can help understand the extraordinary motions of soccer ball, or identify the ideal lace orientation to provide the desired trajectory of a baseball pitch. These types of studies are also of interest to sports equipment manufacturers striving to advance the performance characteristics of their products.

This paper will present the computational aerodynamic analysis of two different soccer balls, a baseball and a volleyball. A commercial CFD package has been used. We first compute the aerodynamics of these balls in their typical play conditions to serve as a baseline data for comparisons. The resulting trajectories have also been evaluated and will be presented. We then perform case studies to examine the aerodynamic forces exerted on each ball for a variety of linear and angular velocities, and ball sizes, that are prompted by how the balls are, or can be, played.

1.1. Literature Survey

Advancements in sporting equipment have been fueled not only by the competitive nature of sport, but also a greater understanding of the physics governing the way sports are played. Metha (1985) devised a series of experiments on cricket balls, baseballs and golf balls. Aerodynamic forces were obtained and reported in terms of the spinning rate of the balls. Pallis and Mehta (2002) performed wind tunnel studies for sporting balls. Asai, Ito, Seo and Hitotsubashi (2010) showed that the critical Reynolds number at which the drag force drops dramatically is remarkably smaller for new types of volleyball, resulting in faster ball speed. In other studies (Mizota et al., 2013; Oggiano & Saetran, 2010; Barber & Carré, 2010; Goff & Carré, 2009, 2010; Asai, Seo, Kobayashi, & Sakashita, 2007; Carré, Asai & Haake 2002), wind tunnel tests and trajectory analyses were conducted for different types of soccer balls, including a spinning 32-panel soccer ball that is akin to the generic soccer ball used in this study. Goodwills, Chin and Haake (2004) performed a similar study and compared spinning and non-spinning tennis balls. Barber, Chin, and Carré (2009) used CFD simulation to study aerodynamic behavior of soccer balls. Alam, Chowdhury, Stemmer, Wang, and Yang (2012), and Alam et al. (2011) conducted experiments in order to study the aerodynamic forces of several commercially available soccer balls. Similar studies were performed by Alam et al. (2011) and Alam et al. (2012) on baseballs.

2. Methods

The flow of air around the sporting balls presented in this study is governed by the Navier-Stokes equations, the solutions of which describe the flow field around the sports balls, and thus their aerodynamics characteristics, such as lift and drag. A numerical method for solving the Navier-Stokes equations involves the use of computer to integrate the differential equations and yield a solution. This approach is commonly referred to as CFD and has grown in popularity with the continuing advancements of computing powcr. Thc ANSYS FLUENT 14 softwarc has bccn applicd in various industries and is used in this study. The creation of a CFD model for each ball requires first building a three-dimensional digital model for both the ball and surrounding field of air. These models are then meshed into discrete sub-volumes defining the numerical domain and the appropriate initial and boundary conditions needed for each case being evaluated. These steps are described in the following sections.

2.1. Geometry

Geometric features play an important role in determining the aerodynamic characteristics of the sporting balls. Manufacturers of soccer balls and volleyballs can vary, to an extent, patch patterns, seam designs and surface roughness. They influence the ball's behavior during flight. For the balls used in this study, the more crucial surface features to investigate are seams, laces and patch patterns. To this end, each ball has been carefully modeled to accurately capture these fine, but aerodynamically important surface features.

2.1.1. Soccer Ball and Volleyball

The regulation volleyball with a diameter of 210 mm and two different soccer balls, namely, a generic soccer ball with 220 mm diameter and the 86-panel soccer ball with 225 mm diameter have been selected for study. In the history of soccer, balls of different pattern, size and weight have been used. We have selected two different designs to study the effects of the geometric features of soccer balls. Their geometries were obtained from an open source solid modeling website, GrabCAD (Thompson, 2012; Niven, 2012). Minor irregularities in the geometry files, such as holes and gaps, are removed. Figure 1(a, b and c) illustrates the final geometries used in the CFD simulations.

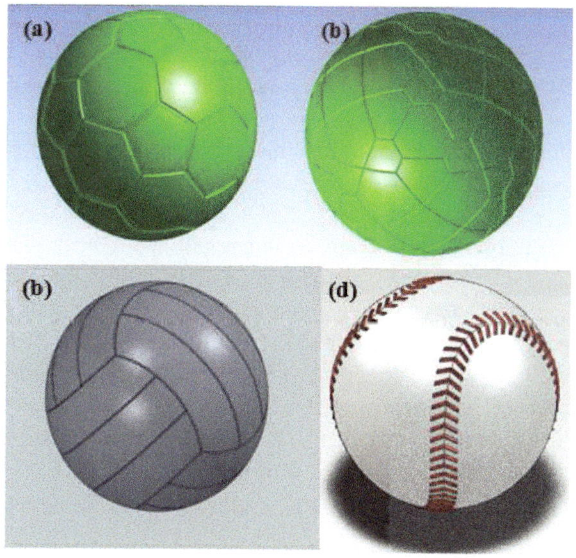

Figure 1. *The generic soccer ball geometry with 220 mm diameter (a), the 86-panel soccer ball geometry with 225 mm diameter (b), the volleyball geometry with 210 mm diameter (c) and the baseball geometry with 73 mm diameter(d).*

2.1.2. Baseball

We created the geometry files for the baseball model using a computer-aided-engineering software. A sphere, 73 mm in diameter was first generated. Then, a three-dimensional sketch was added to the sphere defining the seam pattern. Finally, by generating additional sketch planes, one lace was added to the surface of the sphere and copied using a curve driven pattern command to produce the 108 individual stitches on the surface of the ball, as is shown in Figure 1-d.

2.2. Meshing Generation

Once the geometry was created, the next step was mesh generation in a computational domain, where a computer solution of the Navier-Stokes equations will be sought. Basically, the computational domain must be split into small elements or cells, the collection of which comprises a mesh. Then, the governing equations are discretized for these elements where solutions will be obtained.

2.2.1. General Mesh Structure

Following the successful mesh structure employed by Barber et al. (2009), the general mesh structure we set up is shown in Figure 2.

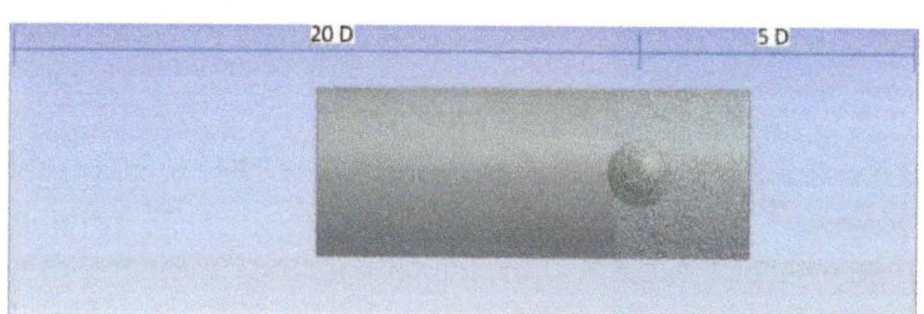

Figure 2. *The chosen general mesh zones including a small sphere, a larger sphere, a cylinder and the enclosure. The ball center was placed 5 diameters from the inlet, 20 diameters from the outlet and 5 diameters from the outer domain boundary sides.*

A ball geometry was imported and a computational domain for the fluid was constructed around the ball by applying a Boolean operation to subtract the ball volume from the surroundings (air). This results in the computational domain for the fluid with a matched fluid-ball boundary. To allow a greater control over the sizes of the mesh elements, three intermediate regions have been used in the computational domain, as illustrated in Figure 2. They include (1) a small sphere immediately surrounding the sporting ball, (2) a larger sphere encompassing the sporting ball and the first sphere, and (3) a cylinder which encloses the ball and the two spheres. The size of the computational domain has been determined in such a way that it reduces the effects of the placement of the outer computational boundaries on the computed flow near the ball.

The process of generating the mesh structures has been utilized for the soccer ball and volleyball, and is only a slightly different from that for the baseball.In this study, the tetrahedron meshing method was used. For the sphere-shaped intermediate regions, the mesh sizes are configured to provide the greatest resolution of the fluid-ball boundary. This is necessary to properly capture the viscous effects of the flow around the rough patches and seams. Meshes were also refined in the cylindrical intermediate region to resolve the flow in the wake of the ball. In the case of the baseball, an additional surface refinement has been applied to the laces to provide sufficient resolution in these regions to capture small-scale flow structures. Figure 3 highlights the finer resolution around the seams and laces for, respectively, soccer ball, volleyball, and baseball.

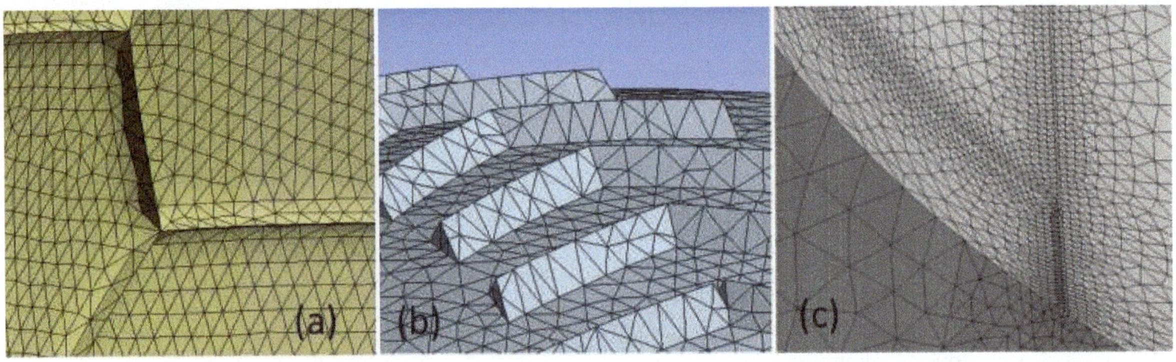

Figure 3. *Meshing near the seams of (a) the 86-panel soccer ball, (b) baseball and (c) volleyball.*

2.2.2. Mesh Quality

To enhance accuracy of the numerical solution, the mesh quality was evaluated. The mesh quality metrics used include the element quality, aspect ratio, Jacobian ratio, warping factor, parallel deviation, maximum corner angle, skewness and orthogonal quality. Each of these quality metrics was assessed for the different sporting ball models and confirmed in accordance with the software's guidelines.

2.3. Setup

After establishing quality meshes, the various CFD runs were properly setup. For this study, a pressure-based, steady-state solver was employed. To include the effect of turbulence in the flow, a realizable k-ε turbulence model was chosen with standard wall treatments. The standard wall-function, near-wall treatment was selected in order to reduce the number of mesh element required near solid surfaces and, thus, the overall mesh counts.

2.3.1. Boundary Conditions

A crucial aspect of properly setting up a CFD model is the definition of the boundary conditions. The primary boundary conditions to consider here are the fluid inlet, fluid outlet, outer fluid boundary, and ball-fluid interface. It should be noted that, although each ball travels with a velocity through the fluid in the physical system, this was modeled as a stationary, rotating ball with the fluid passing around it. In keeping with this change of reference of frame, the inlet (see Figure 2 for reference) was defined having a velocity, normal to the boundary, matching with that specified for the corresponding case being examined. Turbulence at this boundary was specified as having between 0.5% and 1% intensity. A 0.5 m length scale was used, which described low levels of turbulence in the air with relatively large eddy structures, comparing with the sizes of the balls studied. The fluid outlet was described similarly with like turbulence values; however, rather than a velocity, a gauge pressure of 0 Pascal was assigned.

To describe the rotational motion, a moving mesh boundary condition was applied. The moving mesh boundary condition allows the two meshed bodies to slide relative to each other, thereby capturing properly the effects of the rotating surface features, such as laces, seams and patches. The resulting non-conformal mesh is handled by passing fluxes using the non-conformal interface algorithm. An angular velocity about the axis of rotation was specified to match the angular velocity of the corresponding case. The surface roughness of each ball was used to match that of its physical counterpart.

A no-slip shear was applied at the ball surface (wall) and a free-slip shear condition was applied on the outer boundaries of the computational domain.

2.3.2. Solution

The solution process was initialized using the inlet boundary conditions as the initial velocity throughout the fluid domain. Second-order upwinding schemes were employed for the momentum, turbulent kinetic energy, turbulent dissipation, and energy equations.

2.4. Trajectory Analysis

In previous studies (Goff & Carré, 2009, 2010; Carré et al., 2002), sporting ball trajectory was determined from experimetal data. The measured trajectory was then used to obtain drag and lift coefficients. In contrast, in this study, the trajectory is predicted based on the CFD simulated drag and lift forces, and therefore, reflects the simulated aerodynamics of the ball. Figure 4 illustrates a free-body diagram of a ball subjected to the drag, lift and gravitational forces. The ball spins around the horizontal axis perpendicular to the ball's velocity vector and the side force is neglected. With the Newton's second law, the equation governing the motion of the ball can be written as

$$\boldsymbol{F_D} + \boldsymbol{F_L} + m\boldsymbol{g} = m\boldsymbol{a} \quad (1)$$

where m is the mass of the ball, $\boldsymbol{g}$ the vector gravitational acceleration, $\boldsymbol{a}$ ball's vector acceleration. $\boldsymbol{F_D}$ and $\boldsymbol{F_L}$ are drag and lift force vectors, respectively, the magnitudes of which are defined as $F_D=0.5C_D\rho Av^2$ and $F_L=0.5C_L\rho Av^2$, where ρ denotes the air density, A the ball's cross sectional area and v the ball's velocity magnitude. The x and y components of (1) may be written as

$$-\rho Av(C_Lv_y + C_Dv_x) = 2mx'' \quad (2)$$

$$\rho Av(C_Lv_x - C_Dv_y) - 2mg = 2my'' \quad (3)$$

where $v_x=v\cos\theta$, $v_y=v\cos\theta$, $x''=d^2x/dt^2$ and $y''=d^2y/dt^2$. θ denotes the angle between the ball's velocity vector and the horizontal line (x axis), as shown in Figure 4.

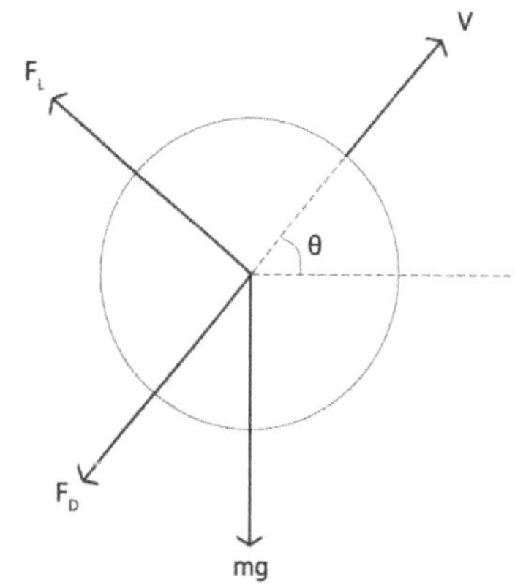

Figure 4. *The free-body diagram of a sporting ball spinning around the axis perpendicular to the page (side view).*

The above system of equations consists of two second order nonlinear ordinary differential equations. The fourth-order Runge-kutta method has been used in a Mathcad (15th version) code to solve the above equations numerically for the x and y coordinates of the ball and, thus, the trajectory. The drag and lift coefficients are assumed constant throughout the ball flight.

3. Results

To study the effects of the prominent features of the balls on their aerodynamics and flights, a number of test cases were developed. Computer simulations of these cases were subsequently performed and the results were analyzed.

3.1. Test Cases

Table 1. *Description of run conditions*

	Volleyball			Soccer ball (The generic and 86 -panel)			Baseball		
Case	Size	Re (×10³)	Spin Rate	Size	Re (×10³)	Spin Rate	Size	Re (×10³)	Spin Rate
1	Actual	250	5 Hz	Actual	250	5 Hz	Actual	250	50 Hz
2	Football	330	5 Hz	Actual	330	5 Hz	Football	330	5 Hz
3	Actual	250	10 Hz	Actual	250	10 Hz	Actual	250	25 Hz
4	-------	-------	-------	Actual	250	25 Hz	Actual	250	25 Hz*

*The rotation axis is a horizontal line perpendicular to the line of the air flow for each case. However, the spin axis was rotated 30 degrees with respect to the vertical line (perpendicular to the air flow line) in case 4 for the baseball in order to show the effect of the lace orientation.

Table 1 presents the cases simulated with varying ball sizes, Reynolds numbers, and spin rates. Each row reflects a set of conditions for the corresponding ball models that highlights a particular feature of the ball, or an in-game scenario. In Case 1, the values of the variables represent that of a typical in-game condition for each sport. Case 2 is designed to compare the effects of the surface pattern and shape on the resulting aerodynamic forces by using an identical diameter (as that of the soccer ball) for all the balls. In Case 3, we vary the typical spin rates seen in the respective games, as depicted in Case 1. Specifically, the spin rates for soccer ball and volleyball were doubled, and that of the baseball halved. Case 4 describes a made-up condition in which the spin rate normally seen in a baseball pitch is applied to a soccer ball. This particular numerical experiment is designed to demonstrate the effects of the size and the surface pattern for a given spin rate.

3.2. Test Results

Table 2. *Drag and lift coefficients computed from test cases*

Case	Volleyball		Soccer ball (The generic)		Baseball	
	C_D	C_L	C_D	C_L	C_D	C_L
1	0.185	0.213	0.211	0.116	0.417	0.141
2	0.096	0.104	0.199	0.095	0.081	0.025
3	0.223	0.216	0.235	0.181	0.410	0.102
4	-------	-------	0.331	0.289	0.410	0.085

Table 2 presents the simulated drag coefficient C_D and lift coefficient C_L for all the cases. Comparing the results of Cases 1 and 3, it can be seen that for the generic soccer ball and volleyball, the higher spin rate in Case 3 increases C_D and C_L. For the baseball, the lower spin rate in Case 3 decreases both C_D and C_L from those of Case 1.

Figure 5 displays the air pressure contours in the vicinity of each ball studied for Case 3. There are noticeable effects of the rotation and ball size on the pressure fields. It is clear that for a ball with a smaller size and higher spin rate, larger pressure differential can been generated, resulting in a larger net force perpendicular to both the axis of rotation and the air flow. Figure 6 shows the streamlines of the simulated air flow around each ball for Case 3. The ball's wake is more clearly shifted with higher spinning rate.

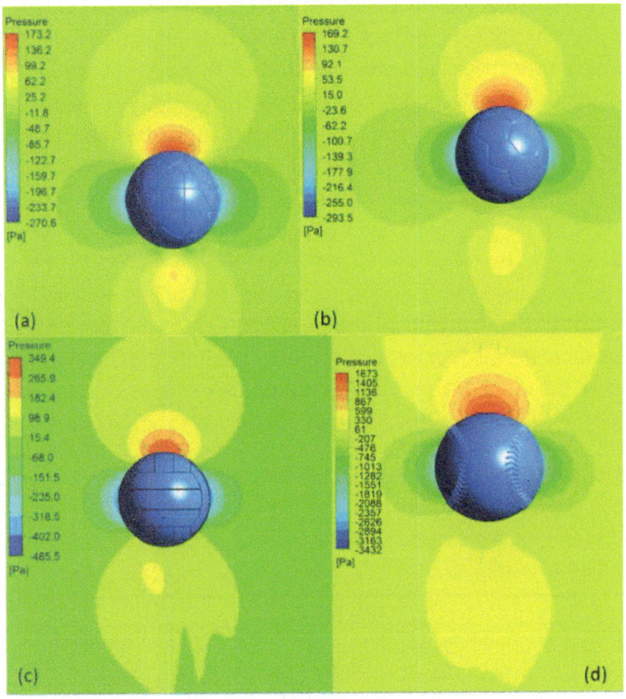

Figure 5. *Pressure contours corresponding to Case 3 for the (a) 86-panel, (b) and generic soccer ball, (c) volleyball and (d) baseball.*

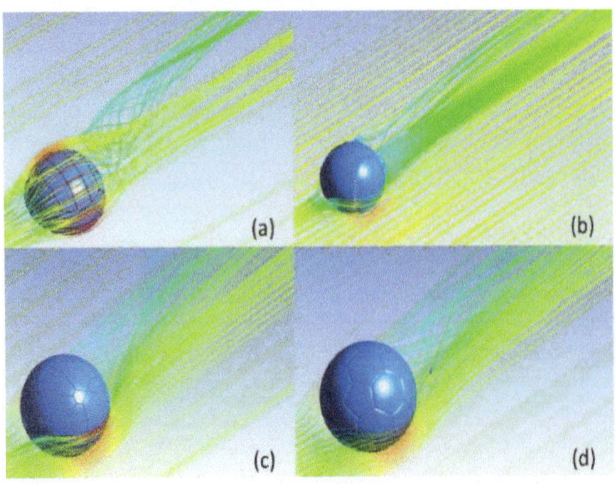

Figure 6. *The streamlines corresponding to Case 3 for (a) volleyball, (b) baseball, (c) the 86-panel football and (d) the generic football.*

The surface shear stress distributions on the balls' surface reveal the importance of seams, patches and surface features. Figure 7 demonstrates that for Case 3, in regions near the seams, wall shear stress changes locally due to the localized small flow structures. This feature of the surface shear stress distribution affects the aerodynamic drag and lift, indicating the potential importance of the ball patterns in the playing and the further development of these sports. Also clear from the figure, the stagnation point, the point on the leading surface of the ball at which the shear stress is zero, is shifted left. This anticipated shift, due to the rotation of the ball is more apparent in the case of baseball where the applied spin rate is the highest.

Using the data collected by Asai et al. (2010), we compared the predicted drag coefficients for the volleyball with the test results. The results showed agreement to within 15%. We also compared the predicted drag coefficients of the modelled generic 32-panel soccer ball with those in previous studies (Barber & Carré, 2010; Goff & Carré, 2009; Asai et al., 2007). The computer simulations under-predict the drag coefficients by about 10%-15%. One of the reasons for the computed drag to digress from test results is likely due to the fact that the simulations are predicted assuming a fully turbulent flow around the ball and use a turbulence model accordingly. In field tests, it has been shown that the air flow around the ball can often be a combination of turbulent and laminar flow in the supercritical region and is not fully turbulent (Barber et al., 2009).

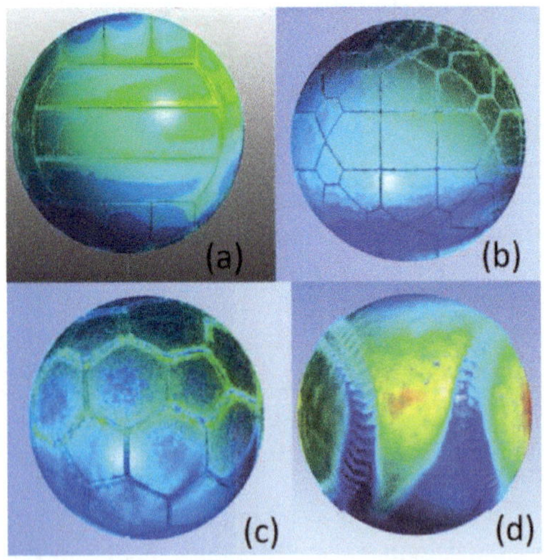

Figure 7. *The surface shear stress distributions corresponding to Case 3 for (a) volleyball, (b) the 86-panel soccer tball, (c) the generic soccer ball and (d) baseball.*

We calculated the trajectory of the generic soccer ball with $\rho=1.225kg.m^{-3}$, $g=9.81m.s^{-1}$. For the generic soccer ball, $m=0.430kg$ and $A=0.0380m^2$. Also, $\theta=20^o$ at $t=0$ s is assumed. The trajectory results are shown in Figure 8. The results indicate that a higher ball's velocity results in a longer horizontal distance a ball can travel and a higher spin rate yields a taller trajectory.

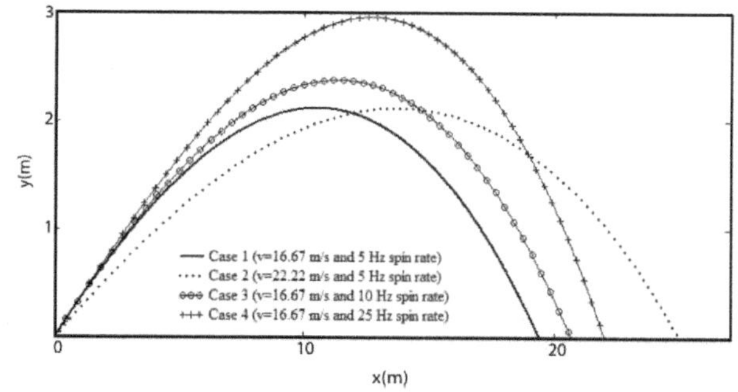

Figure 8. *Computed trajectories for the generic soccer ball.*

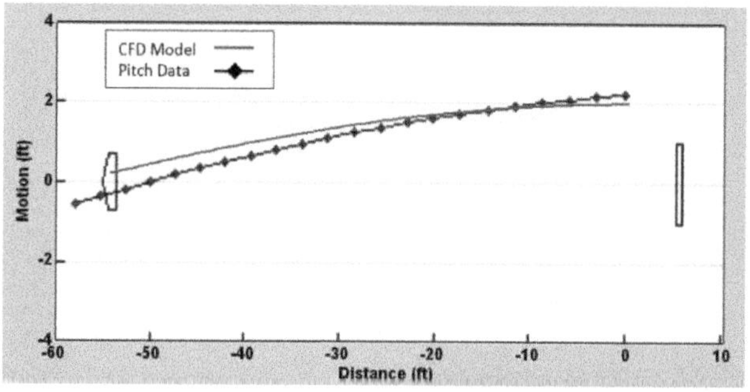

Figure 9. *Comparison of the CFD computed baseball trajectory with the actual pitch data from Somers (2013).*

For the baseball, there exists a vast collection of in-game pitch data recorded by modern pitch tracking systems. A proper reduction of these data, when averaged over a wide range of conditions, for example, provides important information that can be used for validation of computer simulations. For the validation of the baseball simulations, the pitch motion resulting from the model predicted drag and lift forces was compared with the actual pitch motion of an American pitcher, Justin Verlander, of the Detroit Tigers. Curveball data from May 1, 2011 to October 25, 2011 by compiled Somers (2013) were averaged to yield an average spin rate, linear velocity, and trajectory. Using the measured spin rate and the linear velocity as inputs to the CFD model, we compare the total pitch motion and the trajectory results of the simulation with the measurement. The result for the trajectory comparison is shown in Figure 9. As evidenced by Figure 9, the predicted trajectory closely matches with the actual pitch data.

4. Discussion

The results of simulations shown above indicate that both the drag and lift coefficients are highly dependent on the rotational and the linear motions of the ball. For discussions, we employ a non-dimensional spin parameter, $S_p = r\omega/v$ where r denotes the ball radius (m), ω the angular velocity ($rad.s^{-1}$) and v the linear velocity ($m.s^{-1}$). The simulated results obtained here indicate that increasing the value of S_p results in an increase of both the drag and the lift coefficients. In other words, the faster the ball rotates, the more drag and lift forces are exerted on the ball. Not too surprisingly, with decreases of the spin parameter, the predicted lift and drag forces decrease for a given linear velocity. Therefore, it could be advantageous for players to kick the ball to a small spin rate in games, which will result in a lower drag force and, therefore, a longer distance. Naturally, the stabilizing effects of the spinning can decrease with a reduced spin rate, which, in turns, compromises the accuracy of a long kick. Additionally, the results indicate that, compared to the generic soccer ball, the 86-panel soccer ball has higher drag and lift coefficients due to the increased number of panels. There are apparent effects of the geometric features on the aerodynamic characteristics of soccer balls.

In the case of the baseball, the spin parameter has been shown to have a less significant impact on the drag, but a very strong effect on the lift and the overall motion of the pitch. This would imply there is not a significant trade-off, from an aerodynamics standpoint, between linear pitch speed and angular velocity, as it is for soccer ball. In fact, the most advantageous situation would appear to be the case of greatest spin rate. However, it is also necessary to account for the varying human body mechanics between different pitches, which generally dictate the maximum pitch speed achievable. We also highlighted the importance of lace orientation with respect to the total aerodynamic forces generated. Not only does the lace orientation assist a pitcher in applying spin to a pitch, but the laces themselves have a substantial impact on the total motion of a pitch. This study showed that, for a 30 degree change in the lace orientation, the aerodynamic force responsible for the lateral motion dropped by approximately 17% with a 7% increase in the lift.

The travel distance of a volleyball during an actual game can be no longer than 20 meters, which is the diagonal length of a regulation volleyball court. The typical time in the air for a fast ball is about 0.7 seconds. A player must move into position behind the ball during this short period of time to make a play. Wobbling and unpredictable behavior of the ball caused by its axisymmetric surface patterns add to the difficulty for a player to anticipate the ball's trajectory and react accordingly. The critical ball speed associated with the critical Reynolds number, at which the drag coefficient drops dramatically, is an important aerodynamic parameter. For a ball travelling near the critical Reynolds number, the magnitude of the drag force is relatively small and has the least effect on the ball. This makes the motion of the ball smoother and more predictable. The lower drag also increases the ball's speed and consequently the pace of the game. Therefore, it can be advantageous to design the volleyball so that the critical ball speed is close to the speed range of real-world plays. It is shown in Table 2 that the volleyball in Case 2 has small drag and lift coefficients compared to those in Cases 1 and 3. It suggests that the critical Reynolds number is between 250,000 and 330,000, which is in agreement with the results of Asai et al. (2010).

5. Conclusions

This work presented the processes and the results of a computational study of the aerodynamics of soccer ball, baseball and volleyball. We simulated their aerodynamic behaviors and identified a number of important aerodynamics features of each ball. The analysis showed that for the soccer ball and volleyball, the spin parameter plays an important role in determining the resulting aerodynamic forces, provided the Reynolds number is above 200,000. At this point, the lift and drag forces become closely tied to the spin parameter and largely independent of the Reynolds number. Conversely, it was found that, for the baseball, the drag coefficient was not as closely related to the spin parameter, but the forces that generate the vertical and lateral motions were. The orientation of the laces was also shown to have a strong influence on the total aerodynamic forces generated. Finally, by comparing soccer balls of differing patch designs, the ball with the greater number of patches, and thus the greater number of seams, was found to yield higher drag and lift coefficients. Computational aerodynamics methods reported here can be readily applied to other sports. We would recommend future efforts to couple computational and experimental studies to better align the conditions used in the two approaches and to better integrate their merits toward actual playing of the sports.

References

[1] Alam, F., Chowdhury, H., Moria, H., Fuss, F. K., Khan, I., Aldawi, F., & Subic, A. (2011). Aerodynamics of contemporary FIFA soccer balls. *Procedia Engineering, 13*, 188-193.

[2] Alam, F., Ho, H., Chowdhury, H., & Subic, A. (2011). Aerodynamics of baseball. *Procedia Engineering, 13*, 207-212.

[3] Alam, F., Chowdhury, H., Stemmer, M., Wang, Z., & Yang, J. (2012). Effects of surface structure on soccer ball aerodynamics. *Procedia Engineering, 34*, 146-151.

[4] Alam, F., Ho, H., Smith, L., Subic, A., Chowdhury, H., & Kumar, A. (2012). A study of baseball and softball aerodynamics. *Procedia Engineering, 34*, 86-91.

[5] ANSYS, Inc. (2010) ANSYS Meshing User's Guide

[6] Asai, T., Seo, K., Kobayashi, O., & Sakashita, R. (2007). Fundamental aerodynamics of the soccer ball. *Sports Engineering, 10*(2), 101-109.

[7] Asai, T., Ito, S., Seo, K., & Hitotsubashi, A. (2010). Aerodynamics of a new volleyball. *Procedia Engineering, 2*(2), 2493-2498.

[8] Barber, S., Chin, S. B., & Carré, M. J. (2009). Sports ball aerodynamics: a numerical study of the erratic motion of soccer balls. *Computers & Fluids,38*(6), 1091-1100.

[9] Barber, S., & Carré, M. J. (2010). The effect of surface geometry on soccer ball trajectories. *Sports Engineering, 13*(1), 47-55.

[10] Carré, M. J., Asai, T., Akatsuka, T., & Haake, S. J. (2002). The curve kick of a football II: flight through the air. *Sports Engineering, 5*(4), 193-200.

[11] Goff, J. E., & Carré, M. J. (2009). Trajectory analysis of a soccer ball. *American Journal of Physics, 77*(11), 1020-1027.

[12] Goff, J. E., & Carré, M. J. (2010). Soccer ball lift coefficients via trajectory analysis. *European Journal of Physics, 31*(4), 775.

[13] Goodwill, S. R., Chin, S. B., & Haake, S. J. (2004). Aerodynamics of spinning and non-spinning tennis balls. *Journal of wind engineering and industrial aerodynamics, 92*(11), 935-958.

[14] Mehta, R. D. (1985). Aerodynamics of sports balls. *Annual Review of Fluid Mechanics, 17*(1), 151-189.

[15] Mizota, T., Kurogi, K., Ohya, Y., Okajima, A., Naruo, T., & Kawamura, Y. (2013). The strange flight behaviour of slowly spinning soccer balls. *Scientific reports, 3*.

[16] Newton, I. (1672). A new theory about light and colors. *Philosophical Transactions of the Royal Society*, 80, 3075-3087

[17] Niven, L. (2012) https://grabcad.com/library/soccer-ball--2 /files/practice.SLDPRT

[18] Oggiano, L., & Sætran, L. (2010). Aerodynamics of modern soccer balls.*Procedia Engineering, 2*(2), 2473-2479.

[19] Pallis, J. M., & Mehta, R. D. (2002). Aerodynamics and hydrodynamics in sports. *The Engineering of Sport, 4*, 31-39.

[20] Somers, Trip. (2013). Justin Verlander, Detroit Tigers - PITCHf/x Pitcher Profile. http://pitchfx.texasleaguers.com/pitcher/434378/

[21] Thompson,S.(2012),https://grabcad.com/library/86-panel -soccer-ball design /files / 86%20panel%20dome.SLDPRT

5

A comparative study of lung function test between physically trained and untrained adults

Sridip Chatterjee[1], Aloke Sen Borman[2], Aparup Konar[3], Samiran Mondal[4]

[1]Department of Physical Education, Jadavpur University, Kolkata – 700032, West Bengal, India
[2]Seva Bharati Mahavidyalaya, Department of Physical Education, Kapgari – 721505, Paschim Midnapore, West Bengal, India
[3]Director of Physical Instruction, Office of the Sports Board, Jadavpur University, Kolkata – 700032, West Bengal, India
[4]Department of Physical Education, Vinaya Bhavana, Visva Bharati, Santiniketan – 731235, West Bengal, India

Email address:
sritun14@gmail.com (S. Chatterjee), dralokesenorman@gmail.com (A. S. Borman), kaparup@gmil.com (A. Konar), msamiran@rediffmail.com (S. Mondal)

Abstract: Background: The maximum lung function for human being reached around the age of 20-25 years. Studies on lung function indicated a progressive age-related functional change of the respiratory physiology. Regular physical activity throughout the life may delay this deterioration of lung function. Objective of the study: The present study was designed to observe the effect of aging on lung function induced by regular physical activity. Methods: Respiratory function was tested by digital spirometer. 479 persons (Male: 246 and Female: 233) ages between 20-70 years were examined at the department labortory, Jadavpur University, Kolkata. 79 persons were excluded from the study due to acute or chronic respiratory disorders and the history of smoking. All the subject were allotted in the five age category (20-29 yrs; 30-39 yrs;40-49 yrs; 50-59 yrs and 60-70 yrs) to observe the age related changes between the trained (male: 100 and female:100) and untrained (male: 100 and female:100) persons. Mean, Standard deviation and't' test were done to calculate the statistical significance and made a valid conclusion. Result: A slow progressive age related decline were observed in trained group compared to untrained in all the age category for both male and female. Conclusion: From the present study it can be concluded that regular physical activity may delay the age related decline of lung function for all the age groups and promote healthy aging.

Keywords: Aging, Spirometry, Exercise

1. Introduction

During the first two decades of life, the lungs undergo a phase of growth and maturation [1]. The maximum lung function reached around the age of 20-25 years. After birth the individual lungs are continuously being exposed to particles in the air, including smoke, pollen, dust and microorganisms. These external hazards may limit the physiological potentialities of the lungs. Aging is associated with a progressive decline in lung performance. The respiratory system undergoes many physiological modifications during aging are: a decrease in the static elastic recoil of the lung, a decrease in compliance of the chest wall, a decrease in the strength of respiratory muscles, the amount of oxygen diffusing from the air sacs into the blood decreases, the rate of air flow through the airways slowly declines and the numbers of alveoli decreases [1, 2].

Exercise when performed regularly has benefits on the various systems of the body and maintains an overall health status of the individual. Regular physical activity has proved to be beneficial for the human body and the lungs are no exception [3-7]. Pulmonary function is a long-term predictor for overall survival rates in both genders [7]. Efficient lung function is a preventive measure and positively influence by exercise habits. The pulmonary functional capacities of normal sedentary individuals have been studied extensively in India [4]. Sedentary lifestyles could be associated with less efficient pulmonary function [7].

Hence, the present study was undertaken with a view to observe the pattern of progressive age related changes of lung function in different age group and how regular physical activity habit influence the pattern compared to age-sex matched sedentary individuals.

2. Methods

In the present study survey cum experimental design was adopted. Comprehensive respiratory health check up cum awareness camp was jointly organized by the department of physical education, Jadavpur University and Cipla Ltd., Kolkata, India. Total 246 male and 233 female ages between 20 years to 70 years from Jadavpur University community were tested for lung function (spirometry) in the physical education department laboratory. All the subjects willingly register their names to attain the said camp and signed the inform consent form. All the subjects were interviewed and instructed to complete a general health-physical activity form with a view to allotted the subjects in the trained (exerciser) and untrained (non-exerciser) group in the five different age category: 20-29 years; 30-39 years; 40-49 years; 50-59 years and 60-69 years. The subjects in the exercise group maintain a regular exercise habit (3-4 days / weak) for minimum period of five years. The subjects in the non-exercise group basically lead a sedentary life style. 27 male and 19 female were excluded from the study due to acute or chronic respiratory disorders. Another 19 male and 14 female were excluded due to the habit of smoking. Finally 100 male & 100 female in the trained group and 100 male & 100 female in the untrained group were considered for analysis of data. Mean, standard deviation and simple percentage from the mean value were calculated. The difference between the means were compared separately (trained vs untrained group) by using student's 't' test for the five different age groups. The mean differences were considered significant when the p values were <0.05.

3. Spirometry (Lung Function Variables)

Peak Expiratory Flow Rate (PEFR), Forced Vital Capacity (FVC), Forced Expiratory Volume in 1 & 6 Sec (FEV_1, FEV_6), Ratio of FEV_1 and FVC (FEV_1/FVC) and Forced expiratory flow 25%-75% (FEF_{25-75}) were measured by using "digital spirometer" (DT Spiro, Mestros Medline System Ltd., Model No. PoP-10.8). Instrument was calibrated properly before each experimental session and best of two trials were considered as final measurement.

4. Results

Data relating to lung function test of trained and untrained group for both male and female in five different age category are presented in table No. 1. It appears that slow progressive age related decline were observed in trained group (exerciser) compared to untrained (non-exerciser) in five different age category for both male and female. Simple percentages were calculated from the mean value for the entire age category and presented in Table no. 1 and graph no. 1 to 6, to see the quantitative changes between trained and untrained group. Single star (*) in the table no. 1 denote P<0.05, double star (**) denote P<0.01 and triple star (***) denote P<0.001.

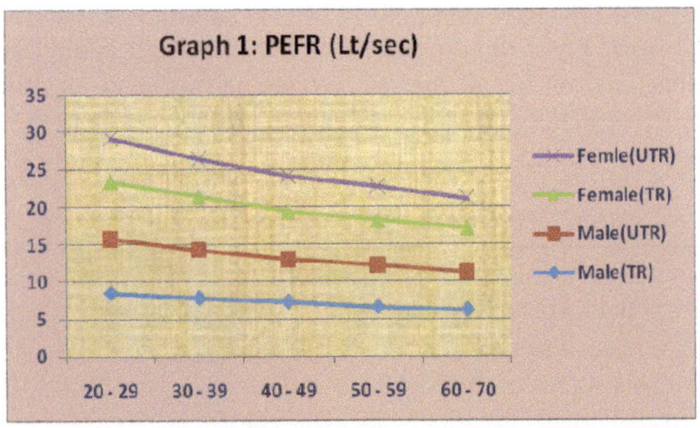

Graph 1: PEFR (Lt/sec)

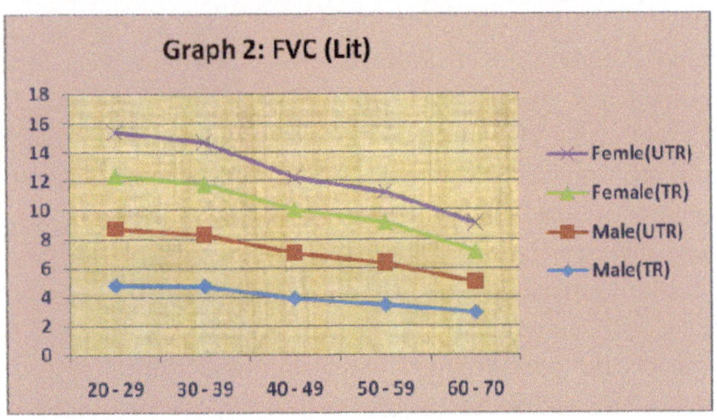

Graph 2: FVC (Lit)

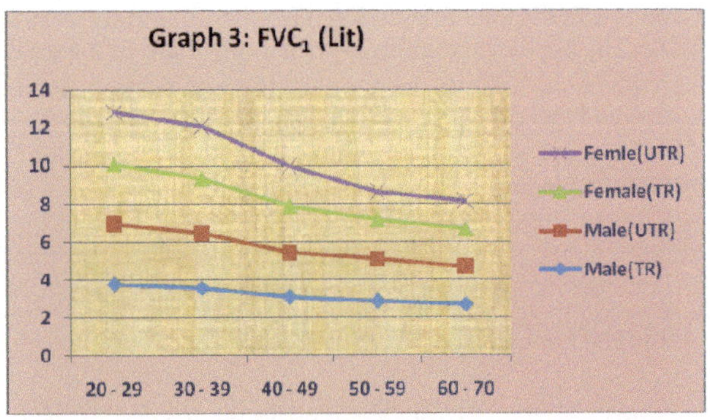

Graph 3: FVC_1 (Lit)

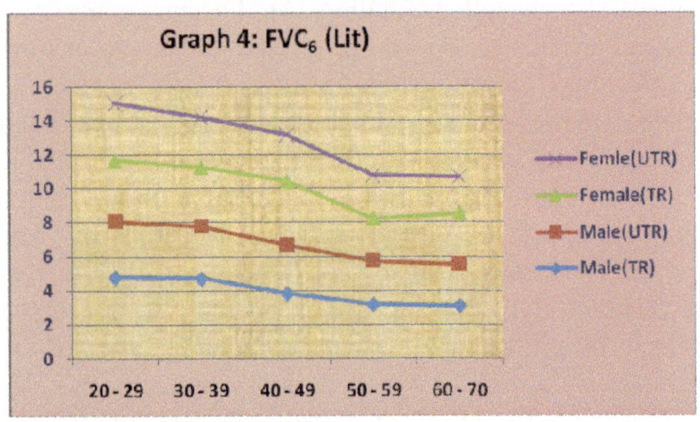

Graph 4: FVC_6 (Lit)

***Table 1.** Status of Lung Function Variables for Trained and Untrained Group*

Age group	Male			Female		
	Trained N= 20	Untrained N= 20	% Change	Trained N= 20	Untrained N= 20	% Change
	Mean ± SD	Mean ± SD		Mean ± SD	Mean ± SD	
PEFR (Lit/Sec)						
20 - 29	8.47 ± 2.02	7.33 ± 1.83	13.46*	7.65 ± 1.54	5.71 ± 1.29	25.36**
30 - 39	7.79 ± 2.30	6.54 ± 1.57	16.05*	7.11 ± 1.81	4.96 ± 1.03	30.24**
40 - 49	7.25 ± 1.83	5.83 ± 0.99	19.59*	6.23 ± 0.78	4.77 ± 0.81	23.44**
50 - 59	6.55 ± 1.47	5.68 ± 0.68	13.288	5.98 ± 0.54	4.45 ± 0.87	25.58**
60 - 70	6.16 ± 1.19	5.07 ± 1.23	17.96*	5.87 ± 0.93	3.98 ± 0.58	32.20**
FVC (Lit)						
20 - 29	4.81 ± 1.27	3.91 ± 1.16	18.71*	3.61 ± 1.09	3.08 ± 1.19	14.68*
30 - 39	4.75 ± 1.12	3.56 + 1.15	25.05**	3.42 ± 1.21	2.97 ± 1.11	13.16*
40 - 49	3.86 ± 1.36	3.16 + 1.24	18.13*	2.97 ± 1.21	2.23 ± 0.73	24.92**
50 - 59	3.43 ± 1.26	2.90 + 1.38	15.45*	2.79 ± 1.24	2.10 ± 0.81	24.73**
60 - 70	2.90 ± 1.04	2.12 + 1.28	7.42	2.10 ± 0.97	1.93 ± 0.87	8.09
FEV_1 (Lit)						
20 - 29	3.76 ± 1.03	3.18 ± 1.37	15.43*	3.16 ± 1.29	2.74 ± 1.13	13.298
30 - 39	3.53 ± 1.14	2.91 ± 1.41	17.56*	2.92 ± 1.24	2.70 ± 1.08	7.53
40 - 49	3.07 ± 1.23	2.33 ± 1.07	24.10**	2.48 ± 1.11	2.07 ± 0.77	16.53*
50 - 59	2.85 ± 0.87	2.23 ± 0.78	21.75**	2.06 ± 0.67	1.48 ± 0.39	28.15**
60 - 70	2.68 ± 0.67	1.99 ± 0.49	25.75**	1.98 ± 0.97	1.46 ± 0.43	26.26**
FEV_6 (Lit)						
20 - 29	4.79 ± 1.05	3.28 ± 1.23	31.52**	3.61 ± 1.12	3.37 ± 1.31	6.64
30 - 39	4.71 ± 1.15	3.09 ± 1.33	34.39**	3.45 ± 1.05	2.97 ± 0.79	19.73*
40 - 49	3.83 ± 0.82	2.89 ± 0.87	24.54*	3.50 ± 0.98	2.77 ± 0.57	19.71*
50 - 59	3.19 ± 0.77	2.53 ± 0.49	20.68*	2.53 ± 0.76	2.53 ± 0.47	14.81*
60 - 70	3.10 ± 0.49	2.47 ± 0.57	20.328	2.97 ± 0.93	2.13 ± 0.39	15.81*
FEV1/FVC (%)						
20 - 29	83.4 ± 7.78	76.7 ± 8.23	8.03	82.8 ± 8.15	78.0 ± 7.79	5.79
30 - 39	82.10 ± 8.37	75.47 ± 8.54	8.07	81.23 ± 7.93	76.91 ± 6.89	5.32
40 - 49	79.25 ± 6.87	73.59 ± 6.42	7.14*	79.50 ± 7.22	75.30 ± 7.44	5.28*
50 - 59	78.07 ± 7.11	71.53 ± 8.37	8.38*	78.74 ± 6.31	75.00 ± 7.41	4.75
60 - 70	77.7 ± 9.17	71.47 ± 5.23	8.02	78.1 ± 5.04	74.23 ± 6.67	4.96
FEV_{25-75} (Lit/Sec)						
20 - 29	4.96 ± 1.51	3.60 ± 1.03	27.41**	4.01 ± 1.43	3.12 ± 1.03	22.19**
30 - 39	4.73 ± 1.71	3.19 ± 1.11	32.56***	3.95 ± 1.28	2.71 ± 0.49	31.39**
40 - 49	3.81 ± 0.79	2.89 ± 0.58	24.15**	3.71 ± 1.01	2.19 ± 0.78	40.97***
50 - 59	3.11 ± 0.29	2.67 ± 0.58	14.15*	3.43 ± 0.79	2.04 ± 0.55	40.52***
60 - 70	3.09 ± 0.47	2.50 ± 0.73	19.09*	2.81 ± 0.67	1.87 ± 0.52	33.45**

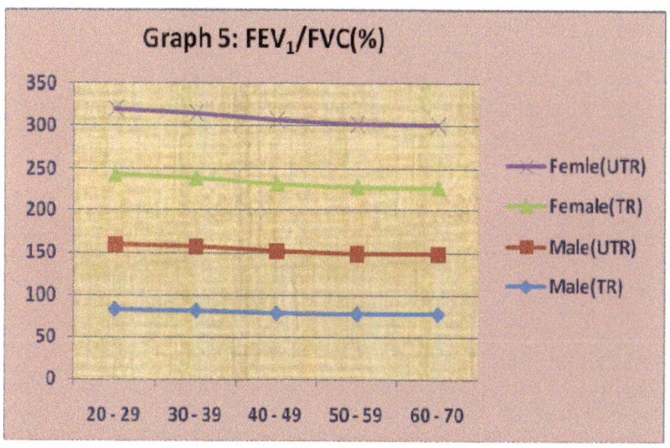

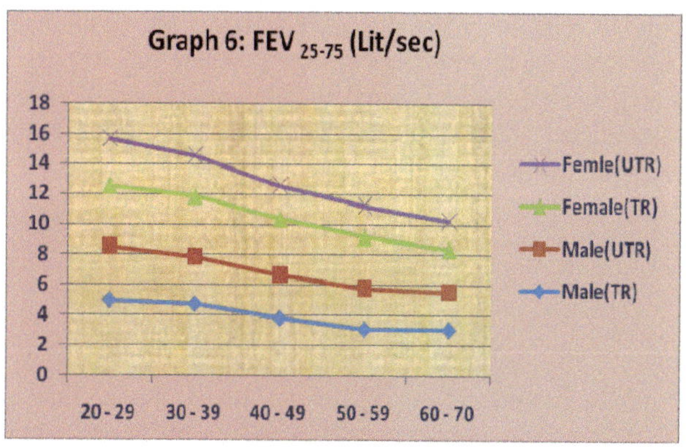

5. Discussion

Age is an unmodifiable risk factor for decrease respiratory function. During childhood and adolescence there is a natural rise in lung function, after which it declines gradually. Regular exercise habit may be a preventive strategy for healthy functioning of the lungs. Previous investigations on lung function variables reported that all the sportspersons or exerciser had a higher value of lung functions compared to the sedentary controls [7-11]. Thus the purpose of the present study was to examine and compare the age related changes of lung function variables in trained and untrained subjects. The results of the present study showed that exercise habit throughout the life had a positive influence on lung function as compared to age-sex matched sedentary controls.

Some limitations of our study could be understood. Firstly, the absolute assessment of physical activity was difficult, so only leisure time physical activity was considered in this study. Secondly we did not able to control the individual life style and social factors which may influence the results.

From the above discussion it may be interpreted that: (i) Involvement in certain physical activities or sports develop respiratory muscle strength and static elastic recoil pressure of the lung [1, 10]. (ii) Exercise is associated with an increased in diaphragm thickness and respiratory muscle mass [6]. (iii) Efficient functioning of the alveoli and gaseous exchange between lungs and blood vessels. (iv) Regular physical activity or exercise positively influences the stretch receptors in the air passages and lungs and chemoreceptors function in the body [14]. (v) Regular forceful inspiration and expiration for prolonged period during exercise leads to strengthening of the respiratory muscles. This helps the lungs to inflate and deflate maximally. This maximum inflation and deflation is an important physiological stimulus for the release of surfactant [14].

6. Conclusion

From the present study it can be concluded that regular physical activity may be a strategy to delay the age related decline of respiratory physiological function for all the age groups and thus promote healthy aging. Therefore, exercise is a nonpharmacological complementary alternative method recommended for efficient functioning of the lung throughout the life.

References

[1] J.P. Janssens, J.C. Pache, L.P. Nicod. Physiological changes in respiratory function associated with ageing. Eur Respir J. 1999, 13: 197-205.

[2] J.P. Janssens. Aging of the respiratory system: Impact on pulmonary function tests and adaptation to exertion. Clin Chest Med. 2005, 26 : 469-484.

[3] P. Hamilton, G.M. Andrew. Influence of growth and athletic training on heart and lung functions. Eur J Appl Physiol Occup Physiol. 1976; 36 (1) : 27-38.

[4] A.K. Ghosh, A. Ahuja, G.L. Khanna. Pulmonary capacities of different groups of sportsmen in India. Brit. J. Sports Med. 1985, 19 (4) : 232-234.

[5] S.M. Hulke, M.S. Phatak. Effect of endurance training on lung function: a longitudinal study. Int J Biol Med Res. 2011, 2 (1) : 443-446.

[6] C. Garber, F.D. McCool. Respiratory muscle strength in the physically active elderly. Lung. 2007, 185 : 315-320.

[7] S. Prakash, S. Meshram, U. Ramtekkar. Athletes, Yogi and individuals with sedentary life styles; Do their lung functions differ? Indian J Physiol Pharmacol. 2007, 5 (1) : 76-80.

[8] P.K. Mehrotra, N. Varma, S. Tiwari, P. Kumar. Pulmonary functions in Indian sportsmen playing different sports. Indian J Physiol Pharmacol. 1998, 42 (3) : 412-6.

[9] M.R. Ide, M.A.V. Belini, F.A. Caromano. Effects of an aquatic versus non-aquatic respiratory exercise program on the respiratory muscle strength in healthy aged persons. Clinics. 2005, 60 (2) : 151-158.

[10] Y.J. Cheng, C.A. Macera, C.L. Addy, F.S. Sy, D. Weiland, S.N. Blair. Effects of physical activity on exercise tests and respiratory function. Br J Sports Med. 2003, 37: 521-528.

[11] K.R. Vincent, R.W. Braith, R.A. Feldman, H.E. Kallas, D.T. Lowenthal. Improved cardiorespiratory endurance following 6 months of resistance exercise in elderly men and women. Arch Intern Med. 2002, 162 : 673-678.

[12] A. Rossi, A. Ganassini, C. Tantucci, V. Grassi. Aging and the respiratory system. Aging (Milano). 1996, 8 (3) : 143-61.

[13] R.J. Shephard. Aging, physical activity and health. Human Kinetics. 1997.

[14] L. Shashikal, R. Sarath. Effect of exercise on pulmonary function test. Indian journal of Fundamental and Applied Life Sciences. 2011, 1(3): 230-231.

The effect of the gender variable on the speeches of the pupils in Handball game in Tunisia

Makram Zghibi[1, *], Nabila Bennour[2], Mohamed Jabri[3], Hajer Sahli[3]

[1]LASELDI, University of Franche-Comté, Besançon, France
[2]UMR EFTS, Le Mirail University, Toulouse II, France
[3]Higher Institute of Sports and Physical Education, Kef, Tunisia, Tunisia

Email address:
makwiss@yahoo.fr(M. Zghibi)

Abstract: In this work, we pass from a behavioral conception that considers the teacher as the only source of information to a constructivist and even a semi-constructivist conception which focuses on the fact that the student is a real actor of the teaching-learning process. The objective is to study the semiotics of language interactions between pupils in Physical Education and Sport sessions and the power balance between girls and boys (Wallian, 2010). Discursive interlocutions of Tunisian pupils in handball are marked by a constant negotiation about domination and by a formulation of action projects (Zghibi, 2009). These language interactions have the advantage of deploying a rich and multifaceted rhetoric which is a sign of dynamic learning.

Keywords: Verbalization, Game, Handball, Speeches, Gender

1. Introduction

This study uses a semio-constructivist approach. It aims to study the verbal exchanges between pupils and the power balance between girls and boys during a football game in order to detect the role of language in PES learning in Tunisia. Such a work can indeed, make a valuable contribution to the science of intervention in terms of PES. The purpose is to take into account pupils opinions and how they co-construct their knowledge in and via action (Zghibi and al, 2013a ; Zghibi and al, 2013b).

In accordance with the works of Gréhaigne and Godbout (1999) and Gréhaigne (2009) on the teaching of team sports, and Wallian's works (2007a and 2007b) on the discursive socio-constructivism, the research approach is original. It uses field practices in order to allow pupils to structure their mutual positioning and to develop their interpretation of the game collectively.

Pedagogically and didactically, this paper involves an essential paradigmatic character. The use of linguistics and especially semiotics in team sports generates a real cultural rupture in the teaching/learning methods. The Physical Education and Sports (PES) is no longer a simple motor response, but also a way of discursive interlocutions between subjects. They build a full meaning via the co-construction of effective strategies in order to implement common projects (Gréhaigne et al, 2004).

2. Methodology

A class of 20 pupils (8 girls and 12 boys) with an average of 15 years old alternates French and Tunisian Arabic as mediums of education. If the pupils' speech appears as determinant in the study, language support and distribution of the speech per gender are also relevant factors in the dynamics of verbal exchanges analysis.

What is the impact of this gender approach it in the dynamics of verbal exchanges and in achieving common projects? What is main language support used by boys and by girls? What is the impact of language choice on the Tunisian educational system and on the cultural context of the pupils?

The research protocol proposed in this work is, therefore, to organize a handball teaching cycle of eight "one effective-hour" sessions (8 hours of motor and verbal practice were observed and recorded). The proposed sessions are all based on game situations on a handball court (40 m X 20 m). Each session includes two game situations separated by a sequence of ideas' debate for 6 minutes (3 minutes under the supervision of the teacher and 3 others in his absence (Gréhaigne and Godbout, 1998; Zghibi, 2013a). The descriptive approach is qualitative and quantitative. The first tends to convey the pupils' language productions through analysis models inspired from linguistics (Austin, 1970). This model distinguishes three speech acts: locutionary act, the illocutionary act, the perlocutionary act. The quantitative model serves to identify the effect of the gender variable over the modalities of decision making.

3. Results

3.1. Quantitative Study of Girls/Boys Power Balance

3.1.1. The Distribution of the Speech Made by Boys/Girls in Presence of the Teacher

Table 1. *The speech made by boys and girls in presence of the teacher*

Sessions	*Session1*	*Session2*	*Session3*	*Session4*	*Session5*	*Session6*	*Session7*	*Session8*	Total
Boys	*4*	*5*	*4*	*4*	*7*	*6*	*5*	*5*	*40*
Girls	*4*	*3*	*3*	*5*	*5*	*7*	*6*	*5*	*38*

We note here that in presence of the teacher, girls intervene in speech (38) as well as boys do (40). No significant difference was noted between the speeches of girls and boys.

3.1.2. The Distribution of the Speech Made by Boys/Girls in the Teacher'S Absence

When the teacher is absent, boys tend to speak more than girls. The difference is significant. The table below shows the number of interventions of both sexes in speech on the absence of the teacher. Indeed, there was a substantial increase in the number of boys' contributions comparing to girls during the times when the teacher is absent. We counted 82 interventions in total, including 53 made by boys and only 29 by girls.

Table 2. *The speech made by both genders in absence of the teacher*

Sessions	*Session1*	*Session2*	*Session3*	*Session4*	*Session5*	*Session6*	*Session7*	*Session8*	Total
Boys	*5*	*4*	*6*	*5*	*7*	*7*	*8*	*9*	*53*
Girls	*2*	*3*	*2*	*3*	*3*	*2*	*4*	*5*	*29*

We can therefore conclude that the boys' participation in the debate of ideas is major. Quantitatively, the number of their interventions is more relevant than girls' verbal productions.

3.1.3. Interpretation

The fact that the intervention of girls in the debate of ideas increase only in the teacher's presence can be explained by the persistence of patriarchal system that dominates the Tunisian society (Borrmans, 1977; EL Khayat, 1985; Belhssen, 1992). This system keeps women through constant supremacy made by men, and in conditions of unequal states. Education received by the Tunisian young child, is mainly issued from Arab-Muslim culture that recognizes the differences between men and women. It passes through socialization, ways of doing, thinking, and acting of each gender: (expl boys dominate in discussions). Since it is the "sport", that was for a long time considered incompatible with women (Oglesby, 1986), the situation of sport is "one of the social situations where men and women can effectively implement differences" (Goffman, 2002). Thus, gender is seen as a collective way of life (Matthew, 1991). Like many other domains, sport is a mirror of the social. Not to mention that our subjects are in an age with huge differences to appear between the two sexes (Bessis & Belhassen, 1992). This refers to a substantial literature about sex differences in educational practices. Barry and al consider that men were relevantly more trained to achievement and independence while the female used to obey and to maternity (Clelland et al, 1953). We can therefore conclude that the presence of the teacher represent the educational institution, supposed as based on equal opportunities for girls and boys. Teachers decrease the boys' dominance. That way, girls feel more encouraged, even protected by the presence of the teacher, they feel more free to participate in conversations and express their opinions.

3.2. Qualitative Study of Girls/Boys Power Balance

In this section we analyze the pupils' speech in the absence of the teacher to see the impact of the gender variable in their verbal productions.

➢ **Session N°1**

- Noureddin (boy): "*We must continue to play in the same way*"
  - ✓ Illocutionary act: assertion
  - ✓ Perlocutionary act: order, injunction
- Nabila (girl): "*The solution ... the solution is to attack with more than two players*"
  - ✓ Illocutionary act: assertion
  - ✓ Perlocutionary act: declaration

In this brief dialogue, we note that the boy dominates the discussion, since he produces an injunctive discourse involving the whole group. Nabila, disagrees with him, since she guides the discussion to another solution adopting an assertive form. As a result, the boy's speech does not exceed the level of proposal that does not oblige anyone. Things would be different if the girl used the same form of speech that her classmate. Her speech would then cancel the first to surpass it.

➢ **Session N°2**

- Naim (boy) : "*We will try to take the initiative and be the first to score*"
  - ✓ Illocutionary act: assertion
  - ✓ Perlocutionary act: order
- Fawzi (boy): "*But are you a defender with us or what?*"
  - ✓ Illocutionary act: interrogation
  - ✓ Perlocutionary act: reproach

  "*Try to get the ball*"
  - ✓ Illocutionary act: injunction
  - ✓ Perlocutionary act: order

  "*It's not acceptable that you are stuck in the same place!*"
  - ✓ Illocutionary act: assertion
  - ✓ Perlocutionary act: reproach

It seems that the power balance is on the side of Naim, since he imposes to his teammates game tactics involving the whole group: he appears then as the strategist of the group. These findings would be confirmed if he did not face the intervention of his teammate Fawzi who just criticized all his plans. Fawzi's speeches were interrogative and assertive and they have the form of reproaches that defy what is already said. These verbal productions are reinforced by injunctive form conveying reproaches. From this brief discussion, we can deduce that there is a tension between members of the same team. Concerning power balance, it is always the boys who dominate.

➢ **Session N°3**

- Nourreddin (boy): "*We must score again*"
  - ✓ Illocutionary act: injunction
  - ✓ Perlocutionary act: order

  "*We have to keep a defender to survey the backside*"
  - ✓ Illocutionary act: injunction
  - ✓ Perlocutionary act: ordre

  "*Provide coverage at the back*"
  - ✓ Illocutionary act: injunction
  - ✓ Perlocutionary act: order

  "*We have to score other goals so we can play at ease*"
  - ✓ Illocutionary act: injunction
  - ✓ Perlocutionary act: order
- Fawzi (boy): "*We have to participate collectively in the ball recuperation*"
  - ✓ Illocutionary act: injunction
  - ✓ Perlocutionary act: order

  "*Since you don't try to pull the ball, we will never be able to win*"
  - ✓ Illocutionary act: assertion
  - ✓ Perlocutionary act: declaration

  "*We have to try collectively to take the ball from them*"
  - ✓ Illocutionary act: injunction
  - ✓ Perlocutionary act: order

  "*It must be done continuously and not occasionally!*"
  - ✓ Illocutionary act: injunction
  - ✓ Perlocutionary act: order

For both Noureddin for Fawzi, they use injunctive sentences conveying orders about how to play. Their verbal exchange offers plans to make in order to score via this use of injunctive forms listing many instructions to be followed by all team members.

➢ **Session N°4**

- Montassar (boy): "*We will try not to throw the ball no matter how*"
  - ✓ Illocutionary act: injunction
  - ✓ Perlocutionary act: order

  "*Try to no more use long passes too*"
  - ✓ Illocutionary act : injunction
  - ✓ Perlocutionary act: order

  "*We will opt for short passes*"
  - ✓ Illocutionary act : injunction
  - ✓ Perlocutionary act: order
- Chayma (girl) : "*We will try to be faster in attack*"
  - ✓ Illocutionary act : injunction
  - ✓ Perlocutionary act: order
- Imed (boy): "*We must get closer because we're leaving them plenty space*"
  - ✓ Illocutionary act: injunction
  - ✓ Perlocutionary act: order

  "We must reduce the gaps by making a man to man defense"
  - ✓ Illocutionary act: injunction
  - ✓ Perlocutionary act: order
- Hamdi (boy) : "*Try not to let them play freely*"
  - ✓ Illocutionary act: injunction
  - ✓ Perlocutionary act: order
- Imed (boy) : "*We must be organized in defense not to concede goals*"
  - ✓ Illocutionary act: assertion
  - ✓ Perlocutionary act: order
- Chawki (boy) : "We need to score more because they always find spaces, and they can score at any moment"
  - ✓ Illocutionary act: injunction
  - ✓ Perlocutionary act: order

Four pupils were involved in this debate: one girl and three boys. Although the speech of Montassar is injunctive offering game prospects, Imed's verbal productions remain more perfectible. Indeed, he does not just gives injunctions that involve everyone, but also, he presents argumentative connectives. He uses the justification of his opinions and of the eventual consequences to convince his interlocutors. In the same way, Chawki, in addition to the injunction, uses justification. For Chayma, reformulating an order is not associated to clear explanation. It is clear that the discourse of boys is more consistent than that of girls. Not only quantitatively (01 girl and 04 boys) but also in terms of contribution to the game improvement. This leads us to conclude that girls are dominated by boys; they do not participate as much as boys in verbal exchanges and are briefs in their interventions.

➢ **Session N°5**

- Noureddin (boy): "*We should concentrate more*"
  - ✓ Illocutionary act: injunction
  - ✓ Perlocutionary act : order
- Nawfel (boy): "*We have to profit on every occasion*"
  - ✓ Illocutionary act: injunction
  - ✓ Perlocutionary act : order

  "*We should not miss any occasion*"
  - ✓ Illocutionary act: injunction
  - ✓ Perlocutionary act: order
- Noureddin (boy): "*let's try to no more play air balls and play as usual*"
  - ✓ Illocutionary act: injunction
  - ✓ Perlocutionary act: order
- Nabila (girl): "*We must wait until we score. Since there are occasions on target, we have chances to score*"
  - ✓ Illocutionary act: injunction
  - ✓ Perlocutionary act: order

  "*It would be better that you passed me the ball because i am in a better position than you*"
  - ✓ Illocutionary act: assertion
  - ✓ Perlocutionary act: declaration

The game's actors continue to produce a speech oriented to game tactics to adopt to get back into the game and lead the score. Paradoxically, the speech of Nabila is the richest. Her injunctions are reinforced by explanatory argumentative structures. She uses argumentation to demonstrate the utility of her proposals. In the other hand, boys' injunctions are short and rigid, without any explanation. Qualitatively, the power balance tends to be reversed in favor of girls.

➢ **Session N°6**

- Montasser (boy): "*I'm also the last defender, I'm the responsible of all the defense so I have to move forward and anticipate*"
  - ✓ Illocutionary act: assertion / injunction
  - ✓ Perlocutionary act: declaration
- Ahmed (boy): "*We have change our organization*"
  - ✓ Illocutionary act: injunction
  - ✓ Perlocutionary act: order
- Nawfel (boy): "*We should use long shots and from all the distances*"
  - ✓ Illocutionary act: assertion
  - ✓ Perlocutionary act: order
- Naim (boy): "*That's why we have to profit on those lost balls*"
  - ✓ Illocutionary act: assertion
  - ✓ Perlocutionary act: declaration
- Riadh (boy): "*We have to carry on playing collectively because it's our strength*"
  - ✓ Illocutionary act: assertion
  - ✓ Perlocutionary act: declaration
- Hanen (girl): "*Now we have to be organized so we can be able to stop them and dominate*"
  - ✓ Illocutionary act: assertion
  - ✓ Perlocutionary act: order

  "*Believe me, we can easily dominate them*"
  - ✓ Illocutionary act: assertion
  - ✓ Perlocutionary act: declaration

In general, all the verbal productions aimed to project orders about how to play collectively. Boys' injunctive discourse is completed by arguments. Whether justificative or consequential, arguments given by boys inform us about the reasons and the expected impact of those decisions. Hanen is involved in the same logic twice. Her presence is unfortunately distorted by the quantitative dimension of the verbal production made by the opposite sex. In this sense, the boys dominate the discourse again.

➢ **Session N°7**

- Noureddin (boy): "*You can score without shooting. Like that, you can place the ball*"
  - ✓ Illocutionary act: assertion
  - ✓ Perlocutionary act: reproach
- Hanen (girl): "*We are not organized*"
  - ✓ Illocutionary act: assertion
  - ✓ Perlocutionary act: reproach

  "*We must be better placed all over the pitch*"
  - ✓ Illocutionary act: injunction
  - ✓ Perlocutionary act: order
- Riadh (boy): "*We must attack stronger than this*"
  - ✓ Illocutionary act: injunction
  - ✓ Perlocutionary act: order
- Fawzi (boy): "We must reverse the situation"
  - ✓ Illocutionary act: assertion
  - ✓ Perlocutionary act: order

  "*Attack instead of defending!!*"
  - ✓ Illocutionary act: injunction
  - ✓ Perlocutionary act: order
- Imed (boy): "*We must circulate the ball before going to attack*"
  - ✓ Illocutionary act: assertion
  - ✓ Perlocutionary act: order
- Leila (girl): "*We have to progress as fast as possible to their target*"
  - ✓ Illocutionary act: assertion
  - ✓ Perlocutionary act: order

Two key moments characterize the verbal exchange: reproach and proposed orders to remedy. On a syntactic level, there are two types of sentences: assertive and injunctive. Except Hanen's speech, all statements, whether assertive or conveying orders, remain laconic offering only solutions to be back in the game. Hanen, not only just reformulate a reproach, but she completes it by the full injunctive structure proposing a solution. This made her speech the more structured compared to her teammates.

➢ **Session N°8**

- Nawfel (boy): "*We must continue to play like this*"
  - ✓ Illocutionary act: assertion
  - ✓ Perlocutionary act: order
- Ahmed (boy): "*We must intercept the ball, if not, we will not fix this problem*"
  - ✓ Illocutionary act: assertion
  - ✓ Perlocutionary act: order
- Nawfel (boy): "*We have to surpass their marking otherwise, we will not win*"

- ✓ Illocutionary act: assertion
- ✓ Perlocutionary act: order
- Montassar (boy): "*We should no more concede goals*" "*We have to call for a pass in the open spaces*"
  - ✓ Illocutionary act: assertion
  - ✓ Perlocutionary act: order
- Nawfel (boy): "*We must take advantage of occasions we have*"
  - ✓ Illocutionary act: assertion
  - ✓ Perlocutionary act: order
- Chawki (boy): "*We have to avoid losing balls stupidly*"
  - ✓ Illocutionary act: assertion
  - ✓ Perlocutionary act: order
- Nabila (girl): "*We have to shoot*"
  - ✓ Illocutionary act: assertion
  - ✓ Perlocutionary act: order
- Chawki : "*We must not shoot, we have to fix the goalkeeper and dribble him, the target is too small to shoot from a long distance*"
  - ✓ Illocutionary act: assertion
  - ✓ Perlocutionary act: order

  "*We have to approach as possible as we can from the goalkeeper before taking any decision*"
  - ✓ Illocutionary act: assertion
  - ✓ Acte perlocutoire : order

  "*We will attack in pairs and each time we change the roles*"
  - ✓ Acte illocutoire : assertion
  - ✓ Perlocutionary act: order

Whether produced by girls or boys, all statements are assertive serving to give orders. They are all instructions to correct the failure. Most are, in fact, accompanied by a brief argument that explains the cause or the consequence of the act. Nabila produced a structured speech but she is dominated by boys who made more. Among all the interventions, Chawki's speech remains the most consistent. Quantitatively, girls are dominated by boys who made more intervention regardless of the presence or absence of the teacher. The number of their interventions exceeds that of girls who participate in the debate relevantly less than their male teammates. This result was confirmed by the qualitative study. Indeed, although the girls seem to take part in the discussion, their interventions remain unimportant. Their analytical verbal productions remain negligible or less perfectible compared to those of the boys. Girls are unable to gain the upper hand over the boys.

4. Conclusion

The semio-constructivist approach applied in the PES didactics, is an innovation. This study starts from a handball game situation played in a Tunisian scholar environment, based on Austin's typology (1970). The language interactions are characterized by deploying a rich and multifaceted rhetoric reflecting learning dynamic. It is up to the teacher to schedule and plan sequences of verbalization in PES programs in order to give the game a reflective dimension. This can be a favorable condition for the collective success for all pupils who participate in the process of co-construction of knowledge via their own experiences lived in the game situations. Such occasions, are required to lead pupils to do analysis and to understand what happens during the game situations.

Verbal exchanges between pupils can help them to build effective action rules collectively. In addition, the teacher can allow girls to better contribute to decisions by giving them more opportunities to participate in conversations by democratizing the distribution of speech between girls and boys. Such an approach can strengthen the position and the role of the girls in the game during a PES session and the role and state of women in Tunisian society in general.

References

[1] Austin J.L. (1970). *Quand dire, c'est faire.* Paris: Seuil.

[2] Clelland, David C. John W. Atkinson, Russel A. Clark, and Edgar L. Lowel. (1953) *The achievement Motiive?* New York, Appleton-Century.

[3] Borrmans, M. (1977). *Statut personnel et famille au Maghreb de 1940 à nos jours.* Paris, Editions Mouton.

[4] Bessis, S. ; Belhassen, S. (1992). Femmes du Maghreb: L'enjeu. Paris : Editions JC Lattès.

[5] El Khayat-Bannai, G. (1985). Le monde arabe au féminin. Paris : Editions L'Harmattan.

[6] Goffman Erving. (2002). L'arrangement des sexes Paris, la disparute, coll. Le genre du monde.

[7] Gréhaigne, J.F., Caty, D., & Wallian, N. (2004). Évaluation authentique et rapport de forces en sport collectif. *Mesures et évaluation en éducation*, 27, (3), 25-39.

[8] Gréhaigne, J.F. & Godbout, P. (1998). Observation, critical thinking and transformation: three key elements for a constructivist perspective of the learning process in team sport. In Feingold, R., Roger Rees *Actes du congrès de l'Actualité de la recherche en éducation et en formation (AREF), Université de Genève, septembre 2010* 10 C., Barette, G.T., Fiorentino, L., Virgilio, S., & Kowalski, E. (eds.). *Education for life. Proceedings of the AIESEP World Sport Science. Congress.* New York: Adelphi University Press, 109-118.

[9] Gréhaigne, JF. (2009). *Autour du temps. Apprentissages, Espaces, projets dans les sports collectifs.* Besançon: PUFC.

[10] Mathieu NC. (1991) L'anatomie politique, catégorisation et idéologie de sexe. Paris, Des femmes.

[11] Oglesby, Carole. (1986). *Le sport et la femme: mythe ou réalité.* Collection sport+enseignement. Vigot.

[12] Wallian, N. & Chang, C.W. (2007a). Language, thinking and action: Towards a semio-constructivist approach in physical education. *Physical Education and Sport Pedagogy, 12(3),* 289-311.

[13] Wallian, N., & Chang, C.W. (2007b). Sémiotique de l'action

motrice et des activités langagières: vers une épistémologie des savoirs co-construits en sports collectifs. In Gréhaigne, J.F. (dir.). *Configurations du jeu, débat d'idées et apprentissage des sports collectifs*. Besançon : Presses de l'Université de Franche-Comté, 146-164.

[14] Wallian, N. (2010). *Semiotics of language interactions between peers in Physical Education and Sports (EPS) reports places and conflicts of interpretation.* Conference Proceedings of the News of the Educational Research and Training (AREF), University of Geneva.

[15] Zghibi, M. ; Guinoubi, Ch. ; Bennour, N. ; Jbeli, M. ; Sahli, F. et Jabri, M. (2013a). Evolution of language productions and action rules extraction: case study of an 8th grade class girls during a Handball cycle. *Creative Education.* Vol.4 No.3 2013

[16] Zghibi, M. ; Sahli, H. ; Bennour, N. ;Guinoubi, Ch. ;Guerchi, M. et Hamdi, M. (2013b). The Pupil's discourse and action projects: the case of third year high school pupils in Tunisia. *Creative Education.* Vol.4 No.3 2013.

[17] Zghibi, M. (2009). *Interactions langagières des élèves et apprentissage en football: le cas de quatre Classes de 9ème Année de Base en Tunisie.* Thèse de Doctorat ès Sciences du Sport, Université de franche compté. Besançon.

The comparison of burnout on the three directions of Y test in the basketball players with ankle instability

Hamid Khorramnezhad[2], Hamid Dehnavi[1], Mahdi Seyed Alhosseini[3], Hamid Hassanpanah[1]

[1]Sama Technical and Vocational Training College, Islamic Azad University, Neyshabur Branch, Neyshabur, IRAN
[2]Department of Sport Injury and Corrective Exercises, School of Physical Education and Sport Sciences, Shahid Bahonar University of Kerman, Kerman, Iran
[3]M.S of Physical Education and Sport Science, Farhangian University, Daneshvar Branch, Neyshabur, Iran

Email address:
h_khorramnezhad@yahoo.com(H. Khorramnezhad)

Abstract: Maintaining dynamic balance in daily activities and desirable sport functions is indeed crucial. The purpose of the present study was to compare the burnout on the three directions of Y test in the basketball players with ankle instability. The subjects in this study Included 28 basketball players who were selectively divided into two groups based on the ankle instability questionnaire. first group (n=16, mean weight 71.31 ± 10.49, mean height 181.75 ± 9.16 cm, mean age 18.12 ± 1.70 years old) were functionally instable on their ankles, the second group (n=12, mean weight 73.66±9.89 kg, mean height 183.25±7.08 cm, mean age 18.41 ± 1.83 years old) were healthy basketball players". Basketball Movement Specific Circuit" protocol was used to achieve basketball-specific fatigue, and Y test was used to quantify postural control. To make sure that fatigue occurred, Borg scale was employed. The result of dependent T test indicated that dynamic postural control decreased after fatigue in both groups($\alpha<0.005$). In addition, the result of the one-way ANOVA demonstrated that there is a statistically significant difference between anterior and posteromedial directions in the group with functional ankle instability and between anterior and posterolateral directions in the healthy group. The results of this study showed that fatigue significantly affected the players with functional ankle instability in posteromedial direction and the healthy players in posterolateral direction.

Keywords: Fatigue, Dynamic Postural Control, Functional Ankle Instability, Y Test, Basketball Players

1. Introduction

Measurement of postural control is an important tool in the assessment of pediatric, geriatric, and athletic populations for establishing levels of neuromuscular function for the purposes of injury prevention and rehabilitation. Keeping balance in a closed kinematic chain depends on kinematic strategies and orchestrated feedbacks among the leg, knee and ankle. The torsion of ankle joint, the most common sport injury, is prevalent in most sport fields requiring running, jumping, cutting movements, and stepping to the sides such as football, volleyball, and basketball (frigg et al., 2007), (Bruce et al., 2002). Basketball is one of the world's most popular physical activities. Nearly 11% of the world's population play basketball regularly. Unfortunately, since the number of young male and female basketball players is rising, the rate of injuries also increases (Harmer, 2005). Due to the nature of this sport field, a high percentage of injuries were reported to have occurred in the lower limb and ankle (Harmer, 2005). Damore et al, (2003) stated that the majority of young basketball players' injuries in the lower limb, which were reported to be between 35/9 and 92 percent, were related to the ankle (Damore et al., 2003). The researchers are still trying to reduce the amount of injuries in basketball players; they have mainly focused on risk factors such as proprioception ability, the level of kinematic development, the level of competition, and fatigue (Harmer, 2005). Fatigue is a common phenomenon that occurs during exercises and impairs an athlete's kinematic function (Millet et al., 2004). In the last decade, sports scientists have considered fatigue as a factor which negatively affects sport performance. They also investigated the relation between fatigue and postural control and concluded that fatigue and the reduction of postural control can result in skeletal-muscular injury in athletes (Pappas et al., 2007). Several studies have been done on the relation between fatigue and postural control. For instance, Gribble et al, (2004) examined the effect of fatigue and chronic ankle instability on dynamic postural control in posterior, medial, and anterior directions through applying Star Excursion Balance Test. They found that the individuals had less ankle flexion angle and less balance in all the three directions in the ankle with chronic instability (Gribble et al., 2004). Sadeghee et al, (2008), in a study entitled "The effect of functional fatigue on dynamic postural control", employed a functional fatigue protocol (20- minute activity at 7 stations) and a Star Excursion Balance Test in order to induce fatigue and evaluate dynamic balance respectively. They concluded that dynamic postural control was impaired after employing the fatigue protocol (Sadeghee et al., 2008). Sedaghat (2008), in a study entitled "The effect of football-specific fatigue on the dynamic postural control of the football players with functional ankle instability", measured the players' dynamic balance through applying simulator football protocol and analyzing data in the pretest and posttest of Star Excursion Balance Test. The result indicated that, at the end of the protocol, the players with functional ankle instability had significantly impaired postural control (sedaghat , 2008). Hosseinimehr et al, (2010) explored the influence of fatigue on the static and dynamic postural control of the athletes' with ankle injury. The participants of the study consisted of 30 males and females (15 subjects in the control group, 15 subjects in the experimental one). In order to measure dynamic balance, measure static balance, and induce fatigue, they used a Star Excursion Balance Test, a test of standing on one foot, and a seven-station functional protocol respectively. The results demonstrated that the healthy athletes' dynamic balance significantly decreased after employing the fatigue protocol (Hosseinimehr et al., 2010).

As it is clear, to investigate the impact of fatigue on the postural control system, most studies used protocols unrelated to exercises and competitions. Furthermore, few studies have been conducted to explore dynamic postural control through functional tests; instead, most of them were carried out to investigate the static postural control system. On the whole, it seems that there is a lack of research into the relationship between dynamic postural control and exercise-induced fatigue and its related concepts. Consequently, it is essential to explore any possible effect of whole body fatigue on dynamic postural control through a functional fatigue protocol which is similar to exercises and competitions and a functional test which measures dynamic postural control.

2. Methodology

The subjects of this study were 28 basketball players who participated in the Youth League in Kerman. Their ages ranged between 16 and 21 years old. The players completed the complacency form, they were handed in Cumberland Ankle Instability Tools (CAIT). In this 30-point questionnaire, the score 0 to 27 indicated ankle instability and the score 27 to 30 represented healthy ankle. Then, the participants were selectively divided in two groups: a group of 16 subjects with functional ankle instability and a group of 12 healthy subjects. To make sure that the two groups are exactly similar in terms of the variables of age, weight, height, maximum oxygen consumption, body mass index, and ankle instability score, independent T-Test was held. In other words, T-Test was used to ensure that the only significant difference between the two groups was ankle instability score. The result of the T-Test is presented in the Table 1.

***Table 1.** The result of T-Test ran to ensure homogeneity of the two groups*

Statistical index / variable	T	df	Sig
Age	-0.43	26	0.668
Weight	-0.60	26	0.553
Height	-0.47	26	0.642
Maximum oxygen consumption	0.18	26	0.851
Ankle instability score	-9.76	26	0.001*
Body mass index	-0.41	26	0.679

The sign * illustrates a significant difference ($\alpha<0.05$) between the groups on the variable

The Y balance test device (Intraclass correlation coefficient ranged from 0.89 to 0.93 for the 3 reach directions: anterior 0.89, posteromedial 0.93, and posterolateral 0.91 directions) was used to assess the participants' dynamic postural control. In this device, three directions are situated just like Y(Plisky et al., 2006; figur1). To normalize data, this test measured the actual length of the leg which stretched from anterior superior iliac spines to the medial ankle (Gribble et al., 2003). After the experimenter explained the test to the participants, the subjects practiced six times to familiar the procedure. The Y test was performed on the premier feet. If the right foot was premier, the test was performed in the counterclockwise direction; otherwise in clockwise direction (Gribble et al., 2003).

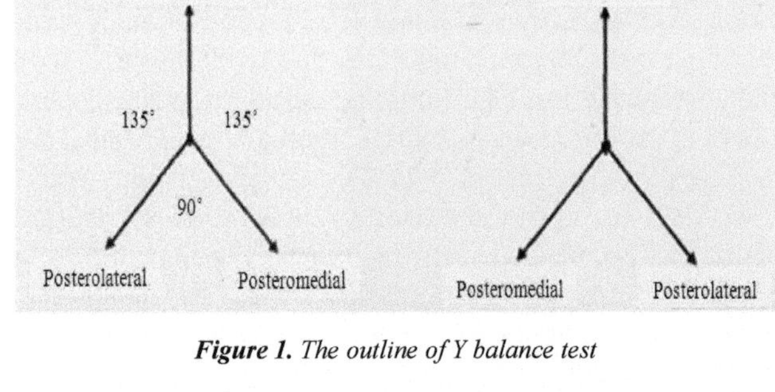

***Figure 1.** The outline of Y balance test*

The player stood on one leg in the center of a grid. While maintaining single-leg stance, the player was asked to reach with the free limb in the anterior, posteromedial, and posterolateral directions in relation to the stance foot. The maximal reach distance was measured by marking the tape measure with erasable ink at the point where the most distal part of the foot reached. The trial was discarded and repeated if the player (1) failed to maintain unilateral stance, (2) lifted or moved the stance foot from the grid, (3) touched ground with the reach foot, or (4) failed to return the reach foot to the starting position. The process was repeated while standing on the other leg. The greatest reach distance of the 3 trials for each direction was used for analysis (Figure2) (plisky et al., 2006). Finally, the mean of the three scores was calculated, and the result was divided by the leg length (cm) and multiplied by 100.

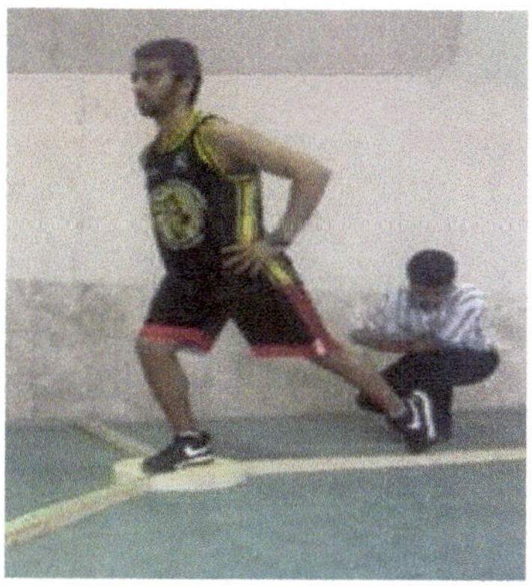

Figure 2. The performance of Y balance test

Basketball-specific fatigue protocol (Basketball Movement Specific Circuit) was employed to induce fatigue (Figure2) (Smith , 2004). This protocol is similar to a basketball game in terms of duration, intensity, and movement patterns. It is applicable in a basketball field. It consists of four 4-minute phases with the heart rate of 90% to 95% HRmax. Between each phase, there is a 3-minute active rest (jogging) with the heart rate of 70% HRmax.

To ensure that adequate fatigue was attained, the clinicians used the 15-point Borg scale to measure each subjects Rating of Perceived Exertion (RPE). After the participants prepared themselves through a brief warm-up (5-10 minutes of jogging and stretching the lower limb), Y test and PRE were administered as pretests. After they finished the protocol, Y test and PRE were held as posttests (Timothy et al., 2006). In order to compare the postural mean scores in every direction and PRE pretest and posttest in each group, dependent T-Test ($p<0.05$) was run. Furthermore, one-way Anova was employed to compare the postural control mean scores in the three directions of Y test in each group. Then, LSD post hoc test was used to find the exact place of difference.

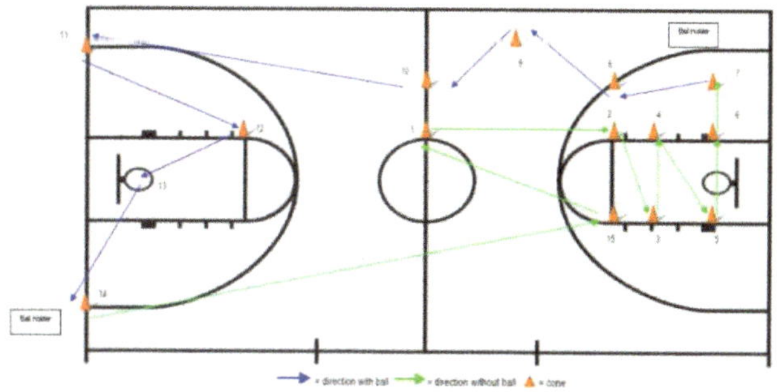

Figure 3. Basketball movement specific training circuit. 1-2 forward sprint; 2 pivot left; 2-3 shuffle left; 3-4 shuffle right; 4-5 shuffle left; 5-6 shuffle right; 6-7 run into vertical jump(collect ball upon landing); 7-10 speed dribble ball around cones; 10-11 speed dribble; 11-12 speed dribble; 12-13 lay-up attempt; 13 lay-up rebound; 13-14 speed dribble(drop ball at 14); 14-15 forward sprint; 15-1 back pedal.

3. Results

The result of dependent T-Test between the pretest and posttest on mean scores of reach distance in the three directions are presented in the Table 1. there is a significant difference ($\alpha=0.05$)in all the three directions. Besides, the results show that the mean scores of postural control in the three directions of the balance test are not equal(tables 2,3). This suggests that there is a significant difference between the mean scores of at least two directions in each group. Tables 4 and 5 list the result of LSD post hoc test. It reveals that there is a statistically significant difference between anterior and posteromedial directions in the group with functional ankle instability and between anterior and posterolateral directions in the healthy group. Moreover, the significant difference ($t= -14.45$, $p=0.000$) between Borg Scale pretest and posttest, achieved through running T-Test, demonstrated that the intended fatigue really occurred (Graph 1).

Table 2. Comparison between postural control mean scores in each direction in the two groups

Directions	Mean score		Std. deviation		Std. error		t value		df		α	
	control	experimental	control	experimental	control	experimental	control	experimental	control	experimental	control	experimental
Anterior Direction	5.56	4.48	3.13	5.03	0.90	1.25	6.25	3.65	11	15	0.000	0.003
Posteromedial Direction	8.58	10.50	6.7	5.34	1.94	1.33	4.41	7.85	11	15	0.001	0.000
Posterolateral Direction	11.51	8.44	5.36	6.78	1.54	1.69	7.44	4.98	11	15	0.000	0.000

Table 3. The summery of the result of one-way Anova conducted on the data obtained from the experimental and control groups

	Group	Sum of squares	Df	Mean squares	F	Sig
Between groups	experimental	299.574	2	149.787	4.498	0.017
	control	206.501	2	103.250	3.689	0.036
Within groups	experimental	1498.651	45	33.303		
	control	923.631	33	27.989		
Total	experimental	1798.225	47			
	control	1130.132	35			

Table 4. The result of one-way Anova ran to check the difference between the pairs of mean scores in the group with functional ankle instability

phase		Group	Mean score difference	Std. deviation of mean score difference	sig	confidence interval (95%) for mean difference minimum	maximum
1	2	experimental	-6.0189*	2.04032	0.005	-10.1284	-1.9095
		control	-2.9312	2.15982	0.184	-7.3254	1.4630
1	3	experimental	-3.9656	2.04032	0.058	-8.0751	0.1438
		control	-5.8666	2.15982	0.010	-10.2608	-1.4724
2	3	experimental	2.0533	2.040332	0.32	-2.0561	6.1627
		control	-2.9354	2.15982	0.183	-7.3296	1.4588

1: anterior direction 2:posteromedial direction 3:posterolateral direction

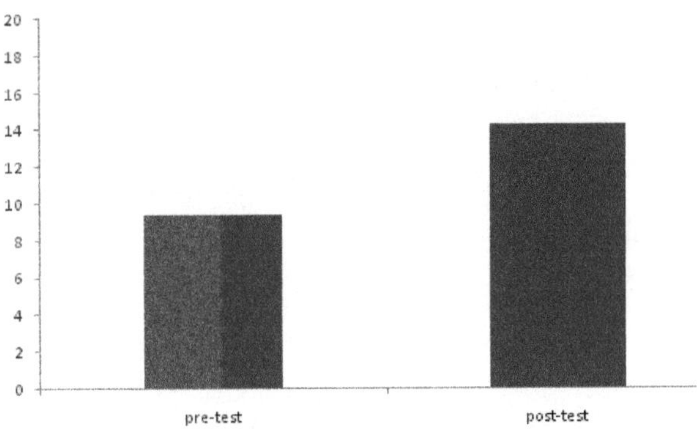

Graph 1. The result of PRE measurement

4. Discussion and Conclusion

The main aim of the present study was the comparison of the effect of the amount of fatigue on the three directions of Y test in the basketball players with ankle instability. The results suggested a relationship between reach operation and time (pretest and posttest). Reach distance in all the three directions in the posttest was lower than the one in the pretest. Besides, the results indicated a significant difference between PRE pretest and posttest mean scores. On the whole, the findings confirm the four research hypotheses: reach distance in all the three directions of the Y balance test in the pretest will be significantly higher than the one in the posttest. The support of the fourth hypothesis, stating that there will be a significant difference between PRE pretest and posttest mean scores, shows that the intended fatigue was induced in the two phases of the fatigue protocol.

The reduction of the reach distance in the three directions of Y test after the application of the fatigue protocol can be attributed to the different roles of each of the lower limb muscles in performing the balance test. In their study, Olmsted et al, (2003) found that the foot on which a person leans while performing the test needs knee flexion, leg flexion, and ankle dorsiflexion. Thus, the lower limb requires adequate motion range, strength, the activity of deep receptors, and neuromuscular control (Gribble et al., 2003), (Olmsted et al., 2003). While an individual performs the reach operation, hamstring and quadric muscles are contracted in all directions. The quadric muscle has its most activities in the anterior direction. This can be accounted on the fact that, while performing reach operation, the individual has to lean back and his body should be extended so that he can maintain his balance. In this situation, the gravitational force acting on the upper part of the body causes high knee flexion torque which should be controlled by the extension torque (eccentric contractions) generated by quadric muscles (Earl et al., 2001). The external broad muscle has its most activities in the posteromedial direction. This is because of the muscular stability which occurs against the muscular forces active to perform the reach operation in this direction (Earl et al., 2001). While an individual performs the reach operation, the biceps are also active. The biceps have their most activities in posteromedial and posterolateral directions. This can be explained in terms of the effect of the gravitational force acting on the body, which causes knee flexion torque. In order to perform activities in the posterior direction, the person should have flexion in his body so that he can open his foot to the back. In this situation, hamstring muscles should be contracted in an eccentric way so that they can resist against the leg flexion torque. Performing an activity in the lateral direction requires severe lateral leg rotation which results in the activity of the upper part of biceps (Earl et al., 2001). Besides, to obtain the highest reach distance while performing the test in posterolateral and posteromedial directions, the participant needs plantar ankle flexion leading to the sever activity of back shank muscles (Earl et al., 2001).

The findings of the present study indicate that the reduction of reach distance in all the three directions of Y test after the induction of fatigue in the different muscles of lower limb depends on the roles that these muscles plays in performing the reach operation. Regarding the preceding discussion, we can attribute the reduction of postural control mean scores in the posttest to reduced muscle strength, impaired joint position sense, delayed neuromuscular responses. The result gained in this study has a consistency with the findings obtained in other similar researches. Mercer et al, (2003), Nyland et al, (1997) and Rahnama et al, (2003) asserted that fatigue reduces muscular strength. In the same vein, Rozzy and Lefart (1999) and Skinner et al, (1986) claimed that joint position sense (proprioception ability) is impaired due to fatigue. Similarly, Gleeson et al, (1998) and Rozzy et al, (1999) believed that, because of fatigue, neuromuscular firing, the reaction of muscles, and neuromuscular responses are postponed.

Considering the directions of SEBT test, many researchers believed that performing an activity is easier in some directions than the others. To put it in more specific words, performing an activity is easiest in posterior, posteromedial, and medial directions but most difficult in anterior, anterolateral, and lateral directions (Gribble , 2003), (Gribble et al., 2003). Post hoc tests demonstrated that, firstly, it is most difficult to perform an activity in the lateral direction; secondly, reach distance is significantly lowest in anterolateral direction (except the lateral direction); and thirdly, reach distance is randomly highest in posterior and posteromedial directions (Gribble , 2003), (Gribble et al., 2003).In the present study, it was concluded that there is a significant decrease in all directions in both groups after the application of the fatigue protocol. Specifically, the post hoc test proved that the healthy participants displayed more significant difference in posterolateral direction and those with functional ankle instability illustrated more significant difference in posteromedial direction.

References

[1] Frigg A, Frigg R, Hintermann B, Barg A, Valderrabano V. (2007). The biomechanical influence of tibio talar containment on stability of the ankle joint. Knee Surg Sports Traumatol Arthrosc. 15(11):1355-62.

[2] Bruce D. Beynnon, Darlene F. Murphy, Denise M. Alosa (2002). Predictive Factors for Lateral Ankle Sprains. J Athl Train. 37(4): 376–380.

[3] Karen P Cote, Michael E Brunet, II, Bruce M Gansneder, Sandra J Shultz. (2005). Effects of pronated and supinated foot postures on static and dynamic postural stability. J Athl Train. 2005 Jan-Mar; 40(1): 41–46.

[4] Damore DT, Metzl JD, Ramundo M, Pan S, Van Amerongen R. (2003).Patterns in childhood sports injury. Pediatr Emerg Care. 19(2):65-7.

[5] Earl JE, Hertel J. (2001). Lower-extremity muscle activation during the star excursion balance tests. Journal of Sport Rehabilitation. Vol. 10 Issue 2, p93

[6] Gleeson NP, Reilly T, Mercer TH, Rakowski S, Rees D. (1998). Influence of acute endurance activity on leg neuromuscular and musculoskeletal performance. Medicine and Science in Sports and Exercise 30 (4), 596–608.

[7] Gribble PA. (2003). The star excursion balance test as a measurement tool. Athl Ther Today;8(2):46- 47.

[8] Gribble PA, Hertel J. (2003). Considerations for the normalizing measures of the star excursion balance test. Measurements Phys Educ Exer Sci;7:89-100.

[9] Gribble PA, Hertel J, Denegar C.R, Buckley EW. (2004). The effects of fatigue and chronic Ankle instability on Dynamic postural control. J of Athletic training. 39 (4): 321-329.

[10] Harmer PA. (2005). "Basketball injuries", Med Sport Sci. Basel. vol 49, pp 31–61.

[11] Hosseinimehr H, Daneshmandi H, Norasteh A. (2010). The Effects of Fatigue and Chronic Ankle Instability on Dynamic Postural Control. Physics International 1 (1): 22-26.

[12] Mercer T.H, Gleeson N.P, Wren K (2003). Influence of prolonged intermittent high-intensity exercise on knee flexor strength in male and female soccer players. European Journal of Applied Physiology 89 (5),506–508.

[13] Millet GY, R Lepers. (2004). Alterations of neuromuscular function after prolonged running, cycling and skiing exercises. Sports Med., 34: 105- 116.

[14] Nyland JA, Shapiro R, Caborn DN, Nitz AJ, Malone TR (1997). The effect of quadriceps femoris, hamstring, and placebo eccentric fatigue on knee and ankle dynamics during crossover cutting. Journal of Orthopaedic & Sports Physical Therapy 25 (3), 171–184.

[15] Olmsted LC, Carcia CR, Hertel J, Shultz SJ. (2003). Efficacy of the star excursion balance tests in detecting reach deficits in subjects with chronic ankle instability. J Athl Train. 37, 501-506.

[16] Pappas E, Sheikhzadeh A, Hagins M, Nordin M (2007). The effect of gender and fatigue on the biomechanics of bilateral landings from a jump: Peak values. J Sports Sci and Med. 6:77-84.

[17] Plisky PJ, Rauh MJ, Kaminski TW, Underwood FB. (2006). Star excursion balance test as a predictor of lower extremity injury in high school basketball players. J Orthop Sports Phys Ther 36: 911–919.

[18] Rahnama N & et al (2003). cc. Journal of sport science, 21:11, 933-942.

[19] Rozzi SL, Lephart SM, Fu FH. (1999). Effects of muscular fatigue on knee joint laxity and neuromuscular characteristics of male and female athletes. Journal of Athletic Training 34 (2), 106– 114.

[20] Sadeghee H, Sershin A, Abbasi A (2008). The effect of functional fatigue on dynamic postural control. Research into Sport Science, 20, 79-94.

[21] Sedaghat M (2008). The effect of football-specific fatigue on the dynamic postural control of the football players with functional ankle instability. Unpublished M.A thesis. Shahid Bahonar University of Kerman.

[22] Smith M. (2004). Basketball skill test for the big men. FIBA Assist Magazine, 07, 59-60.

[23] Skinner H.B, Wyatt M.P, Hodgdon J.A, Conard D.W, Barrack R.L (1986). Effect of fatigue on joint position sense of the knee. Journal of Orthopaedic Research 4 (1), 112–118.

[24] Seliga R, Bhattacharya A, Succop P, Wixhstrom R, Smith D, Willeke K. (1991). Effect of work load and respirator wear on postural stability, heart rate, and perceived exertion. Am Ind Hyg Assoc J;52:417-422.

[25] Timothy A, Kulpa BS. (2006). The Effects of Activity related fatigue on Dynamic postural control as measured by SEBT. Unpublished M.A thesis. Morgantown, West Virginia.

8

Analysis of set shot in basketball in relation with time to perform the course and displacement of center of gravity

Mandeep Singh Nathial

Dept of Higher Education, Government of J&K, Jammu, India

Email address:
bawarayman@yahoo.co.in

Abstract: The purpose of the study was to analysis of the technique of set shot while attempting free throws with the performance, in relation with time to perform the course and displacement of center of gravity. Sixty National level male basketball players of three different height groups i.e. Group I: 5'5" to 5'8",Group II: 5'9" to 6' and Group III: 6' 1" to 6'4",(20 in each group) were selected as subjects for the study. The data was obtained from two given positions (i) Moment of stance in set shot and (ii) Moment of release of ball in set shot. Total ten attempts were given and the successful shots marked as score out of ten as criterion measure of performance. Four Digital Video cameras Sony 2100 series were used in order to register the technique of set shot while attempting set shot. The films were analyzed by using standard motion analyzer. With regard to purpose of the study techniques of product moment correlation and analysis of variance were applied. In order to check the significance, level of significance was set at 0.05. It was found that there is significant relationship between the time to perform the course and the performance in set shot of different height group players in basketball and there is no significant relationship found between the displacement of center of gravity and the performance of set shot of different height group players in basketball and therefore, the selected variable puts no impact on the performance of set shot. It was also concluded that Time to perform the course had lowest impact (7%) in the performance. Further it was concluded that displacement of center of gravity was significantly different in first group (5'5" to 5'8") from the other two groups.

Keywords: Kinematical Analysis, Set Shot, Center of Gravity and Time to Perform the Course of Set Shot

1. Introduction

This study has been taken to analysis of the technique of set shot while attempting free throws with the performance, in relation with time to perform the course and displacement of center of gravity. Of all the animals, man has been the most successful in the constant struggle with the environment. Even though he cannot run as fast as quadriceps, swim as like dolphin, climb as like as apes or fly as birds do. He has been the only creature, able to defy the force of gravity and move into outer space. Now a day, sport has become an essential part of the life. Millions of fans follow different sports events all over the world with enthusiasm and devotion. People participates in sports and games for many reasons, some play for fun, pleasure, happiness, health and fitness while some play as professionalists. Human beings normally run, jump, throw, catch, kick, strike and perform a multitude of basic skills. They learn these first as general skills and latter in modified specified sports skills. Then they combine the skill into patterns of increasingly greater specificity and complexity. [1,3,4]

Ikai M. and Matsumoto Y. (2014) made scientific investigations on the principles underlying the various techniques used in Judo, first analyzed the techniques, and made observations on their kinematics, and further wished to synthesize by adding psychological and physiological investigations. It was found that in the Hiza- guruma velocity was the lowest with 1.95 m/s. Sciences of applied mechanism are fulfilling these demands of high technological knowledge for the enhancement of performance in the field of sports. Physical education reaching new heights and providing equal to expectations of the demand of this profession but still lot more is to be done. [2,5-9,15,16]

Kinematics is the geometry of motion, which includes displacement, velocity and acceleration without regard for the forces acting on the body. Kinematics is the branch of biomechanics that is concerned with describing the motion of bodies. Thus kinematics deals with such things as how far a body moves, how fast it moves and how consistently it moves. It is not concerned at all with what causes a body to move in a way it does. Kinematics is essentially the descriptive geometry of motion with respect to time, ignoring the causes of motion and the concepts of mass, force, momentum and energy. However, the kinematics of a rigid body of finite mass may be analyzed if its mass is to be considered at one point. Kinematic analyses are important in understanding the mechanisms of athlete's injuries. [7,16,19]

The two most common shots that use the above described set up are the set shot and the *jump shot.* The set shot is taken from a standing position, with neither foot leaving the floor, typically used for free throws. The jump shot is taken while in mid-air, when the ball is released near the top of the jump. This provides much greater power and range, and it also allows the player to elevate over the defender. Failure to release the ball before the feet return to the ground is considered a traveling violation.[17] Another common shot is called the *layup.* This shot requires the player to be in motion toward the basket, and to 'lay' the ball 'up' and into the basket, typically off the backboard (the backboard-free, underhand version is called a finger roll). The most crowd-pleasing, and typically highest-percentage accuracy shot is the *slam dunk,* in which the player jumps very high, and throws the ball downward, straight through the hoop. Another shot that is becoming common is the "circus shot". The circus shot is a low-percentage shot that is flipped, heaved, scooped, or flung toward the hoop while the shooter is off-balance, airborne, falling down, and/or facing away from the basket.

2. Objectives of the Study

1. To find out the relational effect of Time to perform the course and Displacement of center of gravity with the performance in set shot.
2. To study the significance of difference in Time to perform the course and Displacement of center of gravity among three different height groups while performing set shot.
3. The study will be designed to prepare an ideal model for the skill of set shot in basketball in relation with Time to perform the course and Displacement of center of gravity of the shooter.

3. Methodology

Selection of subjects and collection of data:

Sixty National level male basketball players of three different height groups i.e.

Group I: 5'5" to 5'8"

Group II: 5'9" to 6'

Group III: 6' 1" to 6'4"

(20 in each group) were selected as subjects for the study. It was ascertained that subjects possess reasonable level of technique. Most of the selected subjects were senior national players and had performed in the National basketball championships.

The age of the subjects ranged between 18 to 30 years. The data was obtained with the help of two given positions of any successful attempt:

(a) Moment of stance in set shot.

(b) Moment of release of ball in set shot.

Criterion Measure:

The criterion measure for this study was the performance of the subjects in set shot in basketball. Total of ten attempts were given to each subject and the successful shots marked as score out of ten. The performance of each trial was judged accurately and total score was recorded.

Analysis of film and collection of data:

Video graphic technique was used in this study. The Videos were recorded and analyzed by using standard motion analyzer software (Motion Pro-Advanced Coach Edition). Only two selected moments were analyzed. Quick snap shots under motion pro software for analysis of variable.

Measuring time to perform the course:

To check the time taken by the performer to perform the set shot, Software set-timer option was used. Time gets started from the moment of stance and stops at the moment of release of ball by the performer (Fig: 01)

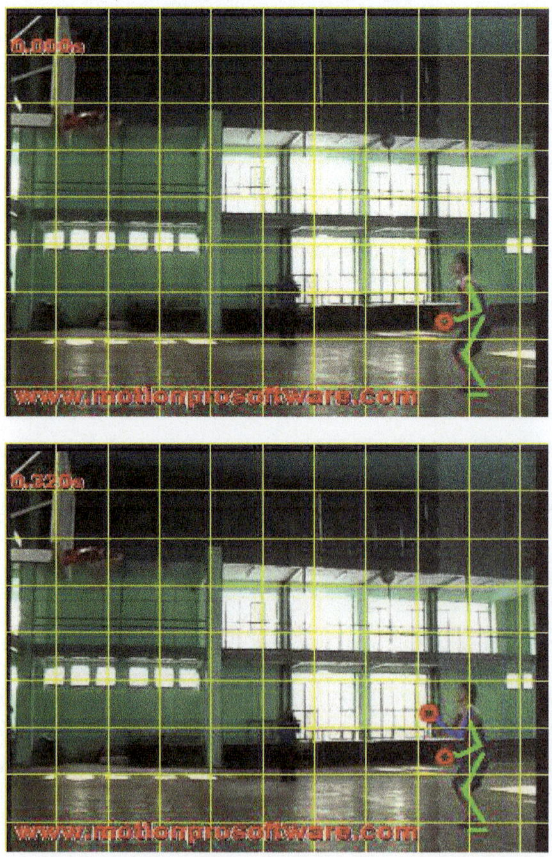

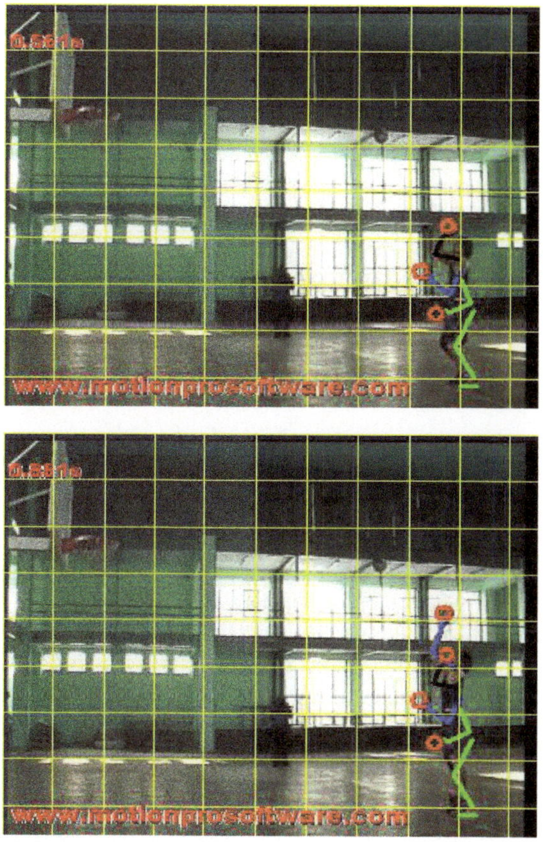

Figure 01. *Display of elapsed time from mark in through motion pro software. (Four snap shots)*

Location of C.G.:

On the basis of Quick snap shot obtained by the software, researcher developed stick figures, with the help of which the location of center of gravity during the moment stance and moment of release of ball in set shot was found.

Statistical analysis of data:

With regard to purpose of the study product moment correlation was calculated between selected kinematical variables with the performance of subjects in set shot in basketball. Analysis of variance (One way ANOVA) was used to study the significance of difference in selected kinematic variables among three different height groups with mean comparisons of different groups through post hoc test while performing set shot. In order to check the significance, level of significance was set at 0.05.

4. Result

Product moment correlation was used to find out the relationship of the selected Kinematical variables with the performance of Basketball players in set shot.

Table 01. *Showing coefficient of correlation of time to perform the course and displacement of center of gravity with the Performance in set shot (N=60)*

Sl.No.	Variables	Coefficient of Correlation
1	Time to perform the course	-.261*
2	Displacement of center of gravity	0.090

Note: * - Significant at 0.05 level

As shown in table 01 the obtained value of coefficient of correlation of the time to perform the course for 58 degree of freedom (-.261) is more than the required value (.250) for 0.05 level of significance, therefore the variable has shown significantly low relationship with the performance in set shot in basketball. However, the selected variable has shown negative correlation with the performance in set shot. This can be stated that there is significant relationship between the time to perform the course and the performance in set shot of different height group players in basketball. Whereas the obtained value of coefficient of correlation of the variable displacement of center of gravity for 58 degree of freedom (0.090) is less than the required value (.250) for 0.05 level of significance, therefore the selected variable has shown no significant relationship with the performance in set shot in basketball.

Table 02. *Showing Regression analysis of time to perform the course (TPC) as independent variable and performance as dependent variable*

Model	R	R square	Adjusted R square	Standardized Coefficients Beta	Sig.
TPC	.261	.068	.052	-.261	.044

Constant: Time to perform the course.

Dependent Variable: Performance.

Table 02 depicts R at .261 and R square at .068. Indicating that 7% variation in the performance was being caused by time to perform the course. The value of Beta coefficient has arrived at -.261 (significant at .05 level), so it signifies that time to perform the course affects performance.

Table 03. *Showing F value of time to perform the course and displacement of center of gravity of three different height groups while performing set shot in basketball.*

	Sources of Variance	SS	Df	MS	F
time to perform the course (TPC)	SS Between	3.386	2	1.693	1.021
	SS with in	94.486	57	1.658	
Displacement of center of gravity (DCG)	SS Between	1120.713	2	560.357	16.304**
	SS with in	1959.024	57	34.369	

There was no significant difference in the time to perform the course of three different height group players while performing set shot. The value of F-ratio for the displacement of center of gravity of three different height groups while performing set shot was significant at .01 level. It indicates that there was significant difference in the displacement of center of gravity of three different height groups while performing set shot.

Table 04. *Showing multiple comparison of different height groups in displacement of center of gravity*

	Group (s)	Group (j)	MD
Displacement of center of gravity	I	II	-6.41250**
	III		-10.50100**
	II	I	6.41250**
	III		-4.08850
	III	I	10.50100**
		II	4.08850

Note: * - Significant at 0.05 level. Height groups: I=5'5" to 5'8", II=5'9" to 6', III=6'1" to 6'4"

Table 04 indicates that first height group players i.e. 5'5" to 5'8" were significantly different from the other two height group players in displacement of center of gravity.

5. Discussion of the Findings

Time to perform the course showed no significant difference among the three different height groups. It was analyzed that 7% of contribution in the performance of set shot was caused by time to perform the course but when we consider players of different heights, time period among different height players may not be different in performing the skill of set shot.

In another previous research study on the relationship of kinematic variables with the performance of standing broad jump (Ruhal A.S. and Ruhal G.S, 2014) it was found that the angle at knee joints and angle at ankle joints were significantly related with the performance in broad jump. In the same study it was also found that the time taken to perform the broad jump was not significantly related with the performance in broad jump. It is felt that executor of any skill, usually take its time according to the personal style of technique. Therefore, the main concentration players put is on performance or accuracy of the technique not on time consumption (it is preferred on the sports where fraction of seconds do not matter much but the accuracy plays important role)

It was also found that the displacements of center of gravity of the shooter have no relationship with the performance of set shot in basketball. Previous study with the purpose to investigate the pattern of motion of the striking arm and muscular/joint activities responsible for it during the arm swing phase of the volleyball spike (Soo Chung, 2013) also showed that the elbow muscles and joint contains no significant value in strengthening respective arm rotation and performance directly. Previous research to develop suitable and feasible criteria for the evaluating different variations of seoi nege and to find out the contributing biomechanical, anthropometric flexibility and motor fitness factors for effective execution of different variation of seoi nage (S. Dhananjoy, 1992) also shown that (i) left elbow joint, right knee joint and center of gravity at the basic stances prefer no correlation with the seoi nege perfecton and (ii) the angle at the ankle joint found not to be significantly correlated with total time as it was less effective too.

6. Conclusions

Based on the analysis and within the limitations of the study following conclusions were drawn:

1. Significant relationship was observed between time to perform the course and the performance of set shot in basketball. Therefore, selected variable puts impact on the performance of set shot.
2. There is no significant relationship found between the displacement of center of gravity and the performance of set shot of different height group players in basketball and therefore, the selected variable puts no impact on the performance of set shot.
3. Time to perform the course had lowest impact (7%) in the performance.
4. Displacement of center of gravity was significantly different in first group (5'5" to 5'8") from the other two groups.
5. Time to perform the course was not significantly different among three groups.

References

[1] Aboub, M.A. (2010). "A Biomechanical Model for the Upper Extremity Using Optimizational Structure of Kinesiology", *Journal of Physical Education*, Pb., Vol. 20, pp.120-121.

[2] Anndrews, J.G. (1995). "Strength Curves for Multiple - Joint Single Degree of Freedom Exercises", *Journal of Biomechanics*, Vol. 18, p.226.

[3] Andrzej W. and Elisaz J. (2004). "Kinematic Analysis of Handball Throws", *Annual Publishing-Poland Polish Air Force Institute of Medicine-II, p.37.*

[4] Asami, Takkaaki, and Toketo (1978). "An Analytical Study on the Position of the Center of Gravity in the Osae-waza (Art of Holding) in Judo". *Bulletin of the Association for the Scientific Studies on Judo*, Repsort V Tokyo: Kodokan.

[5] Aydin, Bergün and Mensure (2009). "Kinematic Analysis of Over Arm Movements for Different Sports", *Journal of Kinsiology*, Vol. 41, pp.105-111.

[6] Barfield, R.W. (2002). "Kinematic Instep Kicking Differences between Elite Female and Male Soccer Players", *Journal of Sports Science and Medicine*, Vol. 72,pp.286-294.

[7] Beach, Clark Richard (1984). "Kinematic Analysis of Spatial and Temporal Errors in Rapid Timing Tasks", *Dissertation Abstract International*, Vol. 44, p.270-A.

[8] Boyson, J.P. (1977). "Interactive Computer Graphics in the Study of Human Body Planner Motion under Free Fall Conditions", *Journal of Biomechanics*, Vol. 10, pp.783-787.

[9] Coh M. (2003). "Cathy Freeman's sprinting Technique", *Track Coach*, pp.4988-4992.

[10] Claessens, A. (1987). "Somatotype and Body Structure of World Top Judoists", *The Journal of Sports Medicine and Physical Fitness*, Vol. 27, pp.105-113.

[11] Cook, E.B. and Wherry, R.J. (1950). "A Statistical Evaluation of Physical Fitness Tools", *Research Quarterly*, Vol. 21, pp.94-111.

[12] Dawson and Lov (1984). "Relationship of Selected Kinematic Variables to in High Jump", *A Review of Literature - Athletic Training*, Vol. 14, pp.161-164.

[13] Dapena, Jesus (1985). "Systematic Error in Three-Dimensional Coordinates within a Large Object - Space when Using DLT & NLT Methods of Three Dimensional Cinematography", *Journal of Biomechanics*, Vol. 18, p.230.

[14] Deol, N.S., S. Mandeep and Gill, M. (2014). "Physical Education for Special People: A Kinematical Analysis", *HPE Forum Bi-annual Professional Journal*, Vol. 08, pp.47-50.

[15] Deusinger, Robert H. (1969). "A Kinetic Analysis of the Book Break Fall and Force of Impact in Judo", *Completed Research in Health, Physical Education and Recreation*, Vol. 11, pp.145-146.

[16] Greenwald, Rosca and Morra (2009). "Assessment of Influence of Contemporary Knee Design on High Flexion", *Human Mov. Sci.*, Vol. 16, pp.457–467.

[17] Greeve, D.w. (1969). "A Device Called The Polon for the Measurement of the Orientation of Parts of the Relative to a Fixed Externalo Axis", *Journal of Physiology*, Vol. 07, p.201.

[18] Guimaraes R. and Cliquet (2009). "Kinematic Analysis of the Knee when Climbing up/down Stairs in Patellofemoral Instability", *Acta. Ortop. Bras.*, pp.157-154.

[19] Huang Chi (2009). "Biomechanics of Standing Long Jump with Handheld Weight", *Journal of Sports Sciences*, Vol. 17, pp.574-575.

[20] Hutto, Louis E. (1938). "Measurement of the Velocity Factor and of Athletic Power in High School Boys", *Research Quarterly*, Vol. 39, p.109.

[21] Ikai, M. and Matsumoto Y. (2014). "The Kinetics of Judo", *Bulletin of the Association for the Scientific Studies on Judo*, Report I Tokyo: Kodokan.

[22] Ikai, M. (1968). "Electromyographic Studies on the Nagewaza (Throwing Techniques) of Judo", *Bulletin of the Association for the Scientific Studies on Judo*, Report II Tokyo: Kodokan.

[23] Kelly McKean (2009). "Kinematic & Kinetic Differences between Male & Female Soccer Players", *ISB XXth Congress - ASB 29th Annual Report*, Cleveland, Ohio, p.458.

[24] Kim L. (1979). "Kinematical Analysis of the Flight Phase in the Long Jump", *Journal of Biomechanics*, Vol. 12, pp.147-157.

[25] Kitagawa, Onishi and Kato (2001). "Kinematical Variables of Underwater Running and Walking", *IEEE Annual Int. Conf. on Systems, Man, and Cybernetics*, Charlottesville, VA.

[26] Lusin, G.F. (1979). Gajdosik, R.L. and Miller, K.E., "Goniometry: A Review of the Literature", *Athletic Training*, Vol. 14, pp.161-164.

[27] Miller, D.I. (1978). "Biomechanics of Running what should the Future Hold", *Canadian Journal of Applied Sport Sciences*, Vol. 3, pp.229-236.

[28] Miura, S. (1970). "An Electrogoniometric Study of a Judo Throwing Technique", *Judo Throwing Technique*, Vol. 42, pp.51-57.

[29] Motoyasu, Koshiyama and Katsumata (2009). "Effects of Joint Movement on the Accuracy of 3-point Shooting in Basketball", *Journal of Sports Sciences*, Vol. 17, pp.85-93.

[30] Murtaugh and Karen (2001). "Initiating Rotation in Back and Reverse Arm Stand Triple Somersault Tuck Dives", *Journal of Applied Sciences*, Vol. 17, pp.21-27.

[31] Nesbit S.M. (2005). "A Kinematic and Kinetic Study of the Golf Swing", *Journal of Sports Science and Medicine*, Vol. 4, pp.499-509.

[32] Rojas F.J., Cepero and Gutierrez (2000). "Kinematic Adjustments in the Basketball Jump Shot against An Opponent", *Annual Ergonomics*, Vol. 43, pp.1651-1660.

[33] S. Mandeep (2010). "Evaluation and Improvement of Sports Techniques through Biomechanical Updated Analyzing Technology", *University News - Special Issue*, Association of Indian University, Vol. 48, pp.54-57.

[34] Soo Chung (2013). "Analysis of Motion of the Striking Arm and Related Muscular/Joint Activities in Volleyball Spike", *Dissertation Abstract International*, Vol. 77, pp.48-49.

[35] Smith R., Bake M. and Fiatarone (2009). "Gait and Posture in Arthritic and Healthy Knees", *Scientia Iranica*, Vol. 3, pp.257-261.

[36] Winter, D.A. (1974). "Measurement anpd Reduction of Noise in Kinematics of Locomotio", *Journal of Biomechanics*, Vol. 7, pp.157-159.

[37] Zernicke, R.F. (1976). "Fitting Biomechanical Data with Cubic Spline Functions", *Research Quarterly*, Vol. 45, pp.9-19.

[38] Zhou Fou (2009). "Kinematical Research on Elite Chine's Male 3m Spring Board Divers", *Human Mov. Sci.*, Vol. 16, pp.259-274.

Form - A new cricket statistics

Parag Shah[1], Mitesh Shah[2]

[1]Dept. of Statistics, H. L. College of Commerce, Gujarat, India
[2]Dept. of Statistics, S.V. College, Gujarat, India

Email address:
pbs1374@yahoo.co.in (P. Shah), m_a_shah73@yahoo.com (M. Shah)

Abstract: Traditionally, evaluation of individual player performances in one-day cricket and T -20 has been based on measures such as batting and bowling averages, and strike and economy rates. Whenever a player's performance statistics are quoted, there is nearly always some verbal qualification that is necessary in order to place the statistics into context. We have found a new statistical measure –FORM, which measures the form of a player. We have used what is known as an *exponentially decaying average (EDMA)*. In this statistic, every score is considered in the calculation, but as you go back in time, each score is discounted by a certain percentage. This means recent score is given highest importance and past scores are given less weightage. Simple logic of short term EDMA and long term EDMA is used for calculating FORM. FORM of individual players is vital as the success of the team depends on the number of players who are in form. It can be used to estimate the total team score.

Keywords: Moving Average, Weighted Moving Average, Exponentially Decaying Averages

1. Introduction

Traditionally, evaluation of individual player performances in one-day cricket and T -20 has been based on measures such as batting and bowling averages, and strike and economy rates. Use of Statistics in sports is not new and cricket is a sport in which statistics features heavily. Cricket has recently experienced a highly-successful intervention from the field of Operational Research in the form of the 'Duckworth-Lewis' method of adjusting target scores in one day matches (Duckworth & Lewis, 1998) which was subsequently adopted by the International Cricket Council (Duckworth & Lewis,2004). Player performance remains of significant interest to cricket team selectors and coaches who are trying to build winning teams from a fixed pool of players or within a limited budget, and this imperative to win will probably lead to developments in the use of cricket statistics – at least among cricket professionals. Measuring cricketers only through their averages is liable to give skewed and unreliable results.

Barr G.D.I. and Kantor B.S. (2004) has discussed a criterion for comparing and selecting batsman in limited over cricket and Kimber A.C. and Hansford A.R. (1993) has given a Statistical Analysis of Batting in Cricket. But it is recognized, within the game of cricket, that such measures have severe limitations in assessing the true performances and abilities of players.

Lewis A.C. (2006) has tried to develop a fairer measure of player's performance in one-day cricket. This measure still does not evaluate the consistency of the batsman.

Lemmer H. H. (2004) in his paper has shown the importance of batsman's consistency. He has discussed the consistency coefficient and also illustrated its importance by showing that a batsman with a high consistency coefficient has a better chance to get a good score than one with a low consistency coefficient. He has also shown how the consistency curve can be used to assess the present form of a batsman. He by making use of a data set consisting of the statistics of a large group of one-day international players, these three measures will be combined into a single measure that can be used to assess the performance of a batsman and to compare different batsmen with each other. A classification scheme with ten classes according to which batsmen can be classified will be given. The best batsmen are those who fall into class one. The same procedure will be used to find a formula for batting performance and a classification table for Test players. Whenever a player's performance statistics are quoted, there is nearly always some verbal qualification that is necessary in order to place the statistics into context.

David Harper (2009) has explained the use of exponentially

weighted moving average in the finance domain particularly on stock market data. Chris P. Tsokos (2010) has discussed K-th Moving, Weighted and Exponential Moving Average for Time Series Forecasting Models.

2. Methodology

In current scenario, runs scored in the innings in which batsman remains not out are considered in the total runs scored by the batsman but while calculating the average that innings is not considered in total number of innings. This actually overestimates the batsman's performance. And if not out runs are considered as out runs, it underestimates the batsman's performance.

To overcome this drawback of existing average, we have considered a new logic for the average.

If not out runs > = average then consider not out runs in his total runs and

If not out runs < average then consider average in his total runs.

This logic will solve the problem of overestimation or under estimation.

To illustrate this logic of new batting average let us consider runs scored by a batsman new to international cricket in ten innings : 25, 15, 55*, 25, 32*, 6, 65, 89, 12, 21. * represent that the batsman is not out in that innings.

Table 1. *Calculation of new batting average.*

Innings	Runs	Runs to be added in total runs	Cumulative Runs	New batting Average
1	25	25	25	25.00
2	15	15	40	20.00
3	55	55	95	31.67
4	40	40	135	33.75
5	32*	34	169	33.80
6	6	6	175	29.17
7	65*	65	240	34.29
8	89	89	329	41.13
9	12*	41	370	41.11
10	21	21	391	39.10

Here in Table 1 you can see that in fifth innings he has scored 32 runs and was not out. Upto four innings his batting average was 33.75. As his runs (32) < his batting average (33.75), runs that will be added in his total runs will be 34 after rounding off to nearest integer. While in seventh innings he scored 65 runs and was not out and upto 6 innings his batting average was 29.17. As his runs (65) > his batting average (29.17), runs that will be added in his total runs will be 65.

The batsman is evaluated on the basis of their batting average only or at most their strike rates. But in this batting average simple average is used which gives equal weightage to runs scored in all innings. But for calculating Form of a batsman, latest score should be given more weightage and weights decreases for the past innings. This can be done with the use of *exponentially decaying average*. In this statistic, every score is considered in the calculation, but as you go back in time, each value is discounted by a certain percentage.

Exponentially decaying Moving Averages (EDMA) are widely used in financial mathematics to track the recent average behavior of stocks. EDMA's are generally used in systems where the first seen value is of little importance compared to the last seen value. So we calculate the average by assigning different weights to the moving average scale. But the underlying awesomeness of EDMA is that it decays exponentially.

Simple avg. = Sum of samples / Number of samples.

EDMA = (current EDMA.) * k / sample * (1.00 – k)

There are several implementations of EDMA of which this is one. Here k = decay factor or constant smoothing factor.

Many times you might have heard commentators saying this batsman is in form or is not in form. But form of a batsman was never quantified. For the first time we are developing a statistics which will quantify FORM of a batsman. These statistics can be used as other statistics like batting average, strike rate etc i.e. at a particular point of time.

FORM of individual players is vital as the success of the team depends on the number of players who are in form. FORM can also be used in predicting the performance of the team. In this paper we have considered batsmen FORM only but similar work can be done for bowlers and wicket-keepers. For calculating the FORM of a batsman we have considered five (short term) and eleven matches (Long term) exponentially decaying moving averages of runs scored. The not-out scores are replaced by the average till that match or the not-out runs whichever is higher.

The FORM of a batsman is given as:

FORM= (Short term EDMA) / (Long term EDMA)*100

We have considered FORM in terms of percentage. So, 100 will be considered as a Base of comparison.

3. Results & Discussion

To illustrate how FORM can be calculated we have taken the data of runs scored by Sachin in last 50 innings from *www.cricinfo.com* website. Here we will assume 4 % decay rate and 5 matches and 11 matches exponentially decaying moving average as short term and long term exponentially decaying moving averages respectively.

Table 2. *Calculation of FORM for Sachin.*

Runs	5 EDMA	11 EDMA	FORM
99			
8			
55			
71			
94			
30			
0			
16			
43			

Runs	5 EDMA	11 EDMA	FORM
79			
47	38.26619	48.54623	78.82423
72	52.33453	47.57898	109.9951
21	51.96442	47.43323	109.5528
4	43.15638	42.09682	102.517
99	48.92318	46.34891	105.5541
29	44.94651	41.06789	109.4444
97	51.44496	48.03338	107.1025
30	52.17704	49.42916	105.5592
10	51.54987	47.42857	108.6895
35	39.58211	46.36686	85.36723
44	42.40861	43.80223	96.81839
32	30.50984	42.27158	72.17578
5	25.07313	36.05251	69.54616
0	22.30368	33.12843	67.3249
2	15.662	31.74215	49.34132
63	20.91192	30.45193	68.67189
117	39.77092	40.12405	99.11991
91	57.01221	41.73566	136.6031
11	57.1149	39.1654	145.83
50	65.30964	42.4216	153.9537
5	52.65139	38.80762	135.6728
6	31.17689	34.81365	89.55365
7	15.37099	31.93684	48.12934
20	17.14602	32.51792	52.72792
61	20.84336	37.962	54.90587
163	54.44075	54.32534	100.2124
46	61.16923	52.79263	115.867
27	63.33551	45.4096	139.4761
138	87.16711	52.43002	166.2542
8	74.63783	50.44111	147.9703
14	45.89107	46.44293	98.81175
4	36.79602	44.67464	82.36443
32	37.48744	46.00249	81.49003
40	20.27598	48.09121	42.16151
175	55.96594	64.10596	87.30223
10	53.42069	58.34264	91.56372
69	65.52628	52.13532	125.685
43	66.56841	51.55819	129.1132
96	77.63823	58.20522	133.3871
8	45.3517	47.02287	96.44605
4	42.63772	45.01967	94.70908
200	72.07371	64.34497	112.0114

** 5 EDMA: Exponentially decaying moving average of 5 matches.
11EDMA: Exponentially decaying moving average of 11 matches.

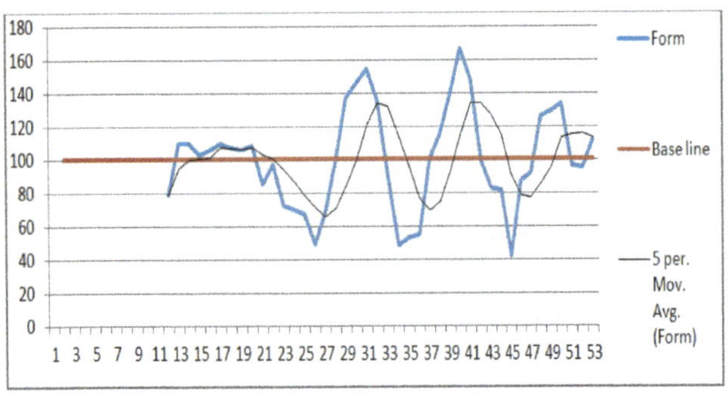

4. Conclusion

In calculating current batting average not out runs are added in total career runs but innings is not counted. This results in overestimation of average. The new batting average that we have developed solves this problem of overestimation.

When short term EDMA is more than long term EDMA it shows that batsman is scoring well in recent matches compared to long past matches. So when this situation arise, the FORM will be more than 100 and we can say that batsman is in good form and when it is less than 100, we say he is not in good form.

It can also be observed that FORM is cyclic in nature. Using the trend analysis, we can also predict the FORM of the batsman. This will help in estimating the expected total runs of the team.

Similar measure can be obtained for the bowlers.

References

[1] Duckworth, F.C. and Lewis, A.J. (1998). A fair method for resetting targets in one-day cricket matches. Journal of the Operational Research Society, 49: 220-227.

[2] Duckworth, F.C. and Lewis, A.J. (2004). A successful operational research intervention in one-day cricket. Journal of the Operational Research Society, 55: 749-759.

[3] Barr, G.D.I. and Kantor, B.S. (2004)."A criterion for comparing and selecting batsman in limited over cricket" Journal of Operation research Society, 55, 1266-1274.

[4] Kimber, A.C. and Hansford, A.R. (1993)"A Statistical Analysis of Batting in Cricket". J.R. Statist. Soc. A, 156, 3, 443-455

[5] Lewis, A.C. (2006)."Towards fairer measure of player's performance in one-day cricket" Journal of operation research society, 56,804-815.

[6] Lemmer, H. H. (2004). " A measure for the batting performance of cricket player "*South African Journal for Research in Sport, Physical Education and Recreation* Vol.26(1) , 55-64

[7] David Harper (2009)." Exploring the Exponentially Weighted Moving Average" Investopedia.

[8] Tsokos, C.P. (2010) "K-th Moving, Weighted and Exponential Moving Average for Time Series Forecasting Models" European journal of pure and applied mathematics, Vol. 3, No. 3, 2010, 406-416

[9] www.cricinfo.com

10

Physiological performance and cardiac function in female ironman- triathletes

Roman Leischik, Spelsberg N., Littwitz H., Dworrak B.

Department of Cardiology, Section Prevention and Sports Medicine, Faculty of Health, School of Medicine, Witten/Herdecke University, Witten, Germany

Email address:
info@dr-leischik.de (R. Leischik)

Abstract: Background: Data about physiological performance of female ironman-triathletes are rare. However, some papers reported endurance sport may cause damage of the right or left ventricle even in females. Aim: The goal of this study was to assess prospectively the right/left ventricular function and physiological performance in female ironman-athletes (middle- and long-distance). Methods: 33 female healthy triathletes were examined using spiroergometry and echocardiography. Inclusion criterion was participation in at least one middle distance triathlon. Results: The triathletes achieved the following results: VO_2max 52.8 ± 5.7 ml/min/kg, Wmax 264.0 ± 26.1, VAT (aerobic threshold) VO2 38.5 ± 7.9 ml/min/kg, 193.0 ± 48.4 Watt. In respect of echocardiographic readings LVEDD (left ventricular end-diastolic diameter) was 4.4 ± 0.3 cm and the left ventricular muscle mass (LVM) was 145.9 ± 31.3 g (LVM index 85.8 g/m² ± 18.7). Conclusions: The performance date of female triathletes can be used as training goals for leisure female triathletes, when middle or long distances in triathlon competitions should be finished. In respect of echocardiographic parameters a right or left ventricular dysfunction could not be found despite of long times of training and finishing of long distance competitions (5.4 ± 2.8 years triathlon competitions non-elite and 7.6 ± 5.8 years elite athletes).

Keywords: Triathlon, Ironman, Cardiac Fatigue, Female Athletes

1. Introduction

Participation in triathlon competitions has increased in the recent years. At the end of 1999, membership (annual and one-day) stood at 127,824. Those numbers had more than doubled to 262,703 by 2005, and USA triathlon continued to experience double-digit annual growth through 2007, when it reached 336,356 members [1]. Performance and echocardiographic data of average female triathletes participating in middle and long distance triathlons are rare. Some papers presumed pathological right ventricular remodelling [2] and "left ventricular fatigue" after middle or long distance triathlons [3]. Cases of sudden death during triathlons were reported [4].

Triathlon is an endurance sport specifically performed in middle and long distance formats (e.g. middle/long distance ironman: 1.9/3.8km swim, 90/180 km bicycle ride and 21.1/42.2 km run), mainly under aerobic conditions [5]. It is particularly important for triathletes to perform at sub-maximal levels over a long period to avoid reaching a state of exhaustion [6]. Elite athletes require 4 to 4.5 hours to complete middle distance events and 8 to 10 hours for long distance events. Amateur athletes typically take periods of 5 to 6.5 hours for middle distance events and 10 to 16 hours for long distance events. Such long periods of stress require both the amateur athletes as well as the top athletes to be adequately trained and to have sufficient aerobic capacity [5, 7]. A number of studies with small cohorts have been published in respect of spiroergometric data [8-13]. Echocardiographic data of triathletes (retrospective analysis, mainly males) have also been reported [14]. All these studies raise the question which types of cardiac changes in function or structure can be found in female triathletes. Further questions are:

- Which performance data can be achieved by mainstream female triathletes participating in middle and full distance competitions?
- Are there signs of cardiac dysfunction (cardiac fatigue) in middle and long distance female triathletes?

2. Patients and Methods

33 female triathletes have been examined by echocardiography and spiroergometry. The echocardiograph produced by General Electric, model Vivid 7 was used for the examinations. The Ergobike 8I produced by Daum and the Metalizer 3B produced by Cortex were used for spiroergometric examination. In order to compare the data from elite triathletes with those of non-elite triathletes, athletes were divided into two groups according to the aerobic capacity (relative $VmaxO_2$/min/kg at the aerobic threshold).

All triathletes were examined during one day using at first echocardiography and later spiroergometry.

2.1. Echocardiography

The echocardiographic analysis and estimation of left ventricular mass (LVM) was conducted according to general recommendations (20). The formula recommended by the American Society of Echocardiography (ASE) was used to calculate the muscle mass. EDV and ESV was determined monoplane (unclear meaning) after the modified Simpson method.

2.2. Spiroergometry

Spiroergometry was performed in the following way: The stress test was conducted in stages after successful gas and volume calibration: 50 W for 3 minutes, 100 W for a further 3 minutes and thereafter increased by another 30 Watt every 3 minutes. The test ended when the subject could no longer maintain the predefined RPM of 90 or if the subject was exhausted.

Spiroergometric analyses were conducted according to literature: VAT was determined as first non-linear increase of the ventilatory equivalent for oxygen without simultaneous increase of the ventilatory equivalent for CO_2 and RCP as simultaneous non-linear increase of both ventilatory equivalents according to recommendations (21). VO_2max was registered as the highest average value of oxygen absorption over 30 seconds.

2.3. Statistics

The entire statistical analysis plan was designed as follows: Stata/IC 13.1 for Windows was used for data preparation and statistical analysis. The Mann-Whitney-U-Test was used for comparing the groups.

3. Results

3.1. Anthropometry

Anthropometric data and general echocardiographic parameters of triathletes are listed in table 1. Systolic blood pressure values at rest were similar: 117.4 ± 8.6 mmHg vs. 121.9 ± 8.4 mmHg (n.s.) in females with LVM >95 g/m^2 vs. LVM <95 g/m^2.

***Table 1.** Anthropometry and echocardiographic parameters.*

	n	Mv	Sd	Min-Max
Age (years)	33	34,3	8,1	20.0 - 53.0
Weight (kg)	33	61,5	7,8	48.7 - 79.6
Size (cm)	33	168,8	6,4	158.0 - 180.0
BMI (kg/m²)	33	21,6	2,28	18.3 - 26.6
BSA (m²)	33	1,7	0,13	1.48 - 1.97
%bodyfat	33	22,8	4,7	12.7 - 32.6
Aorta (cm)	33	2,47	0,24	2.00 - 2.9
Leftatrium (cm)	33	2,35	0,25	1.90 - 2.9
LAESV* (ml)	33	27,4	9,3	14.0 - 55.0
IVS diastolic (cm)	33	1,02	0,17	0.70 - 1.50
IVS systolic (cm)	33	1,44	0,22	0.90 - 1.90
PWD diastolic (cm)	33	1,02	0,16	0.80 - 1.40
PWD systolic (cm)	33	1,48	0,2	1.20 - 2.00
Relative Wallthickness	33	0,47	0,09	0.33 - 0.76
LVEDD (cm)	33	4,4	0,32	3.7 - 5.0
LVESD (cm)	33	2,9	0,27	2.40 - 3.4
LVM (g)	33	145,9	31,3	86.8 - 212.6
LVM (g/m²)	33	85,8	18,7	58.3 - 134.6
LVEDV (ml)	33	105	17,8	79.0 - 148.0
LVESV (ml)	33	38,9	7,1	28.0 - 52.0
SV (ml)	33	66,1	11,3	48.0 - 98.0
EF (%)	33	63	2,7	57.0 - 68.0
LVOT Vmax m/s	32	0,86	0,13	0.63 - 1.17
MV E Max (m/s)	33	0,56	0,12	0.33 - 0.98
MV A Max (m/s)	33	0,38	0,09	0.26 - 0.72
MV E/A Ratio	33	1,54	0,34	0.85 - 2.27
RV parastenal	33	2,4	0,18	2.10 - 2.9
RV AFC%	33	32,2	2,8	24.6 - 38.8

Legend: n = number, Mv = mean value, Sd= standard deviation, Min = minimum, Max = maximum* = of the Mann-Whitney-U-Test, BMI = body mass index, BSA = body surface area, LA = left atrial diameter, LAESV = left atrial endsystolic volume, IVS = intervent. septum, LVPWT = LV posterior wall thickness, RWT = relative wall thickness, LVEDD = LV enddiastolic diameter, LVEDV = LV enddiastolic volume, = diastolic, s=systolic, RV FC%: right ventricular area fractional change.

The first best 15 females were chosen as elite, according to the aerobic capacity (relative VO_2max ml/min/kg at the aerobic threshold). In this group, there was a world ironman champion (age group), a national champion, and participants of the 1st national triathlon league.
The mean time of participation in triathlon for elite athletes was 7.6 ± 5,8 and for non-elite athletes 5.4 ± 2.8 ($p = 0.456$) (table 2). There were no significant differences according to anthropometric data between elite and non-elite athletes, especially with regard to weight or %body fat value (table 2). Only heart rate at rest was significant lower and diastolic wall thickness was minimally increased in elite-females.

***Table 2.** Differences between Elite and Non- Elite female triathletes.*

	p-value	Elite-Females		Non-Elite females	
		Mv	SD	Mv	SD
Age (years)	0.786	33.6	9.2	34.8	7.2
weight (kg)	0.759	60.9	6.8	62.0	8.6
BMI (kg/m²)	0.247	21.1	2.2	22.0	2.3
BSA	0.986	1.69	0.11	1.7	0.14
% bodyfat	0.366	22.1	4.3	23.4	5.0
distance swimm/week	0.185	8.5	3.9	6.1	3.1
distance bike/week/km	0.971	173.0	67.7	164.7	75.2
distance run/week/km	0.085	55.3	9.1	48.3	16.6
HR_{AT}	0.002	160.6	14.5	138.6	19.9

	p-value	Elite-Females		Non-Elite females	
		Mv	SD	Mv	SD
IVSdiastolic cm	0.024	1.09	0.18	0.95	0.12
LVPWd cm	0.034	1.09	0.18	0.97	0.13
IVSsystolic cm	0.042	1.53	0.21	1.37	0.21
EF (Teich) %	0.069	63.7	3.7	61.2	3.9
LVs Mass Index g/m²	0.159	92.3	20.8	80.5	15.4
abs. VO_{2max}	0.006	3,4	0,3	3,1	0,3
rel. VO_{2max}	0.004	56.1	5.7	50.1	4.1
rel. $VO2_{AT}$	0.000	45.5	5.4	32.7	3.8

3.2. Echocardiography

One triathlete showed aortic valve insufficiency, which can be described as mild. All other triathletes showed normal results in respect of their cardiac valves.

There were no significant differences between elite and amateur athletes in respect of echocardiographic parameters.

In the study population concentric changes of the left ventricle characterised the morphology. 17 females (51 %) displayed concentric remodelling and 6 (18 %) concentric hypertrophy. Normal LV-morphology was found in 9 (27 %) females. Eccentric hypertrophy was rare: 1 (3 %) participants of the study.

The classification into the types of hypertrophy followed the criteria of Lang et al. [15]. Right ventricular remodelling or other pathological findings in right ventricle were not found. Left and right ventricular function was excellent in all female triathlete even if they train a lot (Table 3).

Table 3. *Training characteristics for Elite-females and Non-Elite females.*

	Elite Females			Non-Elite Females			
	n	Mv	Sd	n	Mv	Sd	P values*
Swimming time hrs/ week	15	4.0	1.2	18	3.2	1.1	0.072
Swimming dist. km / week	15	8.5	3.9	18	6.6	3.1	0.185
Biking time hrs/ week	15	6.7	2.3	18	6.5	1.9	1.000
Biking dist. km / week	15	173	67.7	18	165	75.2	0.971
Running time hrs/ week	15	5.5	1.3	18	4.8	1.4	0.116
Running dist. km / week	15	55.3	9.1	18	48.3	16.6	0.085
Training time hrs/ week	15	16.5	3.2	18	14.7	3.2	0.059
Triathlete since years	15	7.6	5.8	18	5.4	2.8	0.456

n = number, Mv = mean value, Sd= standard deviation, * = p value of the Mann-Whitney-U-Test

3.3. Spiroergometry

Average maximal relative VO_2max uptake was 52.8 ± 5.7 ml/min/kg, at the aerobic threshold (VAT) 38.5 ± 7.9 ml/min/kg.

Oxygen absorption, ergometer performance and heart rate at VAT, at the anaerobic threshold (RCP) and at peak capacity are shown in table 4, according to the performance data.

Tab 4. *Heart frequency, oxygen uptake and power output depending on performance.*

	Elite females			Non-elite females			
	n	Mv	Sd	n	Mv	Sd	P values *
			VAT (aerobic threshold)				
HR	15	160.6	14.5	18	138.6	19.9	0.002
aVO2	15	2.76	0.35	18	1.99	0.46	0.000
rVO2	15	45.5	5.4	18	32.7	3.8	0.000
%VO2max	15	81.2	7.0	18	64.4	12.9	0.000
W	15	230.0	24.5	18	162.2	41.4	0.000
			RCP (anaerobic threshold)				
HR	15	169.8	12.6	18	152.3	21.0	0.016
aVO2	15	3.06	0.28	18	2.33	0.56	0.001
rVO2	15	46.8	14.9	18	37.4	6.3	0.000
%VO2max	15	91.7	6.7	18	75.3	14.7	0.001
W	15	252.5	23.8	18	195.0	44.0	0.000
			Peak capacity				
HR	15	179.7	10.0	18	179.8	7.6	0.971
aVO2max	15	3.4	0.3	18	3.1	0.3	0.006
rVO2max	15	56.1	5.7	18	50.1	4.1	0.004
Wmax	15	274.0	32.5	18	256.7	16.4	0.097

n = number; Mv = Mean value; Sd = standard deviation, aVO2 = absolute VO2 in L/min, rVO2 = relative VO2 in ml/min/kg, * = of the Mann-Whitney-U-Test, HR = heart rate, W = power output.

Non-elite female triathletes showed maximal performance values comparable to values of recreational female triathletes (50.1 vs. 48.2 ml/min/kg) described by Butts et al. [11]. As expected, the relative oxygen uptake was higher in elite females (abs. and rel. VO_2max), according to the aerobic capacity. The performance data of our long-distance triathlon collective showed lower VO_2max values as compared with data of elite female triathletes from Olympic distance (61.3 ml/min/kg vs. 56.1) [13]. Female triathletes from Olympic distance can obtain even higher values in the range of 65.6 ml/min/kg from treadmill ergometer test [16].

4. Discussion

4.1. General

Most studies of triathlon have focused to male triathletes, this study describes so far the largest cohort of long distance female triathletes using echocardiography and performance data.

4.2. Cardiac Adaptation and Left Ventricular Hypertrophy

The specific endurance training of triathletes leads to physiological changes of the performance parameters [5] and also results in changes of cardiac function or its architecture [17]. This adaptation is linked to the nature and magnitude of the physical exercise [18]. The physiological adaptation is a “harmonic increase in size” of a healthy heart caused by physical activity [19]. The term “athlete`s heart” [18] is known since 1899 [20] and has been a topic of medical and scientific interest since the late nineteenth century [18].

Female athletes have generally less frequently a LVM >220 g. LVM of female endurance athletes was described with 175 ± 38 g [21]. There was a mixed analysis of cyclists, rowers, runners, swimmers and roller skaters.

In our study we found a smaller LVM of 145.9 ± 31.3. Concentric hypertrophy in triathletes has already been described [14].

Douglas et al. [22] published a comparison of 36 male triathletes comprising 17 normal control and 15 high pressure subjects. The authors suggested that triathletes undergo cardiac adaptations like under increased arterial pressure conditions and described a RWD of 0.41. In these triathletes the left ventricular muscle mass was correlated positively with the increased systolic blood pressure during exercise [22]. This problem occurs more often in male triathletes. The present study showed no significant relationship of myocardial thickening to blood pressure values. Hypertension in female triathletes is rare. Neither resulted a correlation between muscle mass and blood pressure values at the aerobic threshold, nor a correlation between increased blood pressure values at rest or at peak capacity. The females of the present study showed no signs of exercise-induced arterial hypertension.

Douglas at al. [14] examined the occurrence of concentric hypertrophy in a retrospective study. Echocardiographic results of 168 male and 67 female Hawaii Ironman triathletes were collected retrospectively and examined from 1985 to 1995. However, in this study concentric hypertrophy was observed only rarely (in 2 % of the triathletes) and eccentric hypertrophy in 7 % of the triathletes.

In other large cohorts of different athletes concentric hypertrophy was also described rarely [23]. However, the meta-analysis described by Pellicia et al. [23] included athletes from 25 different disciplines, so that the results cannot be compared to triathletes. 15 female cyclists of this meta-analysis demonstrated a LVM Index g/m^2 of 115 ± 23.

Cardiovascular adaptations to exercise have been systematically defined and differ depending to the type of conditioning endurance training. Cycling and rowing have the most effects on cavity size and wall thickness. Strength trained athletes showed the highest increase in wall thickness [24].

The main difference between triathletes and cyclist is that triathletes train not only under cycling, but also under running conditions; cycle racing includes more components of strength training. The functional changes of cardiac structures for triathletes resemble the changes in runners [25].

Even though an enlarged atrium should be characteristic for endurance athletes [17], the present study did not show enlarged atria in female triathletes. Highly trained cycle racers however showed an enlarged atrium, which was even larger in older cycle racers than in younger subjects [26].

The systolic and diastolic function in our study was not influenced. The diastolic function in our cohort is not materially impaired.

Sudden cardiac death is more likely in male athletes. [27]. The different causes of sudden cardiac death in athletes were reported: silent coronary disease [28], hypertrophic cardiomyopathy [29] and arrhythmogenic right ventricular cardiomyopathy [30] (table 5).

Table 5. *Distribution of cardiovascular causes of sudden death in young athletes <12-35Years in %.*

	Maron 2007	Corrado 2003	Sollberg 2010	Marijon 2011
Aorticrupture	2,2	1,8	4,3	2
Aorticstenosis/cong. HD	1,8		4,3	6
ARVC	4	22		4
Channelpathies (QT, WPW)	3	1,8	8,7	12
Coronaryarteryanomalies	24	11	3,3	
Coronarydisease	3	18	48	6
Dilatative CM	2	1,8		4
Hypertrophic CM	36	1,8	4,3	10
MVP	4	7,3		2
Myocarditis	5,4	9	22	4
Possible HCM	11,3			4
Riva musclebridge	2,2	3,6		2
Unclear		1,8		36
	n = 1049	n = 55	n = 22	n = 50

4.3. Physiological Performance

An important prerequisite of successful participation in the middle and long distance of triathlon is a sufficient aerobic capacity. It also appears that this is essential to avoid possible damage due to long time endurance training [3]. Well trained endurance athletes do not suffer significant long-term damage [3] even athletes can exhibit momentary “cardiac fatigue“ [3, 31].

The female triathletes examined in the present study showed no signs of pathological right ventricular remodelling or signs of left ventricular dysfunction. The performance data for amateur athletes identified by this study should be assumed as guide values for athletes participating in middle and long distance triathlons.

In the present study female athletes showed a VO_2max of 52.8 ± 5.7 ml/min/kg, the VO_2 uptake at the aerobic threshold was 38.5 ± 7.9 ml/min/kg. This data match with published data of smaller studies. We could not find any value for VO_2 uptake at the aerobic threshold for female triathletes.

The maximum oxygen absorption in the previously published studies had a range of 48.2 up to 61.6 ml/min/kg body weight amongst different groups that have been examined.

In contrast, in studies of groups with, for example, five world class athletes [13] results turn out higher. However, it can be postulated that a VO_2max above 55 ml/min/kg body weight is a good marker for successful participation in an Ironman competition, both in middle and long distance events. The oxygen absorption at the aerobic threshold should be above 35 ml/min/kg body weight for females. In the present study, the examinations always took place using ergometric peak capacity by bicycle; so treadmill data can differ depending on the athletes' background [32]. Bunc et al. [33] proposes VO_2max values for young Olympic triathletes - males an average of above 65 ml/min/kg and females above 60 ml/min/kg. This pertains to elite triathletes. In smaller studies VO_2max values for female athletes [9] were averaged at 57.5 ml/min/kg.

Comparing the performance values of elite and amateur female athletes in the present study, a significant difference can be observed as expected: relative VO_2max 56.1 ± 5.7 vs. 50.1 ± 4 ml/min/kg and VO_2 for VAT 45.5 ± 5.4 vs. 32.7 ± 3.8 ml/min/kg.

5. Limitations and Future Directions

The cross-sectional design of this study does not allow a certain decision about the lack of exercise-induced cardiac fatigue in female triathletes. Although our data suggest normal right and left ventricular function, confirmatory longitudinal work is necessary.

The results of this study support the subjective impression of daily practice and engagement in sports medicine since 15 years that female athletes suffer less frequently from negative-cardiac remodelling as discussed by different authors [31, 34, 35].

6. Summary

The data of the present study on German female triathletes participating in middle and long distance events allow the practical use of this data as a routine part of everyday sports medicine and in classifying the efficiency of performance diagnostic centres. We favour as training goals for successful finishing a middle or long distance triathlon a minimum of aerobic capacity of 35ml/min/kg in female triathletes. In terms of echocardiographic measurement we can expect concentric remodelling /concentric hypertrophy. Concentric hypertrophy can be expected up to 20 % in healthy female triathletes. Valve dysfunctions are possible but in our cohort rare.

We have not found negative long term effects on cardiac structures as proposed for "exercised-induced cardiac fatigue" [35]. In our cohort we have triathletes with a mean time of participation in triathlon competitions of 5.4 years (non-Elite) and 7.8 years (elite). The longest time participating in triathlon competitions was 32 years.

Sudden cardiac death in female athletes is rare (20 x less frequently as in men) [36]. The known problem of arrhythmias in the aged athletes also more often occurs in the male athlete [37].

Adequate screening of triathletes for possible silent diseases based on the different cardiologic diagnostic tools should be considered [38-40]. With regard to our data, we can suggest that long-term adverse cardiac effects of endurance sport in female triathletes seem to be rare [41]. The positive impact of physical activity at the recreational level is not up for discussion [42, 43].

References

[1] Triathlon, U. Demographics, Triathlon participation, growth trends and demographics. 2013 (updated April 2013); Available from: http://www.usatriathlon.org/about-multisport/demographics.aspx.

[2] La Gerche, A., A.T. Burns, D.J. Mooney, W.J. Inder, A.J. Taylor, J. Bogaert, A.I. MacIsaac, H. Heidbüchel and D.L. Prior, Exercise-induced right ventricular dysfunction and structural remodelling in endurance athletes. European heart journal, 2012. 33(8): p. 998-1006.

[3] Douglas, P.S., M.L. O'Toole, W.D. Hiller, K. Hackney and N. Reichek, Cardiac fatigue after prolonged exercise. Circulation, 1987. 76(6): p. 1206-13.

[4] Harris, K.M., J.T. Henry, E. Rohman, T.S. Haas and B.J. Maron, Sudden death during the triathlon. Jama, 2010. 303(13): p. 1255-7.

[5] Suriano, R. and D. Bishop, Physiological attributes of triathletes. J Sci Med Sport, 2010. 13(3): p. 340-7.

[6] Sleivert, G.G. and D.S. Rowlands, Physical and physiological factors associated with success in the triathlon. Sports Med, 1996. 22(1): p. 8-18.

[7] O'Toole, M.L. and P.S. Douglas, Applied physiology of triathlon. Sports Med, 1995. 19(4): p. 251-67.

[8] O'Toole, M.L., D.B. Hiller, L.O. Crosby and P.S. Douglas, The ultraendurance triathlete: a physiological profile. Med Sci Sports Exerc, 1987. 19(1): p. 45-50.

[9] O'Toole, M.L., P.S. Douglas and W.D. Hiller, Lactate, oxygen uptake, and cycling performance in triathletes. Int J Sports Med, 1989. 10(6): p. 413-8.

[10] Kohrt, W.M., D.W. Morgan, B. Bates and J.S. Skinner, Physiological responses of triathletes to maximal swimming, cycling, and running. Med Sci Sports Exerc, 1987. 19(1): p. 51-5.

[11] Butts, N.K., B.A. Henry and D. McLean, Correlations between VO2max and performance times of recreational triathletes. J Sports Med Phys Fitness, 1991. 31(3): p. 339-44.

[12] Sleivert, G.G. and H.A. Wenger, Physiological predictors of short-course triathlon performance. Med Sci Sports Exerc, 1993. 25(7): p. 871-6.

[13] Schabort, E.J., S.C. Killian, A. St Clair Gibson, J.A. Hawley and T.D. Noakes, Prediction of triathlon race time from laboratory testing in national triathletes. Med Sci Sports Exerc, 2000. 32(4): p. 844-9.

[14] Douglas, P.S., M.L. O'Toole, S.E. Katz, G.S. Ginsburg, W.D. Hiller and R.H. Laird, Left ventricular hypertrophy in athletes. Am J Cardiol, 1997. 80(10): p. 1384-8.

[15] Lang, R.M., M. Bierig, R.B. Devereux, F.A. Flachskampf, E. Foster, P.A. Pellikka, M.H. Picard, M.J. Roman, J. Seward and J. Shanewise, Recommendations for chamber quantification. European Journal of Echocardiography, 2006. 7(2): p. 79-108.

[16] Laurenson, N.M., K.Y. Fulcher and P. Korkia, Physiological characteristics of elite and club level female triathletes during running. Int J Sports Med, 1993. 14(8): p. 455-9.

[17] Atchley, A.E., Jr. and P.S. Douglas, Left ventricular hypertrophy in athletes: morphologic features and clinical correlates. Cardiol Clin, 2007. 25(3): p. 371-82, v.

[18] George, K.P., L.A. Wolfe and G.W. Burggraf, The 'athletic heart syndrome'. A critical review. Sports Med, 1991. 11(5): p. 300-30.

[19] Dickhuth, H., A. Hipp, A. Niess, K. Röcker, F. Mayer and T. Horstmann, Differenzialdiagnostik der physiologischen Herzhypertrophie (Sportherz). DEUTSCHE ZEITSCHRIFT FÜR SPORTMEDIZIN, 2001. 52(6): p. 205-210.

[20] Henschen, S., Skilanglauf und Skiwettlauf. Eine medizinische Sportstudie. Mitt Med Klin Upsala, 1899:. 2:: p. 74.

[21] Whyte, G.P., K. George, A. Nevill, R. Shave, S. Sharma and W.J. McKenna, Left ventricular morphology and function in female athletes: a meta-analysis. Int J Sports Med, 2004. 25(5): p. 380-3.

[22] Douglas, P.S., Cardiac considerations in the triathlete. Med Sci Sports Exerc, 1989. 21(5 Suppl): p. S214-8.

[23] Pelliccia, A., B.J. Maron, A. Spataro, M.A. Proschan and P. Spirito, The upper limit of physiologic cardiac hypertrophy in highly trained elite athletes. N Engl J Med, 1991. 324(5): p. 295-301.

[24] Pluim, B.M., A.H. Zwinderman, A. van der Laarse and E.E. van der Wall, The athlete's heart a meta-analysis of cardiac structure and function. Circulation, 2000. 101(3): p. 336-344.

[25] Fagard, R., A. Aubert, J. Staessen, E.V. Eynde, L. Vanhees and A. Amery, Cardiac structure and function in cyclists and runners. Comparative echocardiographic study. Br Heart J, 1984. 52(2): p. 124-9.

[26] Hoogsteen, J., A. Hoogeveen, H. Schaffers, P.F. Wijn and E.E. van der Wall, Left atrial and ventricular dimensions in highly trained cyclists. Int J Cardiovasc Imaging, 2003. 19(3): p. 211-7.

[27] Marijon, E., M. Tafflet, D.S. Celermajer, F. Dumas, M.C. Perier, H. Mustafic, J.F. Toussaint, M. Desnos, M. Rieu, N. Benameur, J.Y. Le Heuzey, J.P. Empana, and X. Jouven, Sports-related sudden death in the general population. Circulation, 2011. 124(6): p. 672-81.

[28] Solberg, E.E., F. Gjertsen, E. Haugstad and L. Kolsrud, Sudden death in sports among young adults in Norway. Eur J Cardiovasc Prev Rehabil, 2010. 17(3): p. 337-41.

[29] Maron, B.J., P.D. Thompson, M.J. Ackerman, G. Balady, S. Berger, D. Cohen, R. Dimeff, P.S. Douglas, D.W. Glover and A.M. Hutter, Recommendations and Considerations Related to Preparticipation Screening for Cardiovascular Abnormalities in Competitive Athletes: 2007 Update A Scientific Statement From the American Heart Association Council on Nutrition, Physical Activity, and Metabolism: Endorsed by the American College of Cardiology Foundation. Circulation, 2007. 115(12): p. 1643-1655.

[30] Corrado, D., C. Basso, G. Rizzoli, M. Schiavon and G. Thiene, Does sports activity enhance the risk of sudden death in adolescents and young adults? J Am Coll Cardiol, 2003. 42(11): p. 1959-63.

[31] Rifai, N., P.S. Douglas, M. O'Toole, E. Rimm and G.S. Ginsburg, Cardiac troponin T and I, echocardiographic [correction of electrocardiographic] wall motion analyses, and ejection fractions in athletes participating in the Hawaii Ironman Triathlon. Am J Cardiol, 1999. 83(7): p. 1085-9.

[32] Hue, O., Prediction of drafted-triathlon race time from submaximal laboratory testing in elite triathletes. Can J Appl Physiol, 2003. 28(4): p. 547-60.

[33] Bunc, V., J. Heller, J. Horcic and J. Novotny, Physiological profile of best Czech male and female young triathletes. J Sports Med Phys Fitness, 1996. 36(4): p. 265-70.

[34] O'Keefe, J.H., R.P. Harshal, C.J. Lavie, A. Magalski, R.A. Vogel and P.A. McCiiough, Potential Adverse Cardiovascular Effects From Excessive Endurance Exercise. Mayo Clin Proc., 2012. 87(6): p. 587-595.

[35] Oxborough, D., K. Birch, R. Shave and K. George, "Exercise-induced cardiac fatigue"--a review of the echocardiographic literature. Echocardiography, 2010. 27(9): p. 1130-40.

[36] Marijon, E., W. Bougouin, M.C. Perier, D.S. Celermajer and X. Jouven, Incidence of sports-related sudden death in France by specific sports and sex. Jama, 2013. 310(6): p. 642-3.

[37] Andersen, K., B. Farahmand, A. Ahlbom, C. Held, S. Ljunghall, K. Michaelsson and J. Sundstrom, Risk of arrhythmias in 52 755 long-distance cross-country skiers: a cohort study. Eur Heart J, 2013.

[38] Leischik, R., B. Dworrak, H. Littwitz and H. Gulker, Prognostic significance of exercise stress echocardiography in 3329 outpatients (5-year longitudinal study). Int J Cardiol, 2007. 119(3): p. 297-305.

[39] Leischik, R. Ugly duckling or Nosferatu ? - marathon running and cardiovascular function How to screen the athletes? 2014; Available from: http://eurheartj.oxfordjournals.org/content/early/2014/01/08/eurheartj.eht502/reply#ehj_el_2040.

[40] La Gerche, A., A.L. Baggish, J. Knuuti, D.L. Prior, S. Sharma, H. Heidbuchel and P.D. Thompson, Cardiac imaging and stress testing asymptomatic athletes to identify those at risk of sudden cardiac death. JACC Cardiovasc Imaging, 2013. 6(9): p. 993-1007.

[41] Pelliccia, A., N. Kinoshita, C. Pisicchio, F. Quattrini, F.M. DiPaolo, R. Ciardo, B. Di Giacinto, E. Guerra, E. De Blasiis, M. Casasco, F. Culasso and B.J. Maron, Long-Term Clinical Consequences of Intense, Uninterrupted Endurance Training in Olympic Athletes. Journal of the American College of Cardiology, 2010. 55(15): p. 1619-1625.

[42] Organisation, W.H. Global Health Risks. 2009; Page 17,18, : Available from: http://www.who.int/healthinfo/global_burden_disease/GlobalHealthRisks_report_full.pdf.

[43] Warburton, D.E., C.W. Nicol and S.S. Bredin, Health benefits of physical activity: the evidence. Cmaj, 2006. 174(6): p. 801-9.

11

Physiological characters in mixed martial arts

Petter Alm, Ji-Guo Yu*

Sports Medicine Unit, Department of Surgical and Perioperative Sciences, Umeå University, 901 87 Umeå, Sweden

Email address:
pettr.alm@gmail.com(P. Alm), jiguo.yu@idrott.umu.se(J-G. Yu)

Abstract: Mixed martial arts (MMA) is a relatively new sport and is a mixture of many different martial arts. Currently, study on the physiological characters in the sport is very limited. The present study evaluated the physiological characters in 5 active male MMA athletes at two occasions with one year between. Aerobic- and anaerobic capacity were estimated through measurement of VO_{2max} and anaerobic threshold using both treadmill running and arm cycling. Muscle strength was evaluated through series measurements. Body composition and personal competition records were also examined. The subjects presented above average aerobic capacity, but rather high anaerobic capacity and threshold levels compared with other similar sports. No significant difference in VO_{2max}, anaerobic threshold or body composition was observed between the two test occasions, despite a decreased tendency in muscle strength/power in the second test compared to the first. The results were interpreted to indicate either the MMA athletes had reached the physiological requirements for MMA or the one year physical training was inefficient in further improving the parameters.

Keywords: Mixed Martial Arts, Physiological Characters, Aerobic Capacity, Anaerobic Capacity

1. Introduction

Modern Mixed Martial Arts (MMA) is a mixture combat sport including boxing, wrestling, Brazilian jiu-jitsu, muay Thai, kickboxing, taekwondo, karate, judo and other styles. MMA allows the use of both striking and grappling while in position of both standing and on the ground. MMA is a new sport with its first authorized competition in 1993 [Ultimate Fighting Championship (UFC)]. However, at that time it was more of human cockfight rather than a real sport, and the participants were from various martial arts with almost no rules. Nowadays, the sport has developed a lot of rules to ensure the safety of the fighters, and has its mainstream audience all over the world.

Even though the popularity of MMA is steadily growing, knowledge of the physiological characters on the sport are relatively few compared with other similar sports like rugby [1], wrestling [2,3,4] or judo [5]. To our knowledge, only one study has examined physiological characteristics in amateur MMA athletes [6]. The study, however, only estimated general physiological demands, not in reveal time MMA competition.

A formal MMA competition consists of 3 rounds with 5 minutes for each round and 1 minute rest between rounds while a title competition usually contains 5 rounds. Therefore, MMA stresses aerobic energy system [7] with respect to the total time of a competition (15 or 25 minutes). However, MMA athletes also utilized lactate energy system during both training and competition [8]. This is reasonable because of the highly competitive actions in each round.

In MMA there are many explosive actions such as kicking and striking, which are often critical for the final result of a competition. Therefore, muscle power of both upper and lower body is especially important in MMA.

In the present study, a group of 5 active male MMA athletes were tested in two occasions with one year in between. The tests included both aerobic and anaerobic systems. Body composition and muscle strength and power of both lower and upper body were also measured. We intended firstly to provide a physiological profile of MMA athletes. Secondly, by comparing the competition record of the subjects with the test results obtained at the two test occasions, we also aimed to evaluate whether the routine physical training was effective to improve competition record and/or physiological parameters.

2. Material and methods

2.1. Subjects

Five elite MMA fighters were recruited for the study. Detailed information of the subjects is listed in table 1.

Table 1. Data for age and anthropometry (Mean ± SD)

Age (Years)	29,6 ± 5,50
Weight (kg)	80,8 ± 11,08
Height (cm)	180,4 ± 9,07

2.2. Experimental Approach

Physiological evaluation on the 5 subjects was performed at two separate occasions with one year in between. One subject did not perform the second test due to injury. All tests were conducted in the laboratory of Sports Medicine Unit at Umeå University.

Using a dual-emission x-ray absorptiometry (GE Lunar iDEXA DPX-L scanner, software version 1, 3y Madison, Wi, USA), all subjects were scan to determine their anthropometrics including bone mineral density, muscle mass, fat mass, fat percentage and muscle percentage . The reliability of the iDEXA has been proved early [9].

To measure VO_{2max}, VO_2 and heart rate at threshold level, the subjects were asked to run on treadmill and perform an arm cycling exercise. After a short standardized warm up, the subjects started running on a treadmill (Rodby, RL2500E, Sweden) with a start speed of 5 km/h. The speed was increased to 7 km/h, 9 km/h, 10,6km/h, 12km/h for every third min till exhausted. If the subjects were still not exhausted at the highest speed, the inclination of the treadmill would be raised by 2% every third minute till exhausted. Personal absolute and relative VO_{2max} and maximal heart rate were recorded during the running. Levels of VO_2 and heart rate were measured at threshold level using ventilation switch point for O_2 [VO_2 at aerobic threshold (AT; vent)], ventilation switch point for CO_2 (VO_2 at AT, Wasserman), respiratory exchange ratio 1 (RER 1; VO_2 at RER1), aerobic lactate threshold (2mMol/l; VO_2 at Lactate 2mMo) and onset of blood lactate accumulation (4mMol/l; VO_2 OBLA). Hemoglobin level and lactate recovery rate after the running were also measured using blood sample (2ml) taken from the right arm vein before every running speed, and at 0, 3, 5 and 10 minutes after the running.

All the tests except the lactate AT tests were repeated using arm cycling. The height of the arm pedals (arm cycle Rodby RE990A, Sweden) was individually standardized to the subjects' intercostale 5. The work load started at 40 watt and increased 30 watt every third minutes till exhausted. For lactate recovery rate, a drop blood sample from the right middle fingertip was taken at 0, 3, 5 and 10 minutes after the arm cycling.

Ventilation AT was measured using mixed chamber analyzer (Jaeger Oxycon Pro, Sweden). Heart rate was measured using a heart rate monitor (POLAR S610i, Finland). Lactate level and hemoglobin values were analyzed using blood analyzer (YSI 2300 STAT Plus, USA) [10].

After 20-30 minutes rest following the treadmill test all subjects were tested for squat jump (SJ), counter movement jump (CMJ), counter movement jump with arm swings (CMJa) and vertical sit-ups. MuscleLab (V8.23) with an infrared contacted mat was used for jump tests.

Personal competition record calculated as percentage of win in total competitions before each test and one year before each test was counted.

2.3. Data Analysis

Statistical analyses were performed using SPSS Statistics (SPSS 20, Inc., and Chicago, IL, USA). Data was presented as mean ± SD. Paired sample t-test was applied to data from the two tests. For the heart rate measurements, an independent sample t-test was used. Statistical significance was set at $p \leq 0.05$.

3. Results

3.1. VO_{2max}, and VO_2 and Heart Rate at Threshold Level

Group values of VO_{2max}, and VO_2 and heart rate at threshold level measured with treadmill and arm cycle for both test occasions were shown in Figure 1-4. No significant difference (P □ 0.05) was observed in any of the variables between the two tests for either treadmill running or arm cycling. However, relative VO_{2max} (ml/min/kg) was significant higher ($p < 0.05$) at the first test compared to the second test for both treadmill running and arm cycling (appendix 1 and 2).

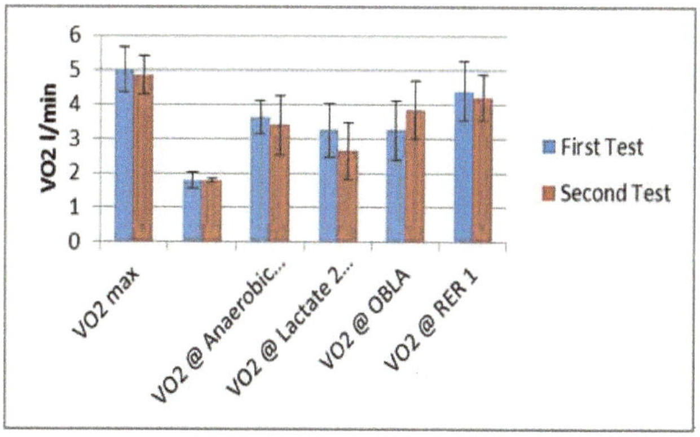

Figure 1. VO_2 @ threshold measured on treadmill

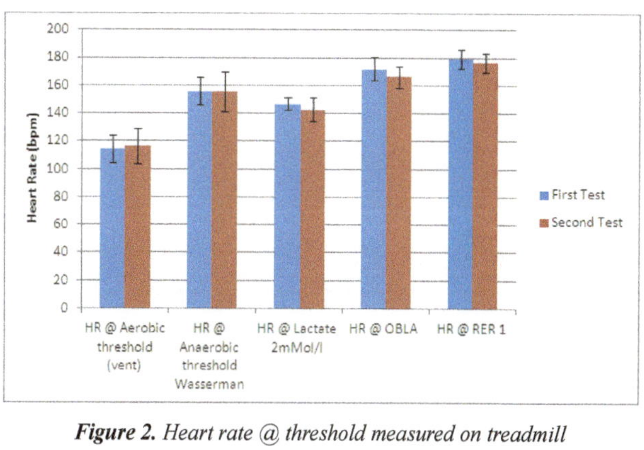

Figure 2. Heart rate @ threshold measured on treadmill

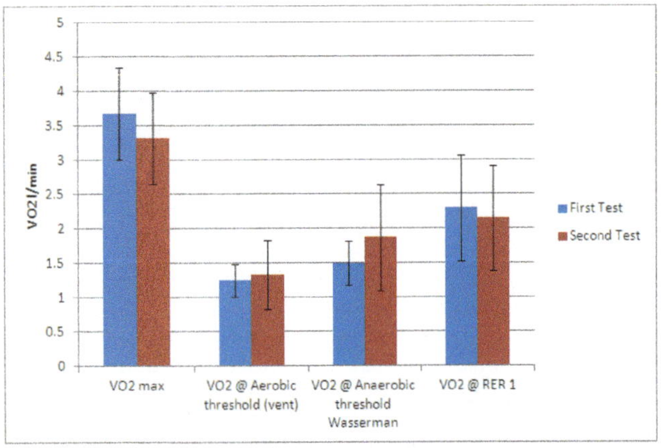

Figure 3. *VO2 @ threshold measured on arm cycle*

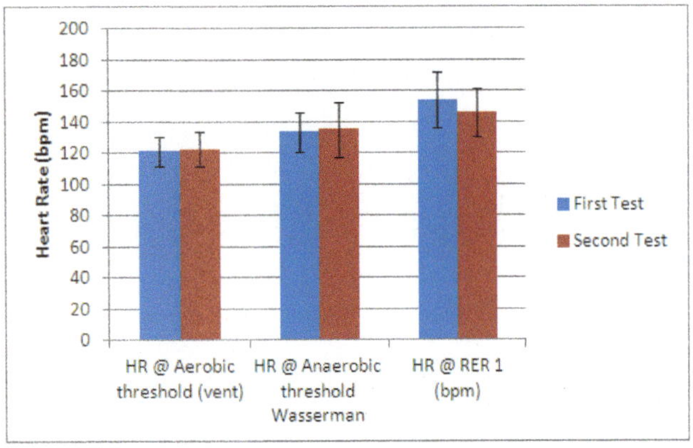

Figure 4. *heart rate @ threshold measured on arm cycle*

3.2. Lactate Recovery Rate

Results of lactate recovery rate were shown in Figure 5. Between the two test occasions, significant difference in lactate level [La] was only observed at 0 min after treadmill running (Figure 5; $p < 0.05$). When comparing [La] values between the two test methods for both test occasions, significant difference ($p < 0.05$) was only observed after the first test occasion at 10 min.

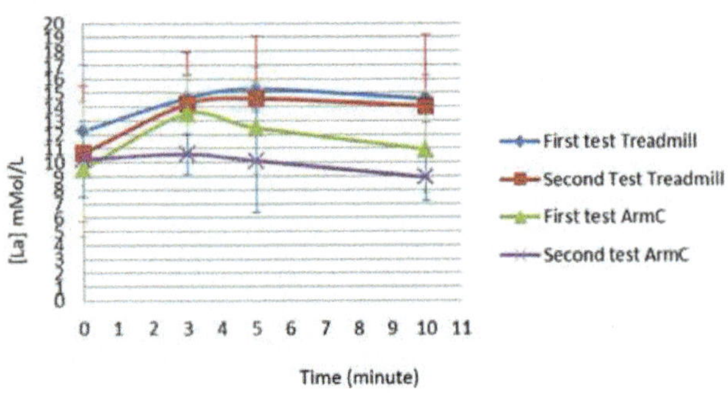

Figure 5. *Lactate [La] recovery rate after the the two test ocasions with both treadmill and arm cykle*

3.3. Strength and Power Tests

Results of the strength and power tests were shown in Table 2. Between the two test occasions, squat jump (cm) and counter movement jump with arm swing (cm/kg) were significant higher ($p < 0.05$) at the first occasion than the second, and all the other measurements showed no significant difference between the two test occasions.

Table 2. *Comparison of strength/power (Mean ± SD)*

	First test	*Second test*	P-value
SJ (cm)	40,3 ± 3,78	36,23 ± 3,59	0,02□
CMJ (cm)	43,1 ± 5,07	41,25 ± 2,13	0,46
CMJa (cm)	50,18 ± 5,63	47,2 ± 1,6	0,31
Vertical sit-ups (reps)	22,25 ± 3,78	23,5 ± 3,1	0,34
Hang Clean (kg/kg)	1,09 ± 0,07	1,06 ± 0,11	0,22
Deadlift (kg/kg)	2,2 ± 0,19	2,12 ± 0,3	0,43
Relative SJ (cm/kg)	0,51 ± 0,05	0,46 ± 0,05	0,85
Relative CMJ (cm/kg)	0,55 ± 0,04	0,52 ± 0,07	0,15
Relative CMJa (cm/kg)	0,63 ± 0,4	0,59 ± 0,09	0,003*

*significant difference between the two tests

3.4. Body Composition

Results of body composition were shown in Table 3. None of the measurements showed significant difference between two the two test occasions.

Table 3. *Comparison of body composition (Mean ± SD)*

	First test	Second test	P-value
Bone mineral density (%)	113,75 ± 4,57	117,25 ± 6,95	0,21
Muscle Mass (kg)	67,18 ± 11,79	66,83 ± 11,22	0,53
Fat mass (kg)	9,9 ± 2,02	10,9 ± 1,64	0,32
Muscle percentage (%)	83,21 ± 0,82	82,68 ± 2,11	0,72
Fat percentage (%)	12,25 ± 0,54	14,18 ± 1,91	0,19

3.5. Personal Competition Record

Personal competition record was shown in Table 4. At group level, the one year physical training did not significantly change personal competition record.

Table 4. *Personal competition record (win percent)*

	Before first test	Before second test	One year before the first test	One year before the second test
Subject 1*	80	81	75	50
Subject 2*	80	80	100	-
Subject 3*	59	73	50	100
Subject 4*	57	56	66	50
Subject 5*	100	100	-	-
Average*	77 ± 0.16	76 ± 0.16	78	75

4. Discussion

The present study revealed the physiological characters of MMA athletes. The one year routine physical training did not significantly improve either the physiological parameters or the personal competition record.

4.1. Aerobic Capacity

The full length of a MMA competition is 15 or 25 minutes, a typical aerobic sport [7]. However, MMA athletes often execute short duration of series intensive actions such as punches, kicks, knees. The energy supply of MMA has been suggested to be similar with repeated sprints; lactate system contributed 40% of the energy at the first sprint but dropped to 9% when repeated 10 times. In the meanwhile, the oxidative metabolism contributed <10% energy at the first sprint but accounted for 40% of the energy needed at the last sprint [11]. Similarly, energy supply switch from initial anaerobic system to aerobic system has also been observed in Muay Thai fighters [12].

Because MMA athletes often execute short duration of series intensive actions, therefore, it highly stresses the lactate energy system [8]. However, if the system is stressed too much and/or too early during a competition, it may cause accumulation of metabolites like [H+] [13, 14] and subsequent acidosis [15], leading to the athletes "gas out".

As shown in Fig. 5, fully lactate recovery takes more than 10 minutes. Because the rest period between two consecutive rounds in MMA is only 1 minute, a primary utilization of the lactate energy system indicates no chance of lactate recovery between rounds, thus fatigue early and loss of competition. Therefore, even though anaerobic capacity is very important in MMA, high aerobic capacity guarantees to sustain an intensive competition.

In the study, the relative VO_{2max} for the five subjects was around 60 ml/min/kg (on treadmill). Currently, there is no available study on MMA to compare our results; however this value is higher than amateur MMA fighters (55.5 ± 7.3 ml/min/kg; [6]) and wrestlers (56.8 ± 3.8 ml/min/kg; [17]), but resembles senior amateur boxers (61.7 ± 9 ml/min/kg) [16].

In addition to VO_{2max}, the percentage of VO_{2max} usage (threshold) is another important parameter in evaluating aerobic capacity. High VO_{2max} level but low threshold indicates recruitment of the lactate energy system too early and too much, thus early fatigue in competition. In contrast, high VO_{2max} level and high threshold will postpone the activation of the anaerobic system, thus, less fatiguing metabolites accumulation and prolonged highly competition.

As shown in Fig. 1 and 3, the VO_2 at AT level was around 1.5 to 4.5 l/min, around 40 to 90% of VO_{2max} (appendix 3 and 4), depending on threshold measurements and test methods (treadmill running or arm cycling). The threshold level observed in the study was similar to the level of physically active individuals, but lower than high aerobic training athletes [18].

Variation in heart rate at AT level followed the same trend as VO_2 at AT level for both test methods (treadmill running and arm cycling). Between the two test occasions, neither VO_2 nor heart rate at AT level showed any significant difference. The results together with the VO_{2max} measurements indicate the one year routine physical training did not further improve the aerobic capacity in the MMA athletes or the MMA athletes had already reached their optimal aerobic level required for MMA.

4.2. Anaerobic Capacity

The anaerobic energy system, especially the ATP-phosphocreatine (PCr) energy system is very important for MMA athletes because a powerful take-down or strike in MMA often means the end a competition. The results of strength and power tests (Table 2) showed a trend of decrease in the second test occasion compared with the first one, although only in two parameters. Similar as the aerobic capacity, the anaerobic test results may also indicate that the MMA athletes had already reached their optimal anaerobic level required for MMA or the energy system was not further improved by the one year training.

As shown in Fig. 5, immediately after both test occasions using both treadmill and arm cycle, all subjects reached high blood lactate levels (9- 12 mm/L), and by 2-3min after the tests, blood lactate levels were even higher. In addition, all subjects reached OBLA level (4 mm/L) and could keep working for extended periods, indicating that the subjects had a high anaerobic and acidosis tolerance/buffering capacity.

The AT values were higher measured on treadmill in both test occasions compared to values measured using arm cycle. Nevertheless, the AT level measured on arm cycle still reached around 60% of VO_{2max}, indicating a high buffering capacity/acidosis tolerance in upper bodies of the MMA athletes.

4.3. Body Composition

The muscle mass was not significantly changed by the one year training; however, the bone density and fat mass were significantly increased in the second test compared to the first test. The increased fat mass might contribute to the decreased relative strength and power, and affect AT as well. At present it is unclear whether the changes in body composition were associated with personal competition record, but it is worth notice that MMA fighters are used to body composition changes of either long or short term before a competition.

In summary, the subjects in the study presented above average aerobic capacity, but rather high anaerobic capacity and threshold levels compared with other similar sports. The one year routine physical training did not significantly improve the physiological parameters, which was consistent with personal competitive records. This may indicate that the subjects had already reached their optimal physiological level required for MMA or the one year physical training was not effective enough to induce significant improvement in the physiological parameters.

We have to notice that MMA athletes usually don't have a standardized on/off season as other sports, suggesting that they might be in different stages of preparation for upcoming competitions. This probably exerts high impact on the test results. The author recognized the low numbers of subjects as a limitation of the study design.

5. Conclusions

On basis of the current results, the following conclusions were made:

1) The MMA-fighters had above average aerobic capacity (VO_{2max} of 60ml/min/kg) and a high lactate tolerance and H+ buffering capacity.

2) The one year regular physical training did not result in significant improvement in the physiological parameters, a consistent result with the personal competition records.

***Appendix 1.** Threshold values using treadmill*

	First test (Mean ± SD)	Second test (Mean ± SD)	P-value
VO_{2max} (l/min)	5 ± 0,65	4,85 ± 0,57	0,18
Relative VO_{2max} (ml/min/kg)	62,75 ± 4,86	60,5 ± 5,07	0,018*
Hb (mg/l)	147,25 ± 6,56	155 ± 11,58	0,22
[La] 0min aw (mMol/l)	12,27 ± 4,8	10,66 ± 4,91	0,002*
[La] 3min aw (mMol/l)	14,63 ± 1,66	14,2 ± 3,71	0,76
[La] 5min aw (mMol/l)	15,27 ± 1,59	14,59 ± 4,53	0,74
[La] 10min aw (mMol/l)	14,57 ± 1,71	14,02 ± 5,16	0,81
VO_2 @ Aerobic Threshold (vent) (l/min)	1,8 ± 0,23	1,78 ± 0,05	0,86
VO_2 @ Anaerobic threshold Wassermann (l/min)	3,63 ± 0,48	3,4 ± 0,86	0,4
VO_2 @ Lactate 2 mMol/l	3,25 ± 0,78	2,65 ± 0,83	0,2
VO_2 @ OBLA	4,1 ± 0,86	3,85 ± 0,85	0,06
VO_2 @ RER 1	4,4 ± 0,87	4,2 ± 0,66	0,44
HR @ Aerobic threshold (vent) (bpm)	114,2 ± 10,09	116,25 ± 12,58	0,3
HR @ Anaerobic threshold Wasserman (bpm)	155,6 ± 10,02	155,25 ± 14,5	0,17
HR @ Lactate 2mMol/l (bpm)	146,8 ± 4,44	142,75 ± 8,34	0,1
HR @ OBLA (bpm)	172 ± 8,49	166,25 ±7,93	0,79
HR @ RER 1 (bpm)	179,5 ± 6,86	176,75 ± 6,9	0,91

* - statistical significant

***Appendix 2.** Threshold values using arm cycle*

	First test (Mean ± SD)	Second test (Mean ± SD)	P-value
VO_{2max} (l/min)	3,68 ± 0,67	3,32 ± 0,61	0,07
Relative VO_{2max} (ml/min/kg)	45,8 ± 2,87	41,15 ± 4,06	0,02*
VO_2 @ Aerobic threshold (vent) (l/min)	1,25 ± 0,24	1,33 ± 0,5	0,63
VO_2 @ Anaerobic threshold Wasserman (l/min)	1,5 ± 0,32	1,87 ± 0,77	0,23
VO_2 @ RER 1 (l/min)	2,3 ± 0,77	2,15 ± 0,76	0,51
[La] 0min aw (mMol/l)	9,53 ± 4,88	10,23 ± 2,77	0,64
[La] 3min aw (mMol/l)	13,49 ± 2,84	10,59 ± 1,43	0,32
[La] 5min aw (mMol/l)	12,49 ± 3,35	10,12 ± 3,77	0,22
[La] 10min aw (mMol/l)	10,9 ± 3,13	8,9 ± 1,71	0,07
HR @ Aerobic threshold (vent) (bpm)	121,2 ± 9,2	122,5 ± 11,09	0,49
HR @ Anaerobic threshold Wasserman (bpm)	133,4 ± 12,68	135 ± 17,7	0,465
HR @ RER 1 (bpm)	154,2 ± 18,06	146 ± 15,44	0,87

* - statistical significant

***Appendix 3.** Threshold using treadmill (relative to the maximum)*

	First test (Mean ± SD)	Second test (Mean ± SD)	P-value
Aerobic threshold (vent) (% mHR)	63,19 ± 7,7	63,04 ± 9,1	0,916
Anaerobic threshold Wasserman (% mHR)	82,22 ± 7,22	83,79 ± 6,34	0,76
Lactate 2mMol/l (% mHR)	78,94 ± 5,15	77,15 ± 4,83	0,42
RER 1 (% mHR)	94,75 ± 2,1	94,17 ± 1,29	0,647
OBLA (% mHR)	92,34 ± 1,64	89,8 ± 3,37	0,091
Aerobic threshold (vent) (% mVO_2)	35,8 ± 0,96	37,13 ± 5,3	0,635
Anaerobic threshold Wasserman (% mVO_2)	72,43 ± 7,63	69,48 ± 11,69	0,598
Lactate 2mMol/l (% mVO2)	63,99 ± 11,44	54,01 ± 13,65	0,237
RER 1 (% mVO_2)	90,59 ± 6,46	89,25 ± 1,63	0,68
OBLA (% mVO_2)	80,99 ± 8,8	81,40 ± 9,07	0,762

(%mHR) – percent of maximal HR
(%mVO_2) – percent of maximal VO_2

***Appendix 4.** Threshold using arm cycle (relative to the maximum)*

	First test (Mean ± SD)	Second test (Mean ± SD)	P-value
Aerobic threshold (vent) (%mHR)	64,82 ± 7,04	66,37 ± 8,16	0,255
Anaerobic threshold Wasserman (%mHR)	69,37 ± 6,52	73,71 ± 12,49	0,284
RER 1 (%mHR)	81,58 ± 10,01	79,37 ± 11,70	0,736
Aerobic threshold (vent) (%mVO_2)	34,07 ± 4,17	39,29 ± 8,71	0,269
Anaerobic threshold Wasserman (%mVO_2)	41,57 ± 5,95	54,84 ± 12,15	0,111
RER 1 (%mVO_2)	58,63 ± 16,47	63,6 ± 11,46	0,583

(%mHR) – percent of maximal HR
(%mVO_2) – percent of maximal VO_2

References

[1] C. P. McLellan, D. I. Lovell and G. C. Gass, Performance analysis of elite Rugby League match play using global positioning systems. J Strength Cond Res. 2011, vol. 25, Jun,

pp. 1703-10.

[2] J. Yoon. Physiological profiles of elite senior wrestlers. Sports Med. 2002, vol. 32, pp. 225-33.

[3] W. J. Kraemer, A. C. Fry, M. R. Rubin, T. Triplett-McBride, S. E. Gordon, L. P. Koziris, et al., Physiological and performance responses to tournament wrestling. Med Sci Sports Exerc, 2001, vol. 33, Aug, pp. 1367-78.

[4] B. Mirzaei, D. B. Curby, F. Rahmani-Nia and M. Moghadasi. Physiological profile of elite Iranian junior freestyle wrestlers. J Strength Cond Res, 2009, vol. 23, Nov, pp. 2339-44.

[5] E. Franchini, F. B. Del Vecchio, K. A. Matsushigue and G. G. Artioli, Physiological profiles of elite judo athletes. Sports Med, 2011, vol. 41, Feb. pp. 147-66.

[6] M. Schick, L. Brown, J. Coburn, W. Beam, E. Schick and N. Dabbs, Physiological Profile of Mixed Martial Artists. Medicina Sportiva, 2010, vol. 14, pp. 182-187.

[7] P. O. Åstrand, K. Rodahl, H. A. Dahl and S. B. Strömme, Textbook of Work Physiology, 4th edition. Human Kinetics. Champaign, USA. 2003.

[8] J.A. Amtmann, K.A. Amtmann and W.K. Spath, Lactate and rate of perceived exertion responses of athletes training for and competing in a mixed martial arts event. Journal of Strength & Conditioning Research, 2008, vol. 22, pp. 645-7.

[9] R. B. Mazess, H. S. Barden,J. P. Bisek and J. Hanson, Dual-energy x-ray absorptiometry for total-body and regional bone-mineral and soft-tissue composition. Am J Clin Nutr, 1990, vol. 51, Jun, pp. 1106-12.

[10] P. Butudom, J. H. Foreman, K. H. Kline and E. L. Whittem, Validation and comparison of two methods of measuring lactate in equine plasma. Equine Vet J, 2010, vol. 42, Nov, Suppl., pp. 155-60.

[11] O. Girard, A. Mendez-Villanueva and D. Bishop. Repeated-sprint ability - part I: factors contributing to fatigue. Sports Med, 2011, vol. 41, Aug, pp. 673-94.

[12] A. Crisafulli, S. Vitelli, I. Cappai, R. Milia, F. Tocco, F. Melis and A. Concu, Physiological responses and energy cost during a simulation of a Muay Thai boxing match. Appl Physiol Nutr Metab, 2009, vol. 34, Apr., pp. 143-50.

[13] D. Bishop, S. Lawrence and M. Spencer. Predictors of repeated-sprint ability in elite female hockey players. J Sci Med Sport, 2003, vol. 6, Jun, pp. 199-209.

[14] S. Ratel, C. A. Williams, J. Oliver and N. Armstrong, Effects of age and recovery duration on performance during multiple treadmill sprints. Int J Sports Med, 2006, vol. 27, Jan, pp. 1-8.

[15] K. Sahlin, R. C. Harris, B. Nylind and E. Hultman, Lactate content and pH in muscle obtained after dynamic exercise. Pflugers Arch, 1976, vol. 28, Dec, pp. 143-9.

[16] G. L. Khanna and I. Manna, Study of physiological profile of Indian boxers. Journal of Sports Science and Medicine, 2006, vol. 5, pp. 90-98.

[17] I. Barbas. G. Fatouros, I. I. Douroudos, A. Chatzinikolaou, Y. Michailidis, D. Draganidis and et al., Physiological and performance adaptations of elite Greco-Roman wrestlers during a one-day tournament. Eur J Appl Physiol, 2011, vol. 111, Jul., pp. 1421-36.

[18] D. L. Wilmore and J. H. Costill. Physiology of sport and exercise. 2nd edition. Champaign (IL): Human Kinetics, 1999.

12

A comparison of internal/external rotation strength and range of motion in the shoulder joint between zurkhaneh athletes and non-athletes

Hamid Dehnavi[1], Hassan Daneshmandi[2], Mohammad khajehpoor Glosalari[3], Hossein Shahrokhi[4]

[1]Sama Technical and Vocational Training College, Islamic Azad University, Neyshabur Branch, Neyshabur, Iran
[2]Associate professor of Guilan University, Iran
[3]Msc Student of sport injury and corrective exercise, Islamic Azad University Khorasgan(Isfahan) Branch, Iran
[4] PhD student of Kharazmi University, Iran

Email address:
Hamiddehnavi@ymail.com (H. Dehnavi)

Abstract: Zurkhaneh as one the oldest sport is include many overhead movements. The purpose of this study was comparison between ratio of strength and range of motion in internal and external rotation in the shoulder joint's zurkhaneh athletes with Non-athletes. The subjects in this study included 29 zurkhaneh athletes with mean age (23.51±2.04) and mean years of sport history (8.75±4.47) and 30 non-athletes athletes with mean age (24.8±1.56). Data were collected through questionnaires, and subjects' strength was measured by "Hand-held dynamometer" and ROM was measured by "Leighton flexometer"(r=0.90–0.99) in both upper extremities. Data were analyzed by paired samples t-test and independent samples t-test. The results of this study showed significant degrees at internal/external rotation ROM ratio of zurkhaneh athletes than the non-athletes group ($p \leq 0.05$). some result also was found in strength ratio in internal/external rotators in this group ($p \leq 0.001$). Therefore repeated pattern of movements in the zurkhaneh sport at the long time causes imbalance in strength and range of motion shoulder joint that need to corrective exercise. It can be included due to specific demands such as repeated rotational movements in shoulder joint, they need a compensatory corrective exercises.

Keywords: Zurkhaneh, Strength, Range of Motion, Shoulder Joint

1. Introduction

The physical demands of sport performance on the athletes' body cause certain musculoskeletal adaptation. Professional athletes spend most of their sporting life in training and competition (Crockett et al., 2002). Load placed on the musculoskeletal system may be generally classified as tensile or compressive. Repeated demands on a musculotendinous unit may cause it to shorten, decreasing normal joint range of motion (Daneshmandi et al., 2010). Musculoskeletal adaptation and some special side effects due to his or her physical demands and movement patterns in professional athletes are very important subjects in sport sciences. The musculoskeletal adaptation at this point is called maladaptation, reducing joint range of motion, changing biomechanical patterns, decreasing the efficiency of force production, and increasing the chance of injuries to the musculoskeletal system (Anderson et al., 2002). Athletes involved in repetitive overhead activities place unique demands on the shoulder girdle (Arroyo et al., 1997). Overhead activities such as throwing, tennis, or volleyball place the athlete at considerable risk of overuse injuries (Burkhart et al., 2003). The glenohumeral joint is inherently unstable, and stability is provided predominantly by the ligamentous, capsular, and muscular structures and by the relative position of the glenoid and the arm through all arm motions (Wilk et al., 2002).

The internal rotator (IR) and external rotator (ER) muscles of the shoulder play a critical role in providing stability and mobility to the glenohumeral joint, particularly in overhead athletes (Ramsi et al., 2004).

Repetitive muscular exertion in the upper extremity required during performance of overhead activities specific movement patterns, leads to the development of sport specific muscular adaptation in overhead players. Muscular imbalance in rotator cuff and scapular musculature, coupled with inadequate muscular endurance and improper stroke biomechanics, can lead to overuse injury in the glenohumeral joint of overhead activity players (Ellenbecker et al., 2003).

Zurkhaneh as traditional sport is unique and very popular in Iran and also few countries, this sport includes many physical activities and skills which performed with and without specific instruments. Most activities performed by overhead movements in shoulder. Despite of this popularity, there are no more academic research in this sport.

Therefore, the main purpose was to study the ratio of strength and range of motion (ROM) in internal and external rotation of shoulder joint's zurkhaneh athletes and compare the data with Non-athletes.

2. Methodology

The subjects of this study were members of league teams with more than 3 years of play in league competitions which voluntary participated in investigation. The total subjects of this study were include 59 men with mean age (24.16±1.91). The groups of athletes included 29 zurkhaneh players with mean age (23.51±2.04) and mean years of sport history (8.75±4.47) and 30 non-athletes athletes with mean age (24.8±1.56). The players completed sport injury risk factor questionnaires which asked about shoulder injuries and the causes of them during last two years. Demographics data also was gathered.

2.1. Range of Motion Test

Duration of dominant and non-dominant glenohumeral joints were made by Leighton flexometer (r=0.90–0.99)(figure 1) in standard position. Goniometric measurement of the glenohumeral join is difficult because of the multi-join nature of the shoulder complex. In general, the literature would appear to indicate that the Leighton flexometer is a reliable measuring tool, especially when used by a single experienced tester.

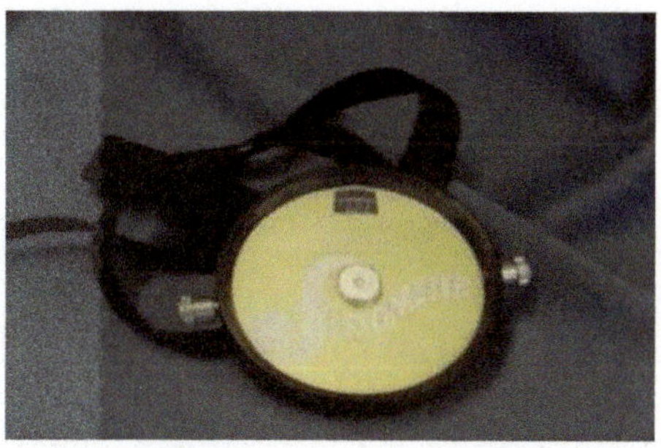

Figure 1: *Leighton flexometer*

All ROMs of subjects were measured in the morning and before play or participating in warm-up drills. No goniometric measurements were taken in the afternoon or after participating in play or warm-up drills to minimize the effect of intense activity or play on range of motion. All testing took place with the subject in a standard position in special bar and plastic cast and stabilized scapula by three special wide tapes on the hip, chest and head areas. Shoulder external and internal rotations were measured with the arm positioned in 90° of glenohumeral abduction and 90° of elbow flexion(figure 2). During testing, the subjects were asked to actively move the joint as far as possible through the range of motion. For each direction, three measurements were taken and the mean measurements were calculated. We performed t-test on dominant versus non-dominant hands of subjects for all measurements. Correlation coefficients were computed to determine the strength of the relationships among variables (Daneshmandi et al., 2010).

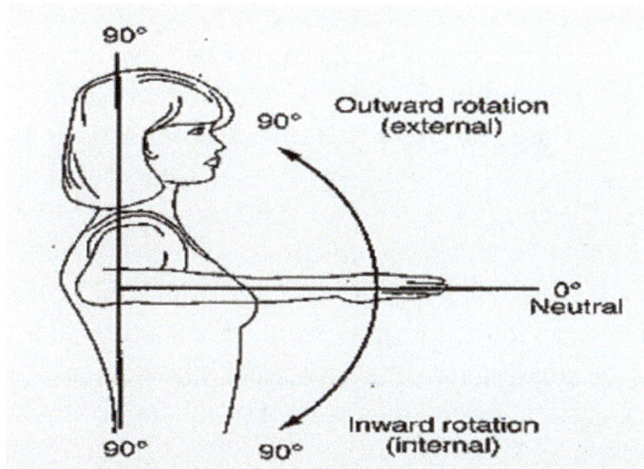

Figure 2: *Measurement of internal/external ROM*

2.2. Isometric Strength Muscle Test

Isometric force was measured with the JTech Power track II™ hand-held dynamometer (figure 3). A variety of shoulder positions have been described for isometric strength testing. Some authors (Kuhlman et al., 1992)have tested in the scapular plane instead of the coronal plane, suggesting it decreases stress on the capsular-ligamentous-tendinous complex, increases the congruity between the humeral head and glenoid and keeps an optimal length-tension relationship for the abductors and rotators. The scapular rotator plane has been defined as the arm at 45° of forward elevation in the sagittal plane and at 30° anterior to the frontal plane (Leroux et al., 1995). Some studies (Greenfield et al., 1990), (This et al., 1996)have suggested that higher torques are produced by subjects with and without shoulder pathology in this position; although others have found that there is minimal (Hartsell et al., 1997) or no difference(Whitcomb et al., 1995) in subjects without shoulder pathology.

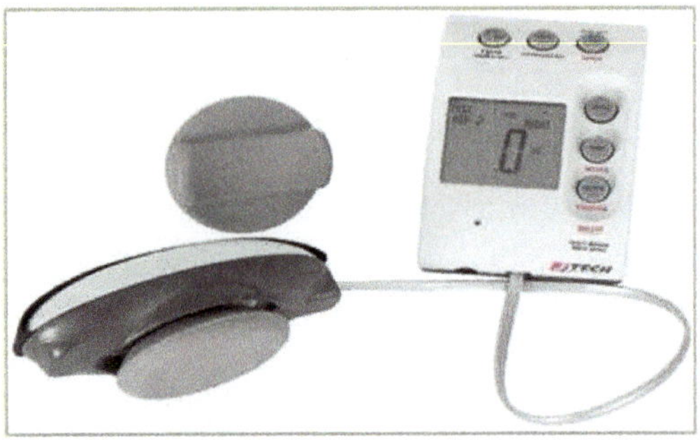

***Figure 3:** JTech Power track II™ hand-held dynamometer*

In the present study all strength tests were performed in the prone position with the designated arm positioned in 90° of abduction and 0° of rotation with the elbow flexed to 90° (Beach et al., 1992), (Magnusson et al., 1995). The humerus was stabilized distally against the plinth, and subjects used the opposite arm to hold o to the side of the testing table for support. A JTech Powertrack II™ hand-held dynamometer was placed just proximal to the ulnar styloid process on the posterior surface of the forearm to assess external rotation strength. The dynamometer was positioned using the same anatomical landmarks on the anterior surface of the forearm to assess internal rotation strength (Beach et al., 1992), (Magnusson et al., 1995). Two maximal isometric contractions were performed, the duration of which was approximately 6-7_S and 30_S rests was given between trials. Subjects were instructed to hold the contraction against maximal examiner pressure and peak isometric muscle force was recorded (Cadogan et al., 2010).

3. Results

The results of this study showed that the strength of internal rotation of zurkhaneh athletes were more than non-athletes, but this deference were less in external rotation ($p<0.001$) (Graph 1).

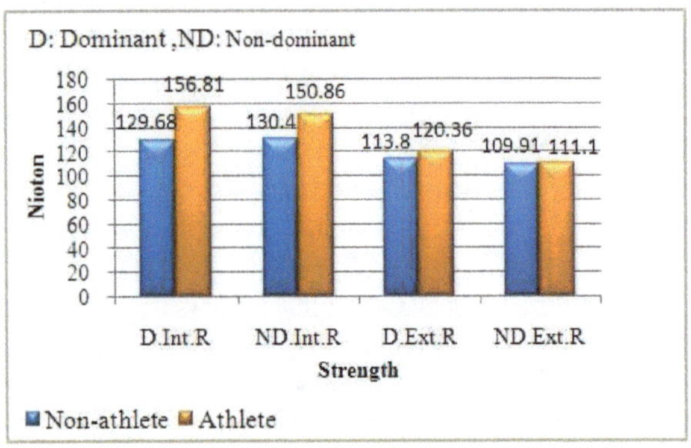

***Graph 1:** Internal/external rotation shoulder strength*

Also the results showed that range of motion of athletes were less than non-athletes for internal rotation ($p<0.001$) (Graph 2).

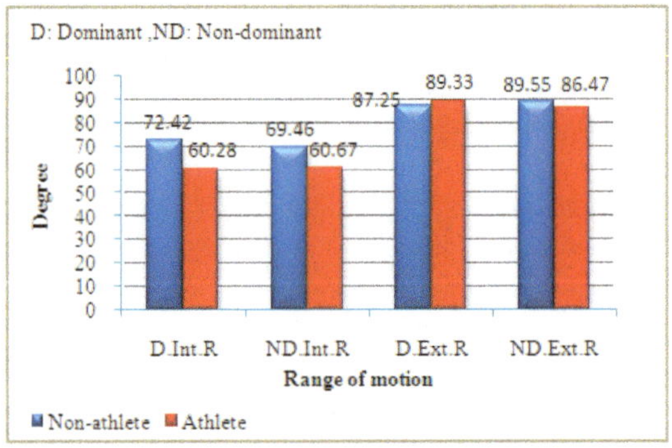

***Graph 2:** Internal/external rotation shoulder Range of motion*

The results of this study showed significant differences at internal/external rotation ROM ratio between zurkhaneh athletes and non-athletes group ($p<0.05$)(Graph 3). Likewise, the results of this study showed significant degrees at internal/external rotation strength ratio between zurkhaneh athletes and non-athletes group ($p<0.001$)(Graph 3).

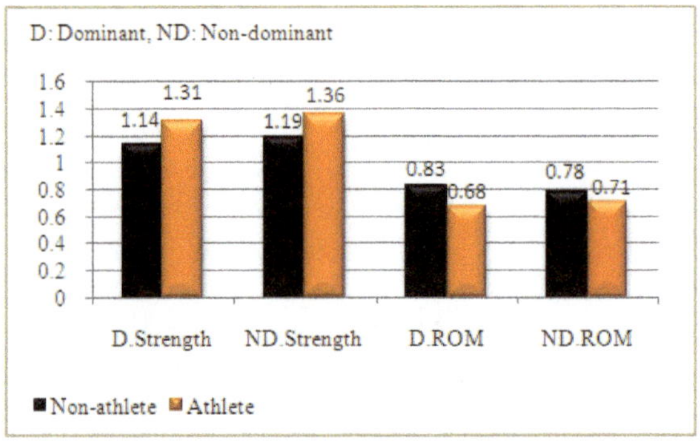

***Graph 3:** Internal/External strength and ROM ratios*

4. Discussion

There is controversy in the literature as to whether absolute strength or the IR:ER strength ratio should be used to quantify optimal levels of dynamic shoulder stability, particularly in overhead athletes (McMaster, 1992) Although similar studies have examined strength values of various levels of overhead athletes, this is the first study to examine ratio of strength and range of motion over the zurkhaneh athletes. The increased strength of IR without comparable increases in ER strength has been found in tennis players (Chandler, 1990), swimmers (Ramsi, 2004),water polo players (McMaster, 1992) and baseball pitchers (Brown, 1998) and has been attributed to the repetitive IR motions involved in this overhead sports. In our study, IR strength consistently increased throughout repetitive IR motions in zurkhaneh players. The reliance on IR muscles for power, coupled with the high number of repetitions, encourages progressive increases in IR strength over the Shoulder Joint's Zurkhaneh. If a strength imbalance ratio develops between the IR and ER muscles, however, chronic upper extremity overuse pathologies might ensue.

Also In this study, the ratio of range of external and internal shoulder rotations was different in zurkhaneh athletes, which can be related to their specific sport demands and emphasizes this point that flexibility is very specific in any joint, Glenohumeral internal rotation of zurkhaneh athletes was less than other groups in this study. A reduction in shoulder internal rotation, can be explained as an adaptation of the anterior shoulder musculature to the overhead movements in this sport. Current research has convincingly showed that deficits of internal rotation of shoulder occur as the athlete adapts to the demands of the sport. It is unclear whether these are normal adaptations that are beneficial, either locally or throughout the kinetic chain, or whether these are mal-adaptations that create potentially harmful local or kinetic chain biomechanics. Also, the role this adaptation may play in injury causation or risk is unclear. Several recent papers suggest that decreased internal rotation and total rotation may adversely affect shoulder performance, and this effect may increase the risk of injury. There are studies which show that inflexibility is a risk factor for further injury (Chandler, 1990). Achievement of full range of motion is one of the first goals in rehabilitation programs (Wilk, 2002).Most shoulder rehabilitation protocols now emphasize on a corrective exercise for internal rotation of shoulder of athletes. This paper showed degrees of asymmetry in dominant and non-dominant hands of zurkhaneh athletes. If we do not note it carefully and do not use correct stretch exercise program, this imbalance in musculature of shoulder girdle leads the athletes to decrease their performance or an increase in the chance of injury.

5. Conclusion

Elite Zurkhaneh athletes without shoulder injury have shoulder rotation muscle strength imbalances that alter the normal functional ratio between the rotator cuff muscles. These differences in strength do not seem to affect athletic performance, but detection and prevention with exercise programs at an early age are recommended.

References

[1] Anderson M K, Hall S J, Martin M. (2004) Foundations of athletic training: Prevention, assessment and management (3rd ed.). Baltimore, MD: Lippincott, Williams & Wilkins Publishing.

[2] Alderink Gj, Kuck DJ. (1986). Isokinetic shoulder strength of high school and college-Aged pitchers. Orthop Sports Phys Ther. 7(4):163-72

[3] Arroyo JS, Hershon SJ, Bigliani LU. (1997). Special considerations in the athletic throwing shoulder. Orthop Clin North Am. 28(1):69-78.

[4] Beach ML, Whitney SL, Dickoff-Hoffman SA. (1992). Relationship of shoulder flexibility, strength, and endurance to shoulder pain in competitive swimmers. Orthop Sports Phys Ther. 16(6):262-8.

[5] Brown LP, Niehues SL, Harrah A, Yavorsky P, Hirshman HP. (1988). Upper extremity range of motion and isokinetic strength of the internal and external shoulder rotators in major league baseball players. Am J Sports Med. 16(6):577-85.

[6] Burkhart SS, Morgan CD, Kibler WB. (2003). The disabled throwing shoulder: spectrum Of pathology, part I:pathoanatomy and biomechanics. Arthroscopy. 19(4):404–420.

[7] Cadogan A, Laslett M, Hing W, McNair P, Williams M. (2011). Reliability of a new hand-held dynamometer in Measuring shoulder range of motion and strength. Man Ther. 16(1):97-101.

[8] Chandler TJ, Kibler WB, Uhl TL, Wooten B, Kiser A, Stone E. (1990). Flexibility comparisons of junior elite tennis players to other athletes. Am J Sports Med. 18(2):134-6.

[9] Cools M Ann, Witvrouw E Erik, Mahieu N Nele, Danneels A Lieven. (2005). Isokinetic Scapular Muscle Performance in Overhead Athletes with and Without Impingement Symptoms. Journal of Athletic Training. 40(2):104-110.

[10] Daneshmandi H, Rahmaninia F, Shahrokhi H, Rahmani P, Esmaeili S. (2010). Shoulder joint flexibility in top athletes. J. Biomedical Science and Engineering. 3(8):811-815

[11] Ellenbecker T, Robert EP. (2003). Age specific isokinetic glenohumeral internal and external rotation strength in elite junior tennis players. Journal of science and medicine in sport. 6(1):63-70.

[12] Greenfield BH, Donatelli R, Wooden MJ, Wilkes J. (1990). Isokinetic evaluation of shoulder rotational strength between the plane of scapula and the frontal plane. Am J Sports Med. 18(2):124–8.

[13] Hartsell HD, Forwell L. (1997). Postoperative eccentric and concentric isokinetic strength for the shoulder rotators in the scapular and neutral planes. J Orthop Sports Phys Ther. 25(1):19–25.

[14] Crockett HC, Gross LB, Wilk KE, Schwartz ML, Reed J, O'Mara J, Reilly MT, Dugas JR, Meister K, Lyman S, Andrews JR. (2002). Osseous adaptation and range of motion at the glenohumeral joint in professional baseball pitchers. Am J Sports Med. 30(1):20-6

[15] Kuhlman JR, Iannotti JP, Kelly MJ, Riegler FX, Gevaert ML, Ergin TM. (1992). Isokinetic and isometric measurement of strength of external rotation and abduction of the shoulder. J Bone Joint Surg Am. 74(9):1320–33.

[16] Leroux JL, Hebert P, Mouilleron P, Thomas E, Bonnel F, Blotman F. (1995). Postoperative shoulder rotators strength in stages II and III impingement syndrome. Clin Orthop Relat Res. (320):46–54.

[17] Magnusson SP, Constantini NW, McHugh MP, Gleim GW. (1995). Strength profiles and performance in masters' level swimming. Am J Sports Med. 23(5):626-631.

[18] McMaster WC, Long SC, Caiozzo VJ. (1992). Shoulder torque changes in the swimming athlete. Am J Sports Med. 20(3): 323-7.

[19] Pink MM, Tibone JE. (2000). The painful shoulder in the swimming athlete. Orthop Clin North Am. 31(2):247–261.

[20] Ramsi M, Swanik A Kathleen, Straub J Stephen, Mattacola G Carl. (2004). Shoulder-Rotator Strength of High School Swimmers over the Course of a Competitive Season. J Sport Rehabil. 13(1):9-18.

[21] This LL, Maxwell T. (1996). The effect of positioning on shoulder isokinetic measures in females. Med Sci Sports Exerc. 28(9):1188–92.

[22] Whitcomb LJ, Kelley MJ, Leiper CI. (1995). A comparison of torque production during dynamic strength testing of shoulder abduction in the coronal plane and the plane of the scapula. J Orthop Sports Phys Ther. 21(4):227–32.

[23] Wilk KE, Meister K, Andrews JR. (2002). Current concepts in the rehabilitation of the overhead throwing athlete. Am J Sports Med. 30(1):136–151.

13

Match participations, field position, length of team membership: Their impact on team cohesion

Gioldasis Aristotelis, Stavrou Nektarios, Sotiropoulos Aristomenis, Psychountaki Maria

Department of Physical Education and Sport Science, National Kapodistrian University of Athens

Email address:
giold_telis@yahoo.gr (A. Gioldasis)

Abstract: The aim of the current study was to examine the relationship between cohesion and its antecedents (match participations, field position and length of team membership). 173 players of Greek amateur leagues participated in the study. They completed the Greek version of the 18-item Group Environment Questionnaire, and also improvised scales for the other variables in the end of the season 2009-2010. The Cronbach alphas of the Group Environment Questionnaire were satisfied for both task and social cohesion. The MANOVA analyses indicated the existence of statistical significant differences on perceptions of cohesion among players with different number of participations, and length of team membership. However, the MANOVA analysis showed that there were not statistical significant differences on perceptions of cohesion among players of different field position. Specifically, players with less participations perceived lower task and social cohesion than players with more participations. Furthermore, players who were members of their team for shorter period perceived lower social cohesion and higher task cohesion than players who were members for longer. Although the no significant results regarding the relationship between cohesion and field position, some trends showed that goalkeepers and attackers perceived the highest cohesion.

Keywords: Cohesion, Soccer, Position, Status, Performance

1. Introduction

In soccer a group of players co-operate so as to achieve team's goals. The coach manages the team in a way that the members have a tendency to stick together or to be united either physically or logically [1]. The team coach is challenged to create the environment which encourages players to achieve their personal and team goals by working together. The famous soccer coach Sven-Göran Eriksson described how "we" mentality can raise both the individual and team performance [2]. A significant psychological predictor of performance is team cohesion. Most of the studies on relationship between cohesion and performance in sports have shown that teamwork leads to increased effort and performance [3-10]. Carron and his colleagues [11], defined cohesion as "a dynamic process that is reflected in the tendency for a group to stick together and remain united in its pursuit of instrumental objectives and/or for the satisfaction of members' affective needs" (p.213). Sport cohesion is a multidimensional construct as it can be divided into two different types: the task and the social cohesion. Task cohesion corresponds to the desire of group members to work towards the achievement of the team goals, while social cohesion corresponds to the need of group members to form and maintain interpersonal bonds. Based on this proposition, Carron developed the conceptual model of team cohesion that specifies the antecedents and the consequences on both team and individual performance [11, 12]. Environmental, personal, leadership and group factors constitute the antecedents of team cohesion. Environmental factors such as the competition and the team size [13], personal factors such as satisfaction [14, 15], the coach leadership style and the way he contributes to cohesion development [16, 17], and group factors such as team goals [18] have been found to affect the cohesion. Although there are many studies which examine the relationships between a variety of factors and cohesion, soccer team cohesion has not been investigated enough.

One very important factor that seems to affect it is the number of players' match participations. Soccer teams consist of 20 to 25 players that co-operate with each other so as to achieve their goals. However, fewer than half of the team members participate in most of the matches. Therefore the players, who display the highest individual performance, play in most of the matches [19]. But how does this difference affect the feelings of the players? It has been noticed that many players get negative feelings when their role in the team is not as important as others' [20]. The results of a study in volleyball concluded that the players whose role is a substitute one perceive lower task cohesion [21]. Also, in American football the first-team players perceive higher levels of task [17] and total cohesion [22]. One explanation for these findings is that the first-team players develop feelings of belonging to the team and they are more focused to the team goals [19, 23].

The position of the players on the field is another factor that seems to affect the cohesion which the players perceive. In soccer, there are 11 different positions with completely different roles and responsibilities for the players. However, soccer coaches use the defenders in one team and the attackers in the other very frequently during training sessions and practice matches. Furthermore, during tactics groups of players often work in different tasks depending on the position. There are four different categories of players in a soccer team, goalkeepers, defenders, midfielders and attackers. Chelladuray and Carron [24] claimed that the positions of the players are specified by two factors, task dependence and propinquity. Task dependence is a factor that relates to the players' perceived cohesion and refers to the interaction among players of the same team. The higher task dependence, the greater interaction and dependence among players of the same team. The second factor, propinquity, consists of two dimensions, observability (knowledge of the movements of other positions) and visibility (the degree the player is observed by those in other positions). For example, the soccer goalkeeper presents the lowest level of task dependence and also low levels of interaction with the other players but high levels of propinquity. Although, it seems that small group players with similar responsibilities (e.g. defenders) would present same levels of perceptions about team cohesion, the findings of other studies concluded that the relationship between the cohesion and the field position is low [17, 25]. However, there was a minor significance of the results adding that the data were not taken from soccer teams which consisted of many players that work in small groups.

Another factor that seems to be related to players' perceived cohesion is the length of team membership. Players, who are members of the same team for a long time, adopt the team objectives/goals. There are studies which confirm that teams, which stick to the same players, present higher team performance very often [26, 27]. However, there is a lack of knowledge regarding the relationship of the length of time in a club for each player separately and its relation to their perceptions about the soccer team cohesion. The researchers of the study also established a lack of knowledge about the factors which related to the soccer team cohesion. The aim of the current study was to examine the relationship between cohesion and match participations, field position and length of a team membership.

2. Method

2.1. Participants

In the present study participated 173 Greek male soccer players. They were all members of Greek soccer clubs for the season 2009-2010. Participants' age ranged from 13 to 38 (M= 21.91, SD= 5.49). Parents or guardians of the under 18 year's old players were notified of the research procedures, requirements, benefits, and risks before giving informed consent. A university Research Ethics Committee granted approval for the study.

2.2. Design

The researchers measured the cohesion at the end of the season, before the last match of each team. According to the steps of team growth which Tuckman first described [28, 29], the end of the season for a team reflects to the stage before team adjourning. The perceived cohesion at the end of the season reflects the experiences that the players felt during the whole season. The researchers hypothesized that perceived cohesion would be differentiated for players of different roles and responsibilities in the team. They examined the players' field position (goalkeepers, defenders, midfielders, attackers), the length of time that these players were members of their team and the number of match participations of each player (first-team or substitute player).

2.3. Measurements / Questionnaires

2.3.1. Cohesion

The perceptions of team cohesion were assessed with the Greek version of the 18-item Group Environment Questionnaire; GEQ [30-32]. The Group Environment Questionnaire assesses the four dimensions of cohesion. Individual Attractions to the Group-Task (ATG-T) is the factor which identifies team-members individual perceptions with regard to their personal involvement to the task. Individual Attractions to the Group-Social (ATG-S) is the factor which identifies team-members individual perceptions in relation to their personal involvement, acceptance and social interaction to the team as a whole. Group Integration-Task (GI-T) is the factor which identifies the team-members individual perceptions on identity, closeness and bonding within the whole group. Group Integration-Social (GI-S) is the factor which identifies the individual perceptions of the team members on identity, closeness, and bonding within the whole group but with regards to its social aspects. Participants rate their consent to items on a 9-point scale anchored by 1 ('strongly disagree') to 9 ('strongly agree'). The reliability coefficients of the Greek version of the questionnaire with sample of team sports were .69 (ATG-T), .75 (ATG-S), .75 (GI-T) and .79 (GI-S).

2.3.2. Cohesion Antecedents

After each match, the researchers collected the line-ups from the score sheets (also including the players who were substitute). At the end of the season, they counted the total number of participations. The categories were then divided according to the total number of participations of each player from low (0-33% of total participations), to middle (34-66% of total participations), and high (67-100% of total participations).

The players filled in the field position which they played more often in their current team (goalkeeper, defender right/left/center/sweeper, midfielder/winger right/left/center, and forward right/left/center). Then, the researchers divided the players in four categories, goalkeepers, defenders, midfielders, and attackers.

The players answered to the question "How long have you been a member of the current team (adult team only)?". They were divided according to their answers to two different categories, less than one season (<1 seasons) and more than one season (≥1 seasons).

2.4. Procedures

The researchers arranged meetings with the 16-teams coaches which participated in the survey. They described them the aims of the study, the ethics about the participants and the dates of the measurements. They arranged dates which all the players could attend so as to give them the questionnaires and also the consent form before the training session. Before the loan of questionnaires, the researchers explained the aims of the study to the players they offered instructions on how to fill in the questions and they assured of the confidentiality of the survey (e.g. only the total team results would be announced and not the players' names). After the end of the study, the researchers presented the conclusions to the teams' staffs and thanked them and the players for their participation.

3. Results

The Cronbach alpha of the Group Environment Questionnaire was satisfied and is presented to the table 1.

Table 1.*Cronbachalpha of the Group Environment Questionnaire.*

Cohesion	Cronbachα
Task Cohesion	.81
Inter-item correlation	.33 (.11-.56)
Item correlation	.51 (.37-.67)
Social Cohesion	.82
Inter-item correlation	.34 (.16-.55)
Item correlation	.52 (.42-.62)

The figure 1 shows the differences among the players with different number of match participations regarding their task and social cohesion in the end of the season. The MANOVA analysis showed the existence of statistical significant differences in both task and social cohesion among players with different number of participations [Pillai's Trace= .116, $F_{(2,171)}$= 5.267, p< .001, η^2_p= .058]. Specifically, the analyses revealed the existence of significant differences for the task cohesion [$F_{(2,171)}$= 10.777, p< .001, η^2_p= .112] as well as for the social cohesion [$F_{(2,171)}$= 5.837, p< .01, η^2_p= .064]. Soccer players with low number of match participations revealed lower task and social cohesion than the players with middle and high number of match participations.

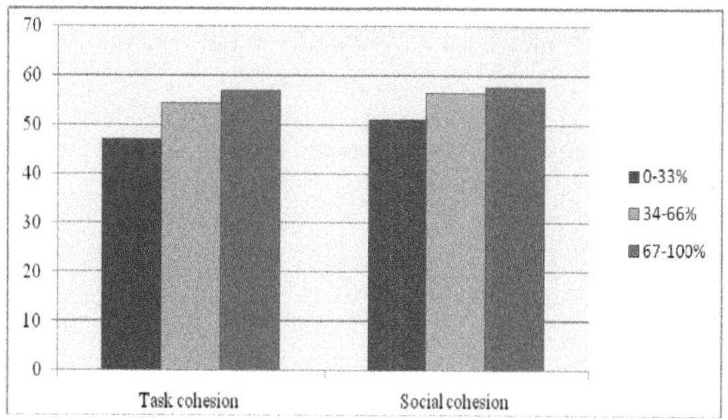

Figure 1. *Match participations and cohesion.*

The figure 2 shows the differences among players of different field position regarding task and social cohesion at the end of the season. The descriptive statistics showed that the goalkeepers and the attackers presented the highest level of task and social cohesion. However, the results of the MANOVA analysis showed that there were not significant differences neither for task nor for social cohesion among players of different field position at the end of the season [Pillai's Trace= .011, $F_{(3,187)}$= .360, ns, η^2_p = .006].

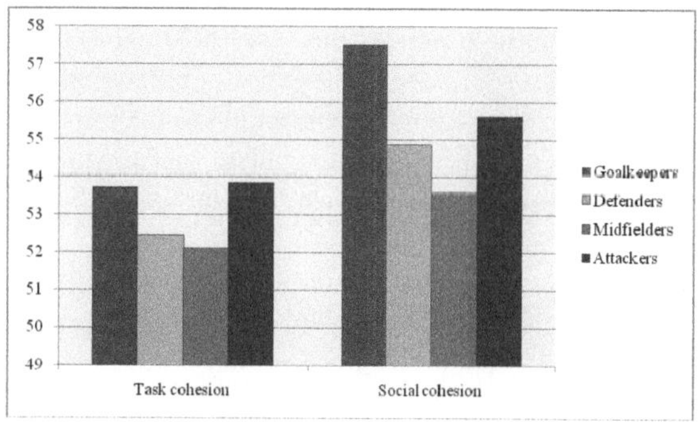

Figure 2. *Position and cohesion.*

The figure 3 shows the differences among players of different length of team membership as far as task and social cohesion at the end of the season. The descriptive statistics indicated that the players with low length of team membership (less than one season) reveal greater task cohesion and less social cohesion than players with high length of team membership. The MANOVA analysis showed the existence of significant differences in both task and social cohesion among players with different length of team membership [Pillai's Trace= .044, $F_{(1,188)}$= 4.350, p<.05, η^2_p= .044]. However, more specific analyses showed that there were not statistical significant differences as far as either task [$F_{(1,188)}$=1.219, ns, η^2_p= .006] or social cohesion [$F_{(1,188)}$= 2.110, ns, η^2_p= .011].

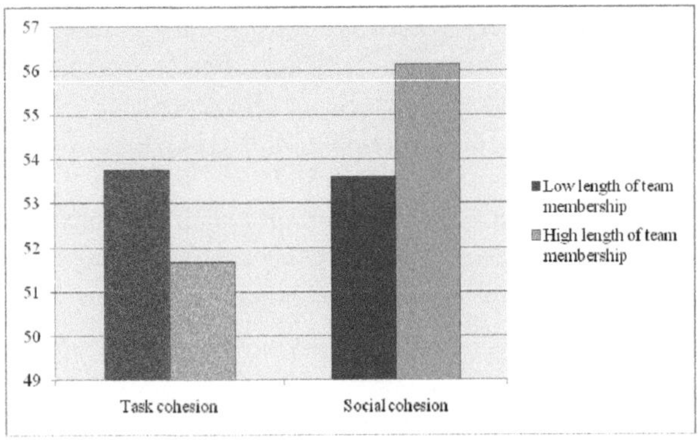

Figure 3. Length of team membershipand cohesion.

4. Discussion

As Carron [12] showed in his conceptual model of group cohesion, many factors affect it which are indirectly related to individual and team performance. According to our expectations, soccer team cohesion is affected by the antecedents which were examined in the current study to a greater or lesser extent. The statistical analyses showed that players with different numbers of match participations displayed differences in their perceptions about team cohesion. Specifically, players with fewer match participations perceived lower levels of task and social cohesion than those with more match participations. Literature supports this finding with regards to the differences to the team cohesion perceptions among players of different playing status [22]. Furthermore, other findings support that the number of match participations is related more to the task cohesion of the team [17]. This finding might be explained because of the sense of belonging to the tasks which the first-team players enjoy as they are more responsible for the achievement of these tasks. Moreover, the first-team players reveal higher commitment to the team tasks [19, 23].

The second factor that was examined with regards to its relationship with cohesion was the players' field position. The differences among the players were not significant although the descriptive statistics showed that goalkeepers and attackers displayed the highest levels of task and social cohesion. Defenders' and midfielders' cohesion ranged to middle levels. Goalkeepers and attackers' high levels of cohesion might be a consequence of the high levels of propinquity that they presented [24]. In total, the finding about no significant relationship between cohesion and position in soccer is supported by sport psychology literature that referred to other sports only [17, 25].

The last factor that the current study examined was the length of team membership. The findings revealed differences between players with short and long length of team membership. Players who were in the team for less than a year perceived higher levels of task cohesion and lower social cohesion than players who were in the team for more years. Other findings support this relationship through the connection of performance and the consistency of the team. Moderator variable for this relationship might be the team cohesion. In addition, players who are in the same team for long, develop more social relationships than the new players who are more oriented to the team tasks [26].

A limitation of the study might be the nature of Greek amateur soccer. In amateur leagues some of the teams pay their players while others not. Even teams that pay some players they do not pay all of them. This probably influences the perceived cohesion of the players. In addition, the amateur participation of the players in training sessions makes it difficult to examine their commitment in teams' schedules (e.g. total number of training sessions that each player was attended).

5. Conclusion

The current study lights the influence of some factors in cohesion of soccer teams. According to our findings, playing status, playing position, and length of team membership, linked to team cohesion. As the relationship between cohesion and performance has already been proved, these findings should be used by the training staff so as to improve cohesion for all the sub-groups of their teams. Coaches should emphasize to players that do not participate in many matches by showing them that they are essential team members. In addition, they should improve the social and task cohesion of players with short and long team membership respectively. It is suggested that future directions in cohesion should be focused on the mediator role of some factors in the relationship between cohesion and performance of soccer teams.

References

[1] Reber, S. A. (1987). *The Penguin dictionary of psychology*. London, UK: Penguin Books.

[2] Eriksson, S. G. (2003). *Sven Göran Eriksson on Football*. Carlton Books, 2003.

[3] Carron, A. V., Bray, S. R., & Eys, M. A. (2002). Team cohesion and team success in sport. *Journal of Sports Sciences, 20*, 119-126.

[4] Carron, A. V., Colman, M. M., Wheeler, J., & Stevens, D. (2002). Cohesion and performance in sport: A meta-analysis. *Journal of Sport & Exercise Psychology, 24*, 168-188.

[5] Chang, A., & Bordia, P. (2001). A multidimensional approach to the group cohesion-group performance relationship. *Small Group Research, 32*, 379-405.

[6] Kozub, S. A., & Button, C. J. (2000). The influence of a competitive outcome on perceptions of cohesion in rugby and swimming teams. *International Journal of Sport Psychology, 31*, 82-95.

[7] Narimari, M., & Ahari, S. S. (2008). A study of the relationship between team cohesion, role ambiguity and athletic performance in football team players. *Research Journal of Biological Sciences, 3*, 47-51.

[8] Pain, M. A., & Harwood, C. G. (2007). The performance environment of the England youth soccer teams. *Journal of Sports Sciences, 25*, 1307-1324.

[9] Singh, R., Kanchan, & Tarandeep (2012). Relationship between team cohesion and performance in ball Games. *Technical & Non-Technical Journal, 3* (5), 191-196.

[10] Tziner, A., Nicola, N., & Rizac, A. (2003). Relation between social cohesion and team performance in soccer teams. *Perceptual & Motor Skills, 96*, 145-148.

[11] Carron, A. V., Brawley, L. R., & Widmeyer, W. N. (1998). *The measurement of cohesiveness in sport groups*. In J. L. Duda (Ed.), Advances in sport and exercise psychology measurement (pp. 213-226). Morgantown, WV: Fitness Information Technology.

[12] Carron, A. V. (1982). Cohesiveness in sport groups: Interpretations and considerations. *Journal of Sport Psychology, 4*, 123-138.

[13] Widmeyer, W. N., Brawley, L. R., & Carron, A.V. (1990). The effects of group size in sport. *Journal of Sport & Exercise Psychology, 12*, 177-190.

[14] Widmeyer, W. N., Carron, A. V., & Brawley, L. R. (1993). Group cohesion in sport and exercise. In J. M. Williams (Ed.), *Applied sport psychology: Personal growth to peak performance* (pp 672-692). Mountain View, CA: Mayfield.

[15] Widmeyer, W. N., & Williams, J. M. (1991). Predicting cohesion in a coacting sport. *Small Group Research, 22*, 548-570.

[16] Gardner, D. E., Shiends, D. L. L., Bredemeier, B. J. L., & Bostrom, A. (1996). The relationship between perceived coaching behaviors and team cohesion among baseball and softball players. *The Sport Pshychologist, 10*, 367-381.

[17] Westre, K. R., & Weiss, M. R. (1991). The relationship between perceived coaching behaviors and group cohesion in high school football teams. *The Sport Psychologist, 5*, 41-54.

[18] Brawley, L. R., Carron, A. V., & Widmeyer, W. N. (1993). The influence of the group and its cohesiveness on perceptions of group goal-related variables. *Journal of Sport & Exercise Psychology, 15*, 245-260.

[19] Heuzé, J. P., Raimbault, N., & Fontayne, P. (2006). Relationships between cohesion, collective efficacy and performance in professional basketball teams: An examination of mediating effects. *Journal of Sports Sciences, 24*, 59-68.

[20] Pain, M. A., & Harwood, C. G. (2008). The performance environment of the England youth soccer teams: A quantitative investigation. *Journal of Sports Sciences, 26*, 1157-1169.

[21] Spink, K. S. (1992). Group cohesion and starting status in successful and less successful elite volleyball teams. *Journal of Sport Sciences, 10*, 379-388.

[22] Granito, V. J., & Rainey, D. W. (1988). Differences in cohesion between high school and college football teams and starters and non-starters. *Perceptual & Motor Skills, 66*, 471-477.

[23] Robinson, T. T., & Carron, A. V. (1982). Personal and situational factors associated with dropping out versus maintaining participation in competitive sport. *Journal of Sport Psychology, 4*, 364-378.

[24] Chelladurai, P., & Carron, A. V. (1977). A reanalysis of formal structure in sport. *Canadian Journal of Applied Sport Science, 2*, 9-14.

[25] Jacob, C. S., & Carron, A. V. (1998). The association between status and cohesion in sport teams. *Journal of Sports Sciences, 16*, 187-198.

[26] Berman, S. L., Down, J., & Hill, C. W. (2002). Tacit knowledge as a source of competitive advantage in the National Basketball Association. *Academy of Management Journal, 45*, 13-31.

[27] Iordanoglou, D. (1992). *Social-Psychological determinants of group performance among professional soccer teams.* Unpublished doctoral dissertation. University of Manchester. England.

[28] Tuckman, B. W. (1965). Developmental sequence in small groups. *Psychological Bulletin, 63*, 384-399.

[29] Tuckman, B. W., & Jensen, M. A. (1977). Stages of small group development revisited. *Group & Organizational Studies, 2*, 419-427.

[30] Carron, A. V., Widmeyer, W. N., & Brawley, L. R. (1985). The development of an instrument to assess cohesion in sport teams: The group environment questionnaire. *Journal of Sport Psychology, 7*, 244-266.

[31] Aggelonidis, I. (1995). *Cohesion of the team and leadership behavior of the coach as factors that affect the performance of volleyball teams.* PhD thesis. Department of physical education and sport sciences. University of Athens.

[32] Ntoumanis, N., & Aggelonidis, Y. (2004). A psychometric evaluation of the Group Environment Questionnaire in a sample of elite and regional level Greek volleyball players. *European Physical Education Review, 10* (3), 261-278.

The effect of fatigue on functional stability in the basketball players with functional ankle instability

Hamid Dehnavi[1], Hamid Khorramnezhad[2], Hamid Hassanpanah[1], Masoud Hajibigloo[1]

[1] Sama Technical and Vocational Training College, Islamic Azad University, Neyshabur Branch, Neyshabur, Iran
[2]Department of Sport Injury and Corrective Exercises, School of Physical Education and Sport Sciences, Shahid Bahonar University of Kerman, Kerman, Iran

Email address:
Hamiddehnavi@ymail.com (H. Dehnavi)

Abstract: The purpose of the present study was to assess the effect of basketball-specific fatigue on the dynamic postural control of the basketball players with functional ankle instability. The subjects in this study included 28 basketball players in the Youth League in Kerman. Their ages ranged between 16 and 21 years old. Based on the results of ankle instability questionnaire (CAIT) and the medical approval, the participants were selectively divided in two groups: a group of 16 subjects with functional ankle instability and a group of 12 healthy subjects. "Basketball Movement Specific Circuit" protocol was used to induce basketball-specific fatigue, and Y test was employed to quantify postural control. Specifically, Y test was administered as a pretest and posttest at the beginning and the end of the fatigue protocol. To make sure that the intended fatigue was really induced, Borg Scale was employed and the participants were asked to express their true feeling about the intensity of the exercise at the beginning and the end of the protocol. The result of analyzing data through dependent T-test indicated that dynamic postural control significantly decreased after the induction of fatigue in both groups. In addition, running independent T-test determined that fatigue equally affected the participants of both groups. This means that the participants in the experimental group coordinated postural control mechanisms with fatigue. Based on the results of this study, it can be concluded that both healthy players and those with functional ankle instability are susceptible to ankle sprain when they feel fatigue due to defect in postural control.

Keywords: Basketball Specific Fatigue, Dynamic Postural Control, Functional Ankle Instability, Test, Borg Scale, Basketball Movement Specific Circuit

1. Introduction

Postural control plays an important role in sport performance. In other words, it has a crucial and decisive role in an athlete's success in all sport fields, both in fields such as shooting which entails the lowest mobility and in those like gymnastics, wrestling, and basketball which require rapid mobility with the highest balance (Huston JL et al., 2005). Basketball is one of the world's most popular physical activities. Nearly 11% of the world's population play basketball regularly. Unfortunately, since the number of young male and female basketball players is rising, the rate of injuries also increases. Due to the nature of this sport field, a high percentage of injuries were reported to have occurred in the lower limb and ankle (Harmer, 2005). The researchers are still trying to reduce the amount of injuries in basketball players; they have mainly focused on risk factors such as proprioception ability, the level of kinematic development, the level of competition, and fatigue (Harmer, 2005). Fatigue is a common phenomenon that occurs during exercises and impairs an athlete's kinematic function (Millet et al., 2004). In the last decade, sports scientists have considered fatigue as a factor which negatively affects sport performance. They also investigated the relation between fatigue and postural control and concluded that fatigue and the reduction of postural control can result in skeletal-muscular injury in athletes (Pappas et al., 2007). To investigate the effect of fatigue on the postural control system, the researchers employed various techniques to exhaust the body and the organs especially the limb. These techniques include isokinetic contractions, repetitive movements, isometric contractions, and functional activities. For example, Nardone et al. (1998) investigated the range of postural volatility in 8 healthy individuals. After the participants ran on a treadmill for 25 minutes, their postural volatility was measured on the dynamometric page. This was done while they put their legs together with both closed and open eyes. They concluded that, 15 minutes after the exercise, postural volatility increased due to fatigue (Nardone et al., 1998). Christina KA et al. (2001) explored the effect of fatigue on ground reaction forces and ankle joint movements in 11 females who were running with the speed of 2.9 meter per second on a treadmill (in the first 50% of stance phase). They investigated dorsiflexor and invertor muscles before and immediately after the induction of fatigue. They concluded that local fatigue in the two groups of muscles had a significant effect on ground reaction forces and ankle motion during walking. Thus, it can play an important role in ankle injuries in trainings and competitions (Christina KA et al., 2001). In addition, Wilkins et al. (2004) studied performance on Balance Error Scoring System (BESS) and investigated how it impairs after fatigue. They made use of a 7-station fatigue protocol to simulate the activity during an exercise. The increase in BESS scores immediately after fatigue indicated that the balance was affected by fatigue (Wilkins JC et al., 2004). Exploring the impact of two types of fatigue on the duration of postural stability defect, Harkins et al. (2005) declared that the higher the amount of fatigue, the greater the defect in postural control system (Harkins et al., 2005). Marco et al. (2007) explored postural control of 20 individuals (15 males and 5 females) on treadmill after they had gone through a series of exhaustive activities. The participants' with mean age (6.3±7.23). The energy page was used to measure the participants' balance. In addition, fatigue was induced through requiring the participants to run on the treadmill (The speed of the treadmill increased every minute). The result proved that there was a significant increase in the body volatility (the reduction of balance) after the application of the fatigue protocol (Marco et al., 2007). Letafatkar et al. (2009) conducted a research on the effect of muscle fatigue induced by exhaustive exercises on professional athletes' functional stability. The participants of this study consisted of 30 professional male athletes with mean age (23±2.1). Biodex device and Running-based Anaerobic Sprint Test (RAST) were employed to measure balance and induce fatigue respectively. The researchers concluded that muscle fatigue reduces functional and lateral stability; however, it is not likely to affect posterior and anterior stability. This can be explained by the fact that when a person suffers from fatigue, CNS compensates for the disturbances created in the functional stability of the body to some extent (Letafatkar et al., 2009).

As it is clear, to investigate the impact of fatigue on the postural control system, most studies used protocols unrelated to exercises and competitions. Furthermore, few studies have been conducted to explore dynamic postural control; instead, most of them were carried out to investigate the static postural control system through functional tests. On the whole, it seems that there is a lack of research into the relationship between dynamic postural control and exercise-induced fatigue and its related concepts. Consequently, it is essential to explore the effects of whole body fatigue on dynamic postural control through a functional fatigue protocol which is similar to exercises and competitions, and a functional test which measures dynamic postural control.

2. Methodology

The subjects of this study were 28 basketball players in the Youth League in Kerman. Based on the results of Cumberland Ankle Instability Tools (CAIT) and medical approval, the participants were selectively divided in two groups: a group of 16 subjects with functional ankle instability and a group of 12 healthy subjects.

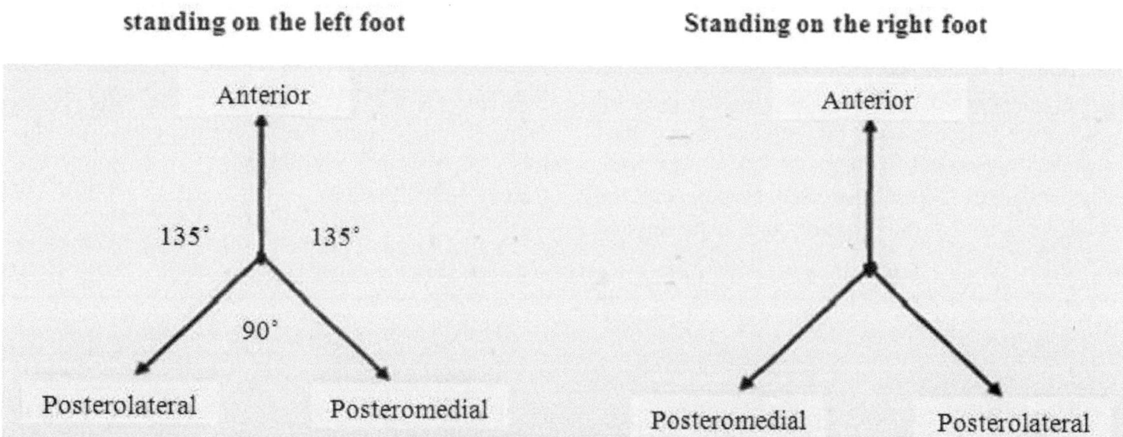

Figure1. *The outline of Y balance test*

The Y balance test device was used to assess the participants' dynamic postural control. In this device, the three directions are situated just like a Y(Plisky et al., 2006; Figure1). To normalize data, this test measured the actual length of the leg which stretched from anterior superior iliac spines to the medial ankle (Gribble et al., 2003). After the experimenter explained the test to the participants, the subjects practiced six times to familiar the procedure. The Y test was performed on the premier feet. If the right foot was premier, the test was performed in the counterclockwise direction; otherwise in clockwise direction (Gribble et al., 2003).

The player stood on one leg in the center of a grid. While maintaining single-leg stance, the player was asked to reach with the free limb in the anterior, posteromedial, and posterolateral directions in relation to the stance foot. The maximal reach distance was measured by marking the tape measure with erasable ink at the point where the most distal part of the foot reached. The trial was discarded and repeated if the player (1) failed to maintain unilateral stance, (2) lifted or moved the stance foot from the grid, (3) touched ground with the reach foot, or (4) failed to return the reach foot to the starting position. The process was repeated while standing on the other leg. The greatest reach distance of the 3 trials for each direction was used for analysis (Figure2) (plisky et al., 2006). Finally, the mean of the three scores was calculated, and the result was divided by the leg length (cm) and multiplied by 100.

Basketball-specific fatigue protocol (Basketball Movement Specific Circuit) was employed to induce fatigue (Figure2) (Smith , 2004). This protocol is similar to a basketball game in terms of duration, intensity, and movement patterns. It is applicable in a basketball field. It consists of four 4-minute phases with the heart rate of 90% to 95% HRmax. Between each phase, there is a 3-minute active rest (jogging) with the heart rate of 70% HRmax.

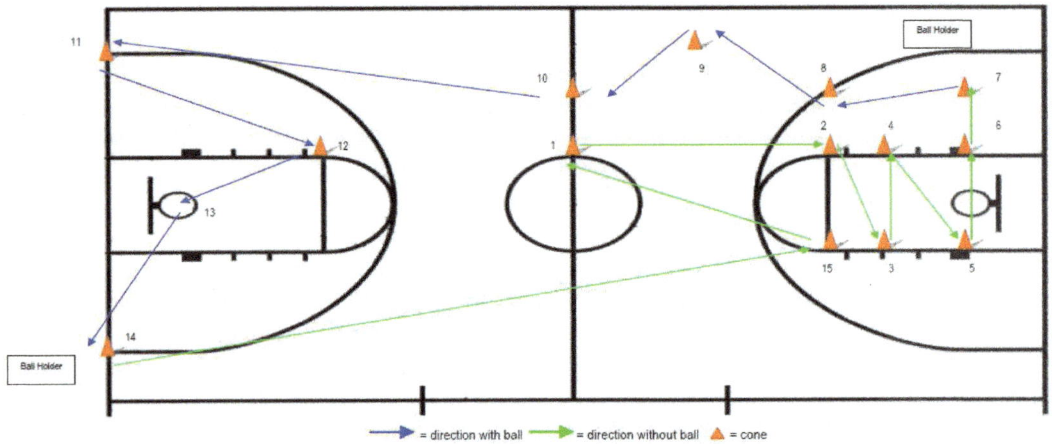

Figure2. *basketball movement specific training circuit. 1-2 forward sprint; 2 pivot left; 2-3 shuffle left; 3-4 shuffle right; 4-5 shuffle left; 5-6 shuffle right; 6-7 run into vertical jump(collect ball upon landing); 7-10 speed dribble ball around cones; 10-11 speed dribble; 11-12 speed dribble; 12-13 lay-up attempt; 13 lay-up rebound; 13-14 speed dribble(drop ball at 14); 14-15 forward sprint; 15-1 back pedal(Smith, 2004).*

To ensure that adequate fatigue was attained, the clinicians used the 15-point Borg scale to measure each subjects Rating of Perceived Exertion (RPE). After the participants prepared themselves through a brief warm-up (5-10 minutes of jogging and stretching the lower limb), Y test and PRE were administered as pretests. After they finished the protocol, Y test and PRE were held as posttests (Timothy et al., 2006). In order to compare the postural mean scores in every direction and PRE pretest and posttest in each group, dependent T-Test ($p<0.05$) was run. Moreover, independent T-Test was used to compare the postural mean scores of the control and experimental groups.

3. Results

The result of dependent T-Test between the pretest and posttest on mean scores of reach distance in the three directions are presented in the Table 1. there is a significant difference ($\alpha=0.05$) in all the three directions. However, the result of independent T-test on the mean difference shows not significant difference between the two group($\alpha=0.05$,Table 2).

Table 1. *Mean scores of dynamic postural control of the healthy and unstable groups*

statistical index variable		N	mean score	Std. deviation	Std. error	t value	df	α
experimental	pretest	16	99.93	6.27	1.56	6.48	15	0.000
	posttest	16	92.11	7.03	1.75			
control	pretest	12	103.20	6.38	1.84	6.84	11	0.000
	posttest	12	94.62	6.18	1.78			

Table 2. Comparison in mean difference of dynamic postural control between the healthy and unstable groups

Group	N	mean score	Std. deviation	Std. error	t value	df	α
unstable group	16	7.81	4.81	1.20	-0.44	26	0.66
healthy group	12	8.58	4.34	1.25			

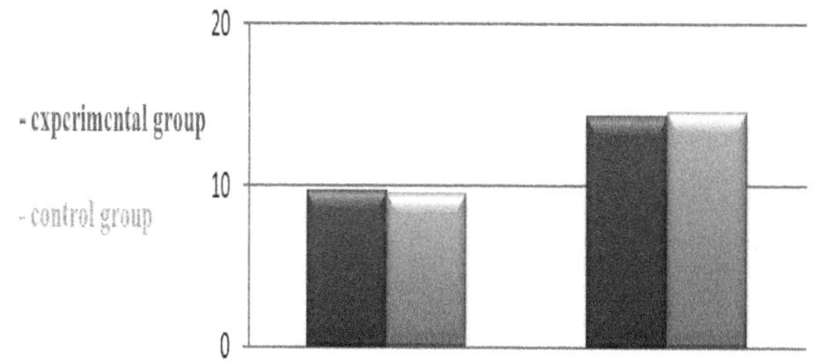

Graph 1. *The mean of the change in the perception of pressure in the control and experimental groups*

4. Discussion and Conclusion

Nardone et al. (1998), Christina KA et al. (2001), Wilkins et al. (2004), Harkins et al. (2005), Marco et al. (2007), and Letafatkar et al. (2009) reported decrease of balance control and increase of body volatility after application of various fatigue protocols. The reduction was attributed to the lack of proper functioning of the muscles and sensory effects of fatigue (Timothy et al., 2006). The application of a fatigue protocol on a part of the body and on the muscles acting on a joint causes the sensory receptors to send messages to the central nervous system. Then, the system, presumably aiming at preventing muscle damage, sends back a message which declares the reduction of the contraction activities of the muscles. Thus, the application of a fatigue protocol results in the reduction of the speed of neural transmission in afferent and efferent neurons ending in a muscle group. This has also been used to explain dynamic balance and reach distance decrease after application of a fatigue protocol (Taylor et al., 2000).

However, Rozzy et al. (1999), found a contradictory result a did not increase the body volatility. One of the reasons for such contradiction results might be due to variation in fatigue-inducing protocols and the test methods employed to measure balance.

In the present study, both groups had impaired postural control after the fatigue protocol; however, there was no significant difference between the two groups. Such results are out of our expectations. We assumed that the experimental group would suffer from more impaired postural control because of the functional ankle instability. Gribble et al. (2004) explored the mixed effects of fatigue and chronic ankle instability on dynamic postural control and drew a conclusion contrary to the present study. they observed that the unhealthy group achieved less reach distance in comparison to the healthy (Gribble et al., 2004). It seems that one of the major reasons for the contradiction between the results of the present study and those of Gribble et al. (2004) is the application of the single-joint fatigue protocol. In the present study, Basketball-specific fatigue protocol was employed whereas in Gribble's study a protocol a single joint movement, not the whole joints of the limb was used.

The result of the present study cannot be attributed to learning effect in the experimental group because both groups performed exactly the Y.

The participants in the experimental group showed less defect than the participants in the control one. The result indicates that the managed to coordinate postural control mechanisms with fatigue. Compared to injured group, the participants in the control group experienced higher defect in postural control. This might be due to the neuromuscular system's discovery-action capacity. The fatigue might induce decreased excitability of the muscular spindles and the nerve cells of the motor cortex. In addition, fatigue interferes with afferent messages. All these changes together lead to more defect in postural control. Nonetheless, while suffering from fatigue, afferent fibers Ia can get more sensitive to the changes in muscle fiber length. Thus, muscular spindles increase their neural firing (Timothy et al., 2006).

Alternatively, the chronic ankle instability might do not affect the functional performance of the limb (Demeritt et al., 2002). As a consequence, fatigue equally impaired the players' postural control in both groups we concluded that although the players suffered from ankle instability, the defects they experienced in their proprioception abilities did not result in the decrease of functional activities.

According to the findings of the present study, sport-induced functional fatigue can affect dynamic postural control; hence; it is likely to results in injuries and the reduction of athletes' sport performance. Thus, making use of proper trainings to improve the athletes' physical fitness and to reduce the experience of fatigue in a specific activity is highly recommended.

References

[1] Damore DT, Metzl JD, Ramundo M, Pan S, Van Amerongen R. (2003) Patterns in childhood sports injury. Pediatr Emerg Care. 19(2):65-67.

[2] Demeritt KM, Shultz SJ, Docherty CL, Gansneder BM, Perrin DH. (2002). Chronic ankle instability does not affect lower extremity functional performance. Journal of Athletic Training. 37(4), 507-511.

[3] Gribble PA, Hertel J, Denegar CR, Buckley EW. (2004).

The effects of fatigue and chronic Ankle instability on Dynamic postural control. J of Athletic training. 39 (4): 321-329.

[4] Gribble PA, Hertel J. (2003). Considerations for the normalizing measures of the star excursion balance test. Measurments Phys Educ Exer Sci;7:89-100.

[5] Harmer PA. (2005). "Basketball injuries", Med Sport Sci. Basel. vol 49, pp 31-61

[6] Harkins KM, Mattacola CG, Uhl TL, Malone TR, McCrory JL. (2005). Effects of 2 ankle fatigue models on the duration of postural stability dysfunction. Journal of Athletic Training. 40(3), 191-196.

[7] Huston JL, Sandrey MA, Lively MW, Kotsko K. (2005). The effects of calf-muscle fatigue on sagittal-plane joint-position sense in the ankle. J Sport Rehabil. (14):168-184.

[8] Christina KA, White SC, Gilchrist LA. (2001). Effect of localized muscle fatigue on vertical ground reaction forces and ankle joint motion during running. Human movement science. 20(3):257-76.

[9] Letafatkar MK, Alizadeh MH, Kordi MR. (2009). The Effect of Exhausting Exercise Induced Fatigue on the Double-Leg Balance of Elite Male Athletes. Journal of Social Sciences. 5 (4): 445-451.

[10] Bove M, Faelli E, Tacchino A, Lofrano F, Cogo CE, Ruggeri P. (2007). Postural control after a strenuous treadmill exercise. Neurosci Lett.18;418(3):276-81

[11] Millet GY, R Lepers. (2004). Alterations of neuromuscular function after prolonged running, cycling and skiing exercises. Sports Med. 34: 105-116.

[12] Nardone A. (1998).Postural adjustments associated with voluntary contraction of leg muscles in standing man. Exp brain research.69(3).469-80

[13] Pappas E, Sheikhzadeh A, Hagins M, Nordin M. (2007). The effect of gender and fatigue on the biomechanics of bilateral landings from a jump: Peak values. J Sports Sci and Med. 6:77-84.

[14] Plisky PJ, Rauh MJ, Kaminski TW, Underwood FB. (2006). Star excursion balance test as a predictor of lower extremity injury in high school basketball players. J Orthop Sports Phys Ther. 36: 911–919.

[15] Rozzi SL, Lephart SM, Fu FH. (1999). Effects of muscular fatigue on knee joint laxity and neuromuscular characteristics of male and female athletes. Journal of Athletic Training. 34 (2), 106–114.

[16] Seliga R, Bhattacharya A, Succop P, Wixhstrom R, Smith D, Willeke K. (1991). Effect of work load and respirator wear on postural stability, heart rate, and perceived exertion. Am Ind Hyg Assoc J. 52:417-422.

[17] Smith M. (2004).Basketball skill test for the big men. FIBA Assist Magazine. 07: 59-60.

[18] Taylor JL, Bulter JE, Gandevia SC. (2000). Changes in muscle afferents, motoneurons and motor drive during muscle fatigue. European journal of applied physiology. 83: 106-

[19] Timothy A, Kulpa BS. (2006). The Effects of Activity related fatigue on Dynamic postural control as measured by SEBT.115.

[20] Wilkins JC, Valovich McLeod TC, Perrin DH, Gansneder BM. (2004). Performance on the balance error scoring system decreases after fatigue. J Athl Train. 39(2):156-161.

15

Effects of an individualized and time based training program on physical fitness and mood states in recreational endurance runners

Kuno Hottenrott[1, 2], Sebastian Ludyga[2], Thomas Gronwald[1, 2], Stephan Schulze[2]

[1]Department of Sport Science, Martin-Luther-University Halle-Wittenberg, Halle, Germany
[2]Institute of Performance Diagnostics and Health Promotion, Martin-Luther-University Halle-Wittenberg, Halle, Germany

Email address:
kuno.hottenrott@sport.uni-halle.de (K. Hottenrott)

Abstract: Previous studies have shown that training guided individually by heart rate variability (HRV) elicits benefits on endurance performance. Meanwhile complex programs, which use HRV assessments to tailor exercise prescriptions to individual needs, are included in portable training computers. However, knowledge on health and fitness benefits of such training programs is still limited. Therefore, the aim of the present study was to investigate effects of HRV-based training included in a portable training computer vs general time-based training on aerobic fitness, half-marathon time as well as mood and mental states. Male (n=10) and female endurance runners (n=10) were recruited and randomly assigned to HRV-based (STAR) and predefined time-based training (TBT). At baseline and after 16 weeks of training an incremental exercise test with spirometry was performed to assess aerobic power. Additionally, mood and mental states were asked. After the training period all subjects took part in a half-marathon. Matched-pairs were selected to compare groups based on similar relative weekly energy expenditure during training. With no differences between groups, STAR and TBT reduced weight (p=0.029), body fat (p=0.002) as well as systolic and diastolic blood pressure ($p \leq 0.001$). Maximal oxygen uptake significantly increased from 43.0 ± 8.3 to 46.1 ± 9.0 $ml \cdot min^{-1} \cdot kg^{-1}$ ($p \leq 0.001$) and 43.2 ± 4.8 to 46.7 ± 4.7 $ml \cdot min^{-1} \cdot kg^{-1}$ ($p \leq 0.001$) in STAR and TBT, respectively. Moreover, both groups improved maximal velocity (TBT: 0.81 + 0.40 $km \cdot h^{-1}$ vs STAR: 0.74 + 0.39 $km \cdot h^{-1}$; $p \leq 0.001$) and completed the half-marathon with similar finish times (01:54:35 ± 00:14:02 [hh:mm:ss] vs. 01:52:42 ± 00:13:45 [hh:mm:ss]; p=0.789). Regarding mood and mental states, no major changes were observed over the training period. In conclusion, both HRV- and time-based training elicited similar improvements in aerobic power and body composition. Consequently, HRV-dependent exercise prescriptions serve as a practical tool for day-to-day periodization of aerobic exercise.

Keywords: Heart Rate Variability, Aerobic Power, Mood States, Endurance Training, Recreational Athletes

1. Introduction

Improved aerobic fitness is associated with a variety of health benefits, such as reduced risk for all-cause mortality and cardiovascular diseases [1,2]. Therefore, recreational athletes seek to follow training programs that promise significant improvements in health-related outcomes. Considerable heterogeneity observed in the training response shows that changes in aerobic fitness do not only depend on training volume and intensity. Even after highly standardized training programs, the magnitude of improvements in maximal oxygen uptake has ranged from none to almost 40 % [3,4,5]. The underlying physiological mechanisms that cause individual differences in the responsiveness to endurance exercise are still not fully understood. To some extent individual differences in age, gender and training status partly explain the variance in the training response [6,7,8]. This might be due to a training stimulus that is not tailored to the individual needs of the athlete. Consequently, exercise scientists face the challenge to provide an effective training program, which allows the repetition of productive exercise without excessive accumulation of stress [9].

A key to initiate desirable changes in the cardiovascular system without compromising the recovery processes might be individualized training based on heart rate variability (HRV), because daily assessment of autonomic nervous system (ANS) activity could serve as an indicator of appropriate physiological condition for aerobic training [3]. Kiviniemi et al. [10] showed that a training guided individually by HRV (based on high frequency power) led to higher increases in maximal running velocity than a predefined training. Especially when there is an increase or no change in instantaneous beat-to-beat variability, a progression of exercise intensity promises enhancements of endurance performance in men and women [11]. The relation between the ANS activity and the responsiveness to specific training stimuli is further emphasized by Vesterinen et al. [12], who found that a high baseline HRV predicts desirable future exercise adaptations. Although HRV is usually assessed with ECG, the results of Gamelin et al. [13] also confirm valid measurements with heart rate monitors.

Due to the technical progress, some portable training computers now feature programs based on regular HRV assessments. This allows the adjustment of exercise prescriptions according to the individual needs of the user. Unfortunately, only a few studies on the effectiveness of such training programs are available. Ring-Dimitrou et al. [14] provide evidence that an exercise telemetry monitored training program elicits higher improvements of running performance at the aerobic threshold compared to a non-exercise telemetry monitored group. Recent findings by Hottenrott et al. [15] support the effectiveness of HRV-based training included in heart rate monitors, as recreational athletes increased their maximal oxygen uptake by 10.3 % after 12 weeks of endurance exercise. However, more studies are necessary to evaluate health and performance benefits of individualized, self-administered training and time-based, predefined approaches.

The aim of the present study was to compare the effects of a standardized, time-based training plan with a training based on individual HRV measurements, which is included in a portable training computer, on aerobic performance, body composition and blood pressure. Additionally, the influence of the training approaches on mood and mental states were assessed. Following the intervention, half-marathon performance was compared between groups.

2. Methods

2.1. Subjects

Table 1. *Subjects' characteristics at baseline.*

	STAR (n=10)		TBT (n=10)		p
	Mean	SD	Mean	SD	
Age [y]	42.3	7.2	40.7	9.9	0.236
Height [cm]	172.2	8.1	170.2	10.8	0.279
Weight [kg]	68.9	10.6	66.1	13.8	0.544
BMI [$kg \cdot m^{-2}$]	23.1	1.9	22.7	2.7	0.401
Body Fat [%]	22.1	7.9	19.8	6.6	0.572
VO_{2MAX} [$ml \cdot min^{-1} \cdot kg^{-1}$]	43.0	8.3	43.2	4.8	0.786

Male (n=10) and female (n=10) recreational endurance runners (Table 1) were recruited for a 16 week intervention period via advert in a local newspaper. Subjects had to fulfill the following inclusion criteria: age 30 to 50 years, non-smokers, weekly running distance of 10 to 20 km within the last 6 months, best 10 km time between 45 and 60 min and best half-marathon time between 2 h and 2 h 30 min. Exclusion criteria were any cardiovascular, metabolic, neurological, pulmonary or orthopedic complications that could limit the performance of the exercises. Prior to the experimental trial recruited subjects underwent a medical check-up, including a personal anamnesis, ECG at rest and measurement of blood pressure. All eligible participants were given full details (except the purposes of the investigation) of the study protocol and any possible risks or discomforts associated with the experimental trial. Afterwards, written informed consent was obtained. The trial received approval by the local Ethics Committee and was in accordance with the Declaration of Helsinki.

2.2. Study Design

For an experimental trial with pre-post design recruited subjects were randomly assigned to either a HRV-based (STAR; n=10) or time-based training program (TBT; n=10). In contrast to TBT, training in STAR was regulated according to the individual response of the autonomic nervous system. At baseline and after 16 weeks of training an incremental exercise test with spirometry was performed to assess aerobic power. Additionally, mood and mental states were asked with the validated BFS scale [16] at baseline, 6 weeks and 16 weeks. One week after completing the post-test assessment all subjects took part in a half-marathon. Matched-pairs were selected to compare groups based on similar relative weekly energy expenditure during training.

2.3. Exercise Testing

Prior to exercise testing, anthropometric data were collected. Following the measurement of weight and body composition with a bio impedance device (Tanita, BC-545, Germany), subjects performed an incremental test with spirometry (Cortex, Metalyzer 3B, Germany) on a treadmill (h/p/cosmos, Pulsar 4.0, Germany). Therefore, the initial speed of 7.0 $km \cdot h^{-1}$ was increased by 1.5 $km \cdot h^{-1}$ per 3 min until volitional exhaustion. During the test, heart rate and respiratory parameters were recorded continuously. Lactate was measured with the enzymatic-amperometric method (Dr. Mueller, Super GL ambulance, Germany) in 10 μl blood taken from an ear lobe after each stage. Collected Data was processed with the software WinLactat 3.1 (Mesics, Germany). Using the Dickhuth model [17], the individual anaerobic threshold was derived from the lactate-velocity curve.

2.4. Training

Subjects assigned to HRV-based training received a training computer (Polar Electro Oy, FT60, Finland) including STAR training program, which is compatible with polarpersonaltrainer.com via Polar FlowLink (Polar Electro Oy, Finland). This training program is based on personal information (weight, height, age, sex), fitness level, activity level as well as training goal and sets intensity and time targets in accordance with the response of the autonomic nervous system. Therefore, data collected from the exercise test were saved in the settings of the portable training computers. For the experimental trial the STAR group trained with the program's option "maximize performance". The STAR program provides three different intensity zones (I=60-70 % HR_{MAX}; II=70-80 % HR_{MAX}; III=80-90 % HR_{MAX}). When the target is set to "maximize performance", the program mainly prescribes exercise in zone II. STAR training is progressive, as weekly training targets are adjusted according to the current fitness level.

Subjects in TBT followed a well-known structured, time-based training plan designed to make non-elite runners finish a half-marathon in less than 2 h [18]. As subjects already had running experience, the first 4 weeks of the original plan were skipped. The training program required two short 30 to 45 min runs (Tuesday and Thursday) and one long run (Sunday) per week. As the training was progressive, time and distance of the endurance exercises were increased over the intervention period.

In both groups training data was recorded with a training computer and followed up online on www.polarpersonaltrainer.com. Within the intervention period the display of the training computer was covered in TBT to prevent subjects from controlling the heart rate.

2.5. Statistics

The statistical analysis was performed with SPSS 21.0 (IBM Statistics, USA) for Windows. Gaussian distribution of the data was tested with the Shapiro-Wilk-Test. By applying a one-way ANOVA, baseline values and half-marathon finish times were compared between groups. Repeated-measures analysis of variance (ANOVA) followed by Bonferroni as post-hoc test was used to assess possible training effects on performance and body composition. For primary outcomes time effects and interactions (time*group) were reported. As mood and mental state variables followed a non-normal distribution, the Wilcoxon test was applied to analyze differences between measurements within groups. For all statistical tests a p level of ≤ 0.05 was considered statistically significant. The following variables were selected to investigate significant changes within and between the groups: maximal oxygen uptake (VO_{2MAX}), velocity at the individual anaerobic threshold (V_{IAT}), maximal velocity (V_{MAX}), blood lactate (La), heart rate (HR), weight, body fat, blood pressure, rating of mood states as well as half-marathon finish time.

3. Results

3.1. Training

Both TBT and STAR had similar relative energy expenditure of 35.2 kcal·(kg·week)$^{-1}$ during training. As displayed in figure 1, mean exercise intensity and duration was different between groups. While runners in STAR had a higher training volume, their mean exercise intensity was lower in comparison to TBT. No differences between groups were observed in training adherence, as STAR and TBT achieved 87 % and 90 % of the weekly training targets, respectively.

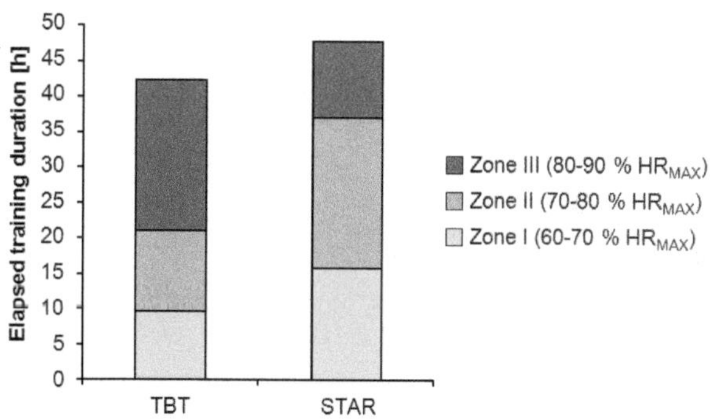

Figure 1. *Training intensity and duration in TBT and STAR.*

Table 2. *Effect of HRV- (STAR; n=5 f / 5 m) vs time-based training (TBT; n=5 f / 5 m) on aerobic performance, blood lactate and heart rate.*

	Group	Pre		Post		Pre vs Post
		Mean	SD	Mean	SD	p
V_{IAT} [km·h^{-1}]	STAR	11.09	1.50	12.01	1.47	≤0.001
	TBT	11.75	0.97	12.55	0.99	≤0.001
V_{MAX} [km·h^{-1}]	STAR	13.87	1.51	14.54	1.53	≤0.001
	TBT	14.65	1.50	15.46	1.53	≤0.001
VO_{2MAX} [ml·min^{-1}·kg^{-1}]	STAR	43.00	8.25	46.12	9.02	≤0.001
	TBT	43.20	4.83	46.70	4.24	≤0.001
La_{MAX} [mmol·l^{-1}]	STAR	8.43	2.45	8.39	2.71	0.864
	TBT	8.59	2.40	9.24	2.29	0.111
HR_{MAX} [min^{-1}]	STAR	185.40	9.95	184.44	11.46	0.578
	TBT	185.40	12.20	185.20	12.67	0.883

3.2. Aerobic Performance and Half-Marathon

Both groups increased maximal oxygen uptake, velocity at individual anaerobic threshold and maximal velocity ($p \leq 0.001$) over the intervention period (Table 2). As there were no significant time*group interactions (VO_{2MAX}: p=0,504, V_{MAX}: p=0.739, V_{IAT}: p=0,540), changes in selected performance parameters did not differ between

STAR and TBT. Furthermore, maximal heart rate (STAR: p=0.578; TBT: p=0.883) and blood lactate concentration (STAR: p=0.864; TBT: p=0.111) was not altered by the exercise intervention. Following the training period, subjects in STAR and TBT completed the half-marathon with similar finish times (01:54:35 ± 00:14:02 [hh:mm:ss] vs. 01:52:42 ± 00:13:45 [hh:mm:ss]; p=0.789).

3.3. Mood and Mental States

Over the training period mood and mental states in STAR were not altered in the assessed dimensions (Table 3). In comparison to baseline, excitation was significantly reduced after time-based training (p=0.047). Furthermore, anger decreased from the intermediate assessment at 6 weeks to post-test in TBT only (p=0.034). Changes in frustration over the intervention period were significantly different between STAR and TBT (p=0.023). For all other domains of mood and mental states no interactions of time and group were observed.

Table 3. *Subjects' mood and mental states at baseline. 6 weeks and 16 weeks of HRV- (STAR, n=5 f / 5 m) and time-based training (TBT; n=5 f / 5m).*

	Group	Baseline		6 weeks		16 weeks	
		MV[2]	SD	MV[2]	SD	MV[2]	SD
Acti-vation[1]	STAR	3.43	0.60	3.20	0.83	3.47	0.70
	TBT	3.57	0.67	3.60	0.53	3.67	0.70
Anger[1]	STAR	1.10	0.23	1.17	0.23	1.13	0.33
	TBT	1.13	0.33	1.33	0.53	1.07[#]	0.13
Positive Mood[1]	STAR	3.53	0.70	3.37	0.97	3.63	0.70
	TBT	3.63	0.90	4.07	0.70	3.67	0.63
Calm-ness[1]	STAR	3.47	0.67	3.30	0.93	3.37	0.97
	TBT	3.60	0.97	4.07	0.57	3.67	0.63
Exci-tation[1]	STAR	1.67	0.63	1.60	0.63	1.77	0.73
	TBT	1.77	0.57	1.63	0.47	1.47*	0.43
Frustra-tion[1]	STAR	1.10	0.23	1.30	0.53	1.10	0.30
	TBT	1.27	0.33	1.07	0.17	1.10	0.17
Fatigue[1]	STAR	1.37	0.47	1.50	0.73	1.37	0.43
	TBT	1.33	0.43	1.40	0.37	1.40	0.60

*$p \leq 0.05$ in comparison to baseline; #$p \leq 0.05$ in comparison to assessment at 6 weeks; [1]5-point scale (1=not correct at all; 5=fully correct); [2]mean values

3.4. Body Composition and Blood Pressure

Training significantly reduced body fat from 19.8 ± 6.9 to 18.5 ± 6.6 % and from 21.3 ± 6.8 to 19.7 ± 6.6 % ($p \leq 0.001$) in TBT and STAR, respectively. Over the intervention period subjects' weight also decreased significantly in both groups (STAR: -0.7 ± 1.7 kg; TBT: -0.9 ± 1.4 kg; p=0.003). Furthermore, the training interventions reduced blood pressure from 139.0 ± 18.2 / 88.5 ± 12.1 to 132.7 ± 17.2 / 83.8 ± 10.4 mmHg in STAR (systolic: p=0.046 ; diastolic: p=0.027) and from 138.5 ± 15.9 / 86.5 ± 10.2 to 127.4 ± 11.4 / 79.9 ± 7.2 mmHg in TBT (systolic: p=0.009 ; diastolic: p=0.028). As there were no interaction effects of time and group, the magnitude of reductions in body fat (p=0.859), weight (p=0.850) as well as systolic (p=0.550) and diastolic blood pressure (p=0.831) were not significantly different between STAR and TBT.

4. Discussion

4.1. Aerobic Performance

Based on a similar relative energy expenditure, both TBT and STAR elicited comparable improvements in aerobic power and maximal velocity after 16 weeks of training, although previous studies have shown that higher exercise intensities are more effective for improving cardiorespiratory fitness [19]. According to Midgley, McNaughton and Wilkinson [20], increased stroke volume due to structural changes of the myocard as well as improved capillarization and oxidative capacity of type II skeletal muscle fibers highly contribute to an enhancement of maximal oxygen uptake. Additionally, metabolic adaptations, which improve rates of fat oxidation and reduce the utilization of muscle glycogen at submaximal exercise ("glycogen sparing effect"), benefit endurance performance [21] and might explain the rightward shift of the lactate velocity curve observed in the present trial.

Whereas the training plan of TBT was designed to make non-elite runners finish a half-marathon in less than 2 h, the STAR program included in the portable training computers was originally not meant to prepare for running events. Nevertheless, subjects assigned to STAR completed the half-marathon with a time comparable to TBT. Previous studies have shown that the training response varies among subjects, because it is influenced by age, gender, stress, rest, prior training and baseline fitness [6,7]. Hence, the effectiveness of the STAR program might be explained by the fact that the training load was regulated in accordance with these factors. Especially the individual optimization of recovery periods was a significant strength of the HRV-based training as the recovery from exercise stress highly influences the training response [3]. In comparison to STAR runners in TBT followed a highly structured training plan, which did not pay attention to individual training needs. Nonetheless, this particular training method fulfilled its purpose, so that subjects were able to finish the marathon in the predefined time. To some extent, this might be due to the structured progression of training loads and a sufficient variability within the intervention period, as subjects performed both endurance runs and interval sessions.

In line with the present findings, Kiviniemi et al. [10] also found similar improvements of cardiorespiratory fitness after an individualized training guided by daily HRV measurements and a structured training. Some authors show that individualized training prescriptions elicit higher improvements in aerobic power [14,22] and foster motivation to subsequent physical activity [23]. To some extent, this heterogeneity among studies might be explained with differences in energy expenditure between the standardized and individualized training approaches. Additionally, the basis for tailoring exercise to individual needs varied among the trials. Especially training prescriptions based on regular assessments of the HRV might be recommended to recreational endurance athletes as A) HRV is a strong predictor of the exercise response [7] and B) prevents insufficient training as well as overtraining [24].

4.2. Mood and Mental States

In elite athletes assessments of mood and mental states are used to detect functional and non-functional overreaching [25]. Especially anger, vigor and fatigue are reliable indicators of overtraining [26] as those mood states correlate with training volume [27]. In TBT and STAR mood and mental states remained relatively stable over the intervention period, although there was a progression of exercise intensity and duration. The absence of major changes implies that both training programs provide a training load, which benefits aerobic performance in recreational runners while overstrain is avoided. However, exercise in TBT and STAR failed to elicit enhancements in positive mood, which are usually associated with endurance training [28]. This might be due to the fact that subjects in both groups already had a very positive mood at baseline and greater exercise benefits are expected among individuals reporting symptoms of depressed mood [29]. Furthermore, a positive mood and mental state might lead to a higher exercise adherence in the long-term. According to Williams et al. [30] the affective response to an acute moderate-intensity exercise stimulus predicts self-reported physical activity 6 and 12 months later. Consequently, the maintenance of a positive mood over the training period in STAR and TBT might be the key for performing exercise on a regular basis after the study.

4.3. Body Composition and Blood Pressure

Exercise leads to improved health benefits by specific biological mechanisms, such as improved body composition (e.g., through reduced abdominal adiposity and improved weight control), enhanced lipid lipoprotein profiles and reduced blood pressure [31,32]. In this respect, the decrease of body fat observed in this study is associated with a lower risk of type 2 diabetes [33] and all-cause mortality [1]. Additionally, HRV-based and time-based training were both efficient in reducing systolic and diastolic blood pressure. Especially the lowering of systolic blood pressure, which is a strong predictor of cardiovascular events, is related to a reduced risk of myocardial infarction and stroke [2]. Thus, training adaptations in both STAR and TBT were associated with relevant health benefits.

5. Limitations

As exercise intensity and duration were different between groups, the comparability of the training programs was limited. Therefore, the authors proceeded with pairs matched for the relative weekly energy expenditure to compare the effects of HRV-based and time-based training on aerobic performance. Unfortunately, this method led to a reduced sample size, which is known to affect the statistical results. Despite this limitation, the effects of the training programs on performance still reached the level of significance. Another methodological concern was the lack of half-marathon finish times at baseline. Nonetheless, the comparison of half-marathon performance after the training period was based on the assumption that finish times at baseline were not different between groups. This is supported by a similar initial aerobic fitness in STAR and TBT.

Regarding mood and mental state, time-based training led to marginal increases in anger and frustration. The lack of further changes might have been due to the limited number of the assessments. In future, more frequent measurements of mood and mental state over the training period could be useful to track differences between groups. Furthermore, the absence of group-related changes could be due to the training adherence in TBT. Subjects were expected to exercise on Tuesday, Thursday and Sunday. In some cases runners in TBT still followed the training prescriptions for time and distance, but rescheduled the training days. Consequently, they individualized training to some extent, although TBT was not meant for own adjustments.

6. Conclusion

Both HRV- and time-based training elicited improvements in aerobic power and body composition, which are associated with a risk reduction for cardiovascular diseases. Although the performance-enhancing effects were similar between the groups, especially the HRV-based training included in portable training computers might be recommended to recreational athletes, as it is more flexible, easy to follow and pays attention to individual needs. Progression of exercise intensity and duration did not affect anger and fatigue, so that HRV-based training prevents overstrain by controlling regeneration processes continuously. Consequently, HRV-dependent exercise prescriptions can serve as a practical tool for day-to-day periodization of aerobic training.

References

[1] Bigaard, J., Frederiksen, K., Tjonneland, A., Thomsen, B.L., Overvad, K., Heitmann, B.L. & Sorensen, T.I.A. (2004). Body fat and fat-free mass and all-cause mortality. *Obesity Res, 12* (7), 1042-1049.

[2] Psaty, B.M., Furberg, C.D., Kuller, L.H., Cushman, M., Savage, P.J., Levine, D., O'Leary, D.H., Bryan, R.N., Anderson, M. & Lumley, T. (2001). Association between blood pressure level and the risk of myocardial infarction, stroke, and total mortality. The cardiovascular health study. *Arch Intern Med, 161* (9), 1183-1192.

[3] Hautala, A.J., Kiviniemi, A.M. & Tulppo, M.P. (2009). Individual responses to aerobic exercise: the role of the autonomic nervous system. *Neurosci Biobehav Rev, 33* (2), 107-115.

[4] Vollaard, N.B., Constantin-Teodosiu, D., Fredriksson, K., Rooyackers, O., Jansson, E., Greenhaff, P.L., Timmons, J.A. & Sundberg, C.J. (2009). Systematic analysis of adaptations in aerobic capacity and submaximal energy metabolism provides a unique insight into determinants of human aerobic performance. *J Appl Physiol,106* (5), 1479-86.

[5] Buchheit, M., Chivot, A., Parouty, J., Mercier, D., Al Haddad, H., Laursen, P.B. & Ahmaidi, S. (2010). Monitoring endurance running performance using cardiac parasympathetic function. *Eur J Appl Physiol, 108* (6),1153-67.

[6] Bouchard, C. & Rankinen, T. (2001). Individual differences in response to regular physical activity. *Med Sci Sports Exerc, 33*, 446–S451.

[7] Hautala, A.J., Mäkikallio, T.H., Kiviniemi, A., Laukkanen, R.T., Nissilä, S., Huikuri, H.V. & Tulppo, M.P. (2003). Cardiovascular autonomic function correlates with the response to aerobic training in healthy sedentary subjects. *Am J Physiol Heart Circ Physiol, 285* (4), H1747-1752.

[8] Hautala, A.J., Kiviniemi, A.M., Makikallio, T.H., Kinnunen, H., Nissila, S., Huikuri, H.V. & Tulppo, M.P. (2006). Individual differences in the responses to endurance and resistance training. *Eur J Appl Physiol, 96*, 535-542.

[9] Friden, J., Lieber, R.I., Hargreaves, M. & Urhausen, A. (2003). *Recovery after training-Inflammation, Metabolism, Tissue Repair and Overtraining, Sports Medicine*. Malden: Blackwell Science, pp. 189-200.

[10] Kiviniemi, A.M., Hautala, A.J., Kinnunen, H. & Tulppo, M.P. (2007). Endurance training guided individually by daily heart rate variability measurements. *Eur J Appl Physiol, 101* (6), 743-751.

[11] Kiviniemi, A. M., Hautala, A. J., Kinnunen, H., Nissila, J., Virtanen, P., Karjalainen, J. & Tulppo, M. P. (2010). Daily exercise prescription on the basis of HR variability among men and women. *Med Sci Sports Exerc, 42* (7), 1355-1363.

[12] Vesterinen, V., Häkkinen, K., Hynynen, E., Mikkola, J., Hokka, L. & Nummela, A. (2013). Heart rate variability in prediction of individual adaptation to endurance training in recreational endurance runners. *Scand J Med Sci Sports, 23* (2), 171-180.

[13] Gamelin, F.X., Berthoin, S. & Bosquet, L. (2006). Validity of the polar S810 heart rate monitor to measure R-R intervals at rest. *Med Sci Sports Exerc, 38*(5), 887-893.

[14] Ring-Dimitriou, S., von Duvillard, S.P., Stadlmann, M., Kinnunen, H., Drachta, O., Müller, E., Laukkanen, R., Hamra, J., Weeks, S. & Peak, K. (2008). Changes in physical fitness in moderately fit adults with and without the use of exercise telemetry monitors. *Eur J Appl Physiol, 102*, 505-513.

[15] Hottenrott, K., Ludyga, S. & Schulze, S. (2013) Evaluierung von unterschiedlichen Trainingsmodellen bei berufstätigen Freizeitläufern. *Sportwiss, 43* (3), 157-165.

[16] Abele, A. & Brehm, W. (1986). Zur Konzeptualisierung und Messung von Befindlichkeit. Die Entwicklung der Befindlichkeitsskalen (BFS). *Diagnostica, 32*, 209-228.

[17] Dickhuth, H.-H., Huonker, M., Münzel, T., Drexler, H., Berg, A. & Keul, J. (1991). Individual anaerobic threshold for evaluation of competitive athletes and patients with left ventricular dysfunction. In N. Bachl, T.E. Graham & H. Löllgen (Hrsg.), *Advances in ergometry* (pp. 173-179). Berlin, Heidelberg: Springer Verlag.

[18] Galloway, J. (2006). *Half-marathon: You Can Do It*. Meyer & Meyer Sport, Oxford, 64.

[19] Gormley, S.E., Swain, D.P., High, R., Spina, R.J., Dowling, E.A., Kotipalli, U.S. & Gandrakota, R. (2008). Effect of Intensity of Aerobic Training on VO2max. *Med Sci Sports Exerc, 40*, 1336-1343.

[20] Midgley, A.W., McNaughton, L.R., Wilkinson, M. (2012). Is there an Optimal Training Intensity for Enhancing the Maximal Oxygen Uptake of Distance Runners? *Sports Medicine, 36*, 117-132.

[21] Yeo, W.K., Carey, A.L., Burke, L., Spriet, L.L. & Hawley, J.A. (2011). Fat adaptation in well-trained athletes: effects on cell metabolism. *Appl Physiol, Nutr Metabol, 36* , 12-22.

[22] Fabre, C., Massé-Biron, J., Ahmaidi, S., Adam, B. & Préfaut, C. (1997). Effectiveness of individualized aerobic training at the ventilatory threshold in the elderly. *J Gerontol A Biol Sci Med Sci, 52* (5), 260-266.

[23] Lafortuna, C.L., Resnik, M., Galvani, C. & Sartorio, A. (2003). Effects of non-specific vs individualized exercise training protocols on aerobic, anaerobic and strength performance in severely obese subjects during a short-term body mass reduction program. *J Endocrinol Invest, 26* (3),197-205.

[24] Mourot, L., Bouhaddi, M., Perrey, S., Cappelle, S., Henriet, M.T., Wolf, J.P., Rouillon, J.D. & Regnard J. (2004). Decrease in heart rate variability with overtraining: assessment by the Poincaré plot analysis. *Clin Physiol Funct Imaging, 24* (1), 10-18.

[25] Rietjens, G.J.W.M., Kuipers, H., Adam, J.J., Saris, W.H.M., van Breda, E., van Hamont, D. & Keizer, H.A. (2005). Physiological, biochemical and psychological markers of strenuous training-induced fatigue. *Int J Sports Med, 26* (1), 16-26.

[26] Grant, C.C., Janse Van Rensburg, D.C., Collins, R., Wood, P.S. & Du Toit, P.J. (2012). Investigation of the Profile of Mood State (POMS) questionnaire as an indicator of Overtraining Syndrome (OTS) in a group of endurance athletes. *AJPHERD*, 23-32.

[27] Pierce, E.F. (2002). Relationship between training volume and mood states in competitive swimmers during a 24-week season. *Percept Mot Skills, 94* (3), 1009-1012.

[28] Peluso, M.A.M. & de Andrade, L.H.S.G. (2005). Physical activity and mental health: The association between exercise and mood. *Clinics, 60* (1), 61-70.

[29] Lane, A.M. & Lovejoy, D.J. (2001). The effects of exercise on mood changes: the moderating effect of depressed mood. *J Sports Med Phys Fitness, 41* (4), 539-545.

[30] Williams, D.M., Dunsiger, S., Ciccolo, J.T., Lewis, B.A., Albrecht, A.E. & Marcus, B.H. (2008). Acute Affective Response to a Moderate-intensity Exercise Stimulus Predicts Physical Activity Participation 6 and 12 Months Later. *Psychol Sport Exerc, 9* (3), 231-245.

[31] Maiorana, A., O'Driscoll, G. & Taylor, R. (2003). Exercise and the nitric oxide vasodilator system. *Sports Med, 33*, 1013-1035.

[32] Warburton, D.E., Gledhill, N. & Quinney, A. (2001). The effects of changes in musculoskeletal fitness on health. *Can J Appl Physiol, 26*, 161-216.

[33] Meisinger, C., Döring, A., Thorand, B., Heier, M. & Löwel, H. (2006). Body fat distribution and risk of type 2 diabetes in the general population: are there differences between men and women? The MONICA/KORA Augsburg Cohort Study. *Am J Clin Nutr, 84* (3), 483-489.

The effects of eccentric training on electromyographic activity and performance in soccer players

Stergios Komsis[1], Georgios Komsis[1], Ioannis Gissis[1], Christos Papadopoulos[1], Dimitrios Patikas[1], Lida Mademli[1], Panagiotis Papadopoulos[2], Vassilis Paschalis[3, 4], Ioannis S. Vrabas[1]

[1]Department of Physical Education and Sports Science at Serres, Aristotle University of Thessaloniki, Greece
[2]Department of Physical Education and Sports Science, Aristotle University of Thessaloniki, Greece
[3]Department of Physical Education and Sports Science, University of Thessaly, Trikala, Greece
[4]Laboratory of Exercise, Health and Human Performance, Research Center, European University of Cyprus, Nicosia, Cyprus

Email address:
igkisis@phed-sr.auth.gr (I. Gissis)

Abstract: The purpose of the present study was to investigate the effects of eccentric training using a multi-joint dynamometer, on the electromyographic activity of rectus femoris, biceps femoris and medial gastrocnemius during counter movement jumps, drop jumps as well as during maximal eccentric actions. Sixteen amateur soccer players was divided into equal sized groups, the control group who participated in their regular training and the training group who performed 16 sessions (in 8 weeks) of eccentric exercise using a multi joint isokinetic dynamometer. The performance of counter movement and drop jumps were evaluated on a force plate. Additionally, maximal isometric, concentric and eccentric force were assessed on the isokinetic dynamometer. After the eccentric training, the electromyographic activity during the concentric phase of counter movement jumps was found to be increased in rectus femoris ($p<0.05$) and reduced in biceps femoris ($p<0.05$). During drop jumps, electromyographic activity of the experimental group found to be increased in the pre-activation phase of gastrocnemius ($p<0.05$). Additionally, during the takeoff phase of the drop jumps smaller angles for hip and ankle joints were observed ($p<0.05$). Finally, the electromyographic activity during eccentric strength evaluation were found to be elevated in rectus femoris ($p<0.05$) and decreased in gastrocnemius ($p<0.05$). The eccentric training which can cause neural adaptations, faster recruitment of motor units as well as changes in the architecture in muscle tendon system may also cause the alterations in electromyographic activity of leg muscles as observed in the present investigation.

Keywords: Contact Time, Isokinetic Dynamometry, Myoelectrical Properties, Soccer players, Stretch-Shortening Cycle, Vertical Jump

1. Introduction

During the most human movement there is an active stretch (eccentric action) of the muscles followed by an immediate shortening (concentric contraction) of the same muscles a condition known as the stretch - shortening cycle (SSC). However, it is also well documented that eccentric muscle actions induce muscle damage which cause delayed onset muscle soreness while deterioration in muscle strength and range of movement is observed [1-4]. Fortunately, it is well established that a repeated bout of eccentric exercise results in markedly reduced symptoms of muscle damage than the initial bout [5, 6].

It is also known that exercise including eccentric muscle actions is more effective in increasing muscle strength compared to concentric muscle contractions [7], probably due to the fact that fast twitch motor units are selectively activated during eccentric muscle actions [8]. Moreover, neuromuscular adaptations induced by eccentric training have been suggested to cause greater strength improvements than concentric training [9]. Lately, the use of the isokinetic dynamometer in resistance training insures pure eccentric muscle actions of maximal intensity through the whole range of motion of the joint [10]. The features of isokinetic muscle activity induces mechanical overload to muscles which may in turn influence gene expression via mechanotransduction pathways [11], leading in muscle hypertrophy, elevation in muscle strength and protection of the muscle against subsequent injury [12, 13].

According to electromyographic (EMG) data, voluntary eccentric muscle actions induce simultaneous activation of the agonist and antagonist muscles [14, 15]. Such a neural mechanism decreases the levels of torque production and stabilizes the joint in response to the high muscle tensions induced by eccentric contractions [16]. It is known that the external torque is the resultant of the torque produced by the agonist muscles minus the torque produced by the antagonist muscles [17]. Interestingly, after eccentric training it was observed a decrease in antagonist EMG activity which means less negative torque output resulting in higher overall torque output [17]. However, no study has examined biomechanical and neural factors after exercise training with eccentric muscle actions of maximal intensity, and their effect on the jumping ability. Therefore, the purpose of the present study was to investigate the effects of eccentric training using a multi-joint dynamometer on EMG activity of major lower limb muscles during counter movement jumps, drop jumps as well as during maximal eccentric muscle action.

2. Material and Methods

2.1. Participants

Sixteen healthy male amateur soccer players with no history of neurological injuries or diseases participated in the present investigation. They were randomly divided in two equal sized groups, the control group (age 22.1±0.3 y, height 174±4 cm, and body mass 86.5±3.5 kg) and the eccentric training group (age 24±0.5 y; height 176±6 cm; and body mass 84.5±5.5 kg). Except for their usual soccer training, subjects did not participate in other organized exercise training programs. They were also instructed not to take anti-inflammatory drugs and abstain from strenuous exercise for 3 days prior to the beginning of the investigation and during the data collection period. Subjects of groups had no experience in organized eccentric training program. The procedures were in accordance with the Helsinki declaration of 1975, as revised in 2000. An informed written consent approved by the local university Ethics Committee was obtained by all participants after they were informed of all risks, discomforts and benefits involved in the study.

2.2. Training Protocol

Participants of the experimental group performed a training protocol using a custom-built multi-joint isokinetic dynamometer (Ydromichaniki SA). The training protocol is described in Table 1. The training protocol was performed during the preseason period. Subjects of the experimental group were performing the sitting leg press exercise two times per week for eight weeks, while between two exercise sessions a recovery period of at least 48 hours was incorporated. During each exercise session, participants were sitting comfortably on the seat of the isokinetic dynamometer placing their legs on a force-plate while their chest and hips were stabilized with straps (Figure 1). During the eccentric exercise sessions the knee joint range of motion was set between 130° to 160° and the linear velocity was set at 0.35 m/s. The first week of the training period served as familiarization period using 70% of the maximal eccentric performance [18-20]. The intensity of the follow up sessions was constantly controlled and readjusted by performing regular assessments of maximal eccentric performance (Table 1). Before each exercise session, subjects performed a warm-up consisting of 6-min cycling on an ergometer at 70 rpm and 50 W followed by 5 min of ordinary stretching exercises of the major muscle groups of the lower limbs.

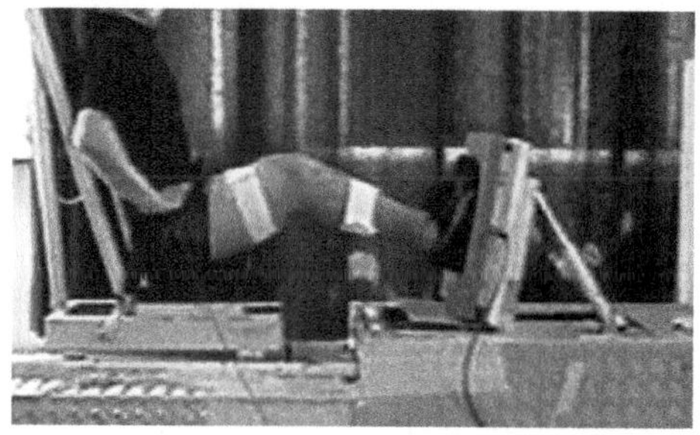

Figure 1. *The multi-joint isokinetic dynamometer*

2.3. Performance Assessments

All the assessments were performed two days before the beginning of the training program and two days after its termination. For the evaluation of strength output the same multi joint isokinetic dynamometer was used. During the assessment 2 trials of isometric maximal strength output (at 120° knee joint angle) were performed and the subjects were instructed to push as hard as possible the force plate and maintain the maximum force for about 4 s. For the assessment of concentric and eccentric force output two trials were performed at a constant velocity of 0.35 m/s while the range of motion for the knee joint was set at 130-160°. The best performance of each exercise mode was recorded for the statistical analysis.

For the assessment of jumping ability, the subjects performed a series of jumps on a force platform (Kistler 9281CA, Instrumente AG, Winterthur, Switzerland) sampling at 1000 Hz. The participants performed 2 jumps with initial acceleration downwards (counter movement jump) and 2 drop jumps, falling from 30 cm height while in both conditions their hands were placed on their waist. In counter movement jumps the best vertical performance measured in cm was recorded while in drop jumps the contact time measured in msec along with the best high performance measured in cm was recorded. During counter movement jump, subjects were instructed to move downwards as fast as possible and to jump as high as possible. During the drop jump, subjects were asked to contact with the ground fast and to execute a vertical jump as high as possible. A 2 min interval was incorporated between the trials. During both counter movement and drop jumps the EMG activity was recorded.

Table 1. Eccentric training protocol. Two exercise sessions were performed each week. Intensity is in % of 1RM.

	Sets × reps	Intensity	Rest (min)
1st week	3X10	70	5
	Evaluation of eccentric power output		
2nd week	5X8	80	3
3rd week	5X8	80	3
	Evaluation of eccentric power output		
4th week	4X5	90	5
5th week	4X5	90	5
	Evaluation of eccentric power output		
6th week	5X6	90	6
7th week	5X6	90	6
	Evaluation of eccentric power output		
8th week	6X6	90	7

2.4. Electromyography

EMG activity was recorded on the dominant leg with surface bipolar (3.5 cm center to center) electrodes (Quinton Quick prep silver/silver chloride) over the rectus femoris, the long head of biceps femoris and the medialis gastrocnemius muscles. These muscles were selected as main contributors to perform vertical jumps [21, 22]. Electrodes were placed according to the SENIAM guidelines [23]. Skin was properly shaved and cleaned with alcohol solution to keep skin impendence below 5kΩ. To ensure consistent placement of the electrodes for each testing session, marks was placed around the circumference of the electrodes with a permanent marker and accordingly the placed electrodes were photographed. For the rectus femoris the electrodes were placed at midpoint between the anterior spina iliaca superior and the superior part of the patella. The biceps femoris electrodes were attached at the half distance between the ischial tuberosity and the lateral epicondyle of the tibia. For the gastrocnemius the electrodes were placed on the gastrocnemius medialis on the most prominent bulge of the muscle. During the assessments the electrodes were not removed and relocated on the subjects' muscles.

The signal was pre-amplified (gain= X400) and sampled at 1000 Hz. Raw EMG was band pass filtered from 8 to 500 Hz with a Butterworth 4th order filter and the root mean square (RMS) for a 20 ms time window was calculated with custom Matlab scripts (version 7, The MathWorks Inc.). According to De Louca [24], the RMS (square root of the integral of the square of the EMG potential with respect to time), has a physical meaning and provides a better strength signal in dynamic muscle activity volitionally produced. The mean of the processed signal was calculated i) during the braking and propulsion phase of the counter movement jump, ii) 100 ms before contact (pre-activation) [25], and during the braking and propulsion of the drop jump, iii) during the whole range of motion throughout the eccentric and concentric phase of the isokinetic movement. All raw signals were synchronized, digitized and saved on an A/D card (AMTI 32channel analog data version 2.02).

2.5. Kinematic Data

The kinematic data during the jumps were analyzed using the 2D Ariel Performance Analysis System (APAS) while the motion captured with a digital camera (Panasonic, PV-900). Five reflective markers (14 mm spheres) were placed at anatomical bony landmarks (i.e. acromion, femoral epicondyle, lateral tibia, lateral malleolus and 5th metatarsal head).

2.6. Statistical Analysis

Two-way ANOVA [group (training and control group) × week (first and eighth week)] with repeated measurements on time were used. If a significant interaction was obtained, pairwise comparisons were performed through simple main effect analysis. t-test was used to compare the anthropometric characteristics between the eccentric training and the control groups. Data are presented as mean ±SEM while the level of significance was set at $\alpha = 0.05$. The SPSS version 15.0 was used for all analyses (SPSS Inc., Chicago, Illinois).

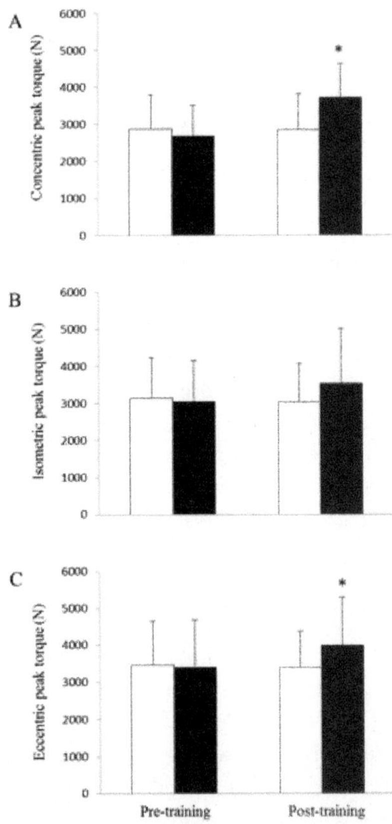

*Figure 2. Concentric (A), isometric (B) and eccentric (C) peak torque pre and post eccentric training for the control (□) and the experimental group (■). *significant different (p<0.05) between pre and post training*

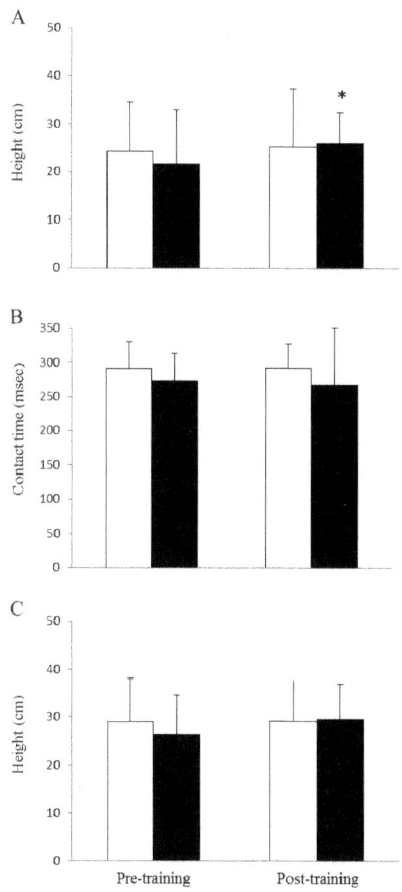

Figure 3. *Height (A) and contact time (B) during drop jump and height during counter movement jump (C) pre and post eccentric training for the control (□) and the experimental group (■). *significant different (p<0.05) between pre and post training*

3. Results

No significant differences in anthropometric characteristics were observed between the two groups. After 8 weeks of eccentric training using a multi-joint isokinetic dynamometer concentric and eccentric muscle strength was elevated only in the experimental group (Figure 2). Regarding the jumping ability no significant alterations were observed in counter movement and the in the contact time of the drop jump for both the control and the experimental group (Figure 3). However, in the experimental group, eccentric training cause elevation in height performance during the drop jumps (Figure 3). Additionally, after the eccentric training, the hip flexion and the dorsiflexion were significantly reduced. Additionally, during the takeoff phase of the drop jump, eccentric training reduced significantly the hip and the ankle angles to 149° from 154° and to 100° from 105°, respectively. The control group at the takeoff phase of the first and the second assessment revealed for the hip joint 144° and 143° respectively and for the angle joint 103° and 106° respectively.

After the eight weeks of eccentric training, EMG activity during counter movement jump significantly elevated in rectus femoris and significantly reduced in biceps femoris during the propulsive phase while EMG activity did not alter during the braking phase (Table 2). After the training period, EMG activity during drop jump significantly elevated during pre-activation phase only in gastrocnemius muscle (Table 2). After the eccentric training the EMG activity during drop jump did not alter in any of the investigated muscles during the braking and propulsive phases.

Table 2. *EMG activity (mV) during the eccentric and the concentric phase of CMJ as well as during the pre-activation, the eccentric and the concentric phase of DJ.*

	Control Group		Experimental Group	
	Pre-training	**Post-training**	**Pre-training**	**Post-training**
CMJ				
Breaking phase				
RF	0.118 ± 0.053	0.080 ± 0.026	0.100 ± 0.056	0.095 ± 0.035
BF	0.071 ± 0.089	0.173 ± 0.197	0.110 ± 0.104	0.032 ± 0.006
GAS	0.040 ± 0.006	0.051 ± 0.019	0.053 ± 0.035	0.071 ± 0.043
Propulsive phase				
RF	0.300 ±0.065	0.185 ±0.086	0.204 ±0.137	0.263 ±0.168*
BF	0.158 ±0.088	0.372 ±0.352	0.184 ±0.038	0.072 ±0.039
GAS	0.219 ±0.058	0.223 ±0.071	0.204 ±0.079	0.237 ±0.120
DJ				
Pre-activation				
RF	0.108 ±0.060	0.064 ±0.010	0.081 ±0.051	0.109 ±0.097
BF	0.074 ±0.043	0.071 ±0.044	0.055 ±0.020	0.039 ±0.015
GAS	0.149 ±0.081	0.158 ±0.087	0.123 ±0.064	0.207 ±0.067
Breaking phase				
RF	0.388 ±0.180	0.190 ±0.115	0.205 ±0.145	0.201 ±0.185
BF	0.220 ±0.378	0.189 ±0.134	0.183 ±0.084	0.079 ±0.031
GAS	0.171 ±0.087	0.195 ±0.087	0.584 ±1.250	0.210 ±0.109
Propulsive phase				
RF	0.344 ±0.170	0.172 ±0.085	0.222 ±0.134	0.149 ±0.099
BF	0.171 ±0.077	0.403 ±0.527	0.188 ±0.083	0.108 ±0.063
GAS	0.242 ± 0.083	0.214 ± 0.083	0.468 ±0.856	0.333 ±0.137

BF, biceps femoris; CMJ, counter movement jump; DJ, drop jump; GAS, gastrocnemius; RF, rectus femoris* significant different (p<0.05) between pre and post training.

After the eight weeks of eccentric training, the EMG activity during the eccentric force assessment, was found to be significantly increased in rectus femoris and significant decreased in gastrocnemius while did not affect in biceps femoris (Table 3). No differences in EMG activity were observed between the control and the experimental group while in the control group no differences were observed between the pre and post training assessments (Table 2).

Table 3. *EMG activity (mV) during maximal eccentric power output of rectus femoris (pre-activation phase), biceps femoris and gastrocnemius (activation phase).*

	Control group	Experimental group
Rectus femoris		
Pre-training	0.057±0.054	0.027±0.070
Post-training	0.056±0.052[#]	0.096±0.018[*]
Biceps femoris		
Pre-training	0.061±0.049	0.024±0.069
Post-training	0.060±0.042	0.069±0.033
Gastrocnemius		
Pre-training	0.074±0.069[#]	0.172±0.044
Post-training	0.075±0.068	0.056±0.128[*]

*significant different ($p<0.05$) between pre and post training
#significant different ($p<0.05$) between the control and experimental group

4. Discussion

The purpose of the present investigation was to evaluate the effects of eccentric training using a multi-joint dynamometer on EMG activity of rectus femoris, biceps femoris, as well as medial gastrocnemius during counter movement jump, drop jump and during maximal eccentric action. As it was expected the control group did not reveal any differences between the pre and post training strength assessment, jumping ability, and EMG activity. On the contrary, in the experimental group the eccentric training affected several of the examined parameters. Specifically, there was significant elevation of concentric and eccentric force while the height of the drop jump was also elevated after the training period. The EMG activity of the examined muscles altered during counter movement jump, drop jump and eccentric isokinetic assessment. However, no difference was observed between the control and the experimental group before or after the eccentric training period.

Isokinetic dynamometers are used in most investigations where eccentric exercise has to be performed. The muscle group that contracts during exercise is isolated in all these isokinetic dynamometers. However, the majority of human movements are multi-joint and recruit a larger number of muscles where agonists enhance movement whereas the co-activation of antagonists results in restriction of speed and amplitude of movement [26]. Taking into account in the present investigation the limitations of the commercially available isokinetic dynamometers, the training protocol as well as the strength assessments were performed on a custom-built multi-joint isokinetic type machine. This device was designed to measure the amount of external work and the linear velocity on the whole range of motion during concentric and eccentric exercise modes.

It is known that eccentric training is associated with higher forces production [27] and larger strength improvements [28] compared to isometric or concentric training. Indeed, in a study where 8 weeks of eccentric or concentric training was performed, eccentric training induced greater increases in baseline eccentric and isometric torque compared to concentric training [29]. Authors suggested that the specific physiological adaptations to resistance exercise are determined by the muscle actions involved [29, 30]. The present finding are in line with previous investigations given the fact that 8 weeks of eccentric training induced notable elevations of peak force compared to the control group.

This could be attributed to the rather lower intensity and the limited number of repetitions that were adopted in the present investigation especially in the first weeks of the training period. Additionally, the fact that the subjects of the control group continued to participate in their regular training may also account for the absence of differences compared to the experimental group.

Eccentric exercise is known to induce modulations in the recruitment order, discharge rate and recruitment threshold of the motor units [31]. It is also known that during an eccentric contraction, the electric activity of a muscle is lower than the one recorded during a concentric contraction for the same level of the force produced [32-34]. However, eccentric training can increase this neuromuscular activation [33, 35]. These could be the case in the present investigation, where the eccentric training, caused increases in EMG activity in the pre-activation phase of gastrocnemius during drop jump which could be further attributed to favorable changes in reflex excitability leading to better facilitation of the myotatic reflex and to depression of the autogenic inhibition generated by the Golgi tendon organs [35]. Additionally, during the takeoff phase of the drop jump, it was found that hip and the ankle angles were reduced. It is suggested that the smaller joint angles are induced by the eccentric training which may cause changes in the architecture in muscle tendon unit [36] and affect both proprioception, force-length and force-velocity relationship [5, 18].

During the counter movement jump, the elevated EMG activity of rectus femoris and the reduced EMG activity of the biceps femoris indicate that eccentric training improved the relationship between agonists and antagonists in favor for the first. Moreover, during the post training eccentric assessment the EMG activity of the rectus femoris and medial gastrocnemius found to be elevated. Indeed, it is known that repeated eccentric training could lead to a progressive recruitment of slow motor units for the better distribution of mechanical stress and may also lead to increase in the discharge frequency of motor units [16, 18, 37, 38]. Caution should be paid however, since the lower EMG activation of the antagonist muscles may induce injuries, since their function is to protect the joint and muscle structures against excessively high tension levels that may occur during eccentric actions [10].

4.1. Conclusion

It is a fact that coaches and athletes seek ways to increase the effectiveness of conditioning programs while eccentric training seems to be the best way for maximizing strength performance. Indeed, eccentric exercise induces structural changes on the muscle-tendon system and adaptations of the nervous central command, causing increases in maximal force production, often higher to those obtained with concentric or isometric training [16]. In the present investigation, it is clear that eccentric training using a multi-joint isokinetic dynamometer may exerts favorable effects of muscle strength and EMG activity of the agonist muscles in amateur young soccer players. Moreover, in competitive sports most muscle strain injuries occur during eccentric muscle actions, and then the training of muscle groups using eccentric exercise may help to diminish the risk of injuries [39]. More research is needed in the area of eccentric training in young athletes using multi-joint isokinetic dynamometers.

References

[1] D. W. Chapman, M. J. Newton, Z. Zainuddin, P. Sacco, and K. Nosaka. Work and peak torque during eccentric exercise do not predict changes in markers of muscle damage. Br J Sports Med. 2008, 42, 585-91.

[2] A. P. Lavender, and K. Nosaka. Changes in fluctuation of isometric force following eccentric and concentric exercise of the elbow flexors. Eur J Appl Physiol. 2006, 96, 235-40.

[3] L. Norrbrand, J. D. Fluckey, M. Pozzo, and P. A. Tesch. Resistance training using eccentric overload induces early adaptations in skeletal muscle size. Eur J Appl Physiol. 2008, 102, 271-81

[4] V. Paschalis, Y. Koutedakis, A. Z. Jamurtas, V. Mougios, and V. Baltzopoulos. Equal volumes of high and low intensity of eccentric exercise in relation to muscle damage and performance. J Strength Cond Res. 2005, 19, 184-8.

[5] T. C. Chen, K. Nosaka, and P. Sacco. Intensity of eccentric exercise, shift of optimum angle, and the magnitude of repeated-bout effect. J Appl Physiol. 2007, 102, 992-9.

[6] V. Paschalis, M. G. Nikolaidis, G. Giakas, A. Z. Jamurtas, E. O. Owolabi, and Y. Koutedakis. Position sense and reaction angle after eccentric exercise: the repeated bout effect. Eur J Appl Physiol. 2008, 103, 9-18.

[7] J. Duclay, A. Martin, A. Robbe, and M. Pousson. Spinal reflex plasticity during maximal dynamic contractions after eccentric training. Med Sci Sports Exerc. 2008, 40, 722-34.

[8] A. Nardone, C. Romano, and M. Schieppati. Selective recruitment of high-threshold human motor units during voluntary isotonic lengthening of active muscles. J Physiol. 1989, 409, 451-71.

[9] M. Roig, K. O'Brien, G. Kirk, R. Murray, P. McKinnon, B. Shadgan, and W. D. Reid. The effects of eccentric versus concentric resistance training on muscle strength and mass in healthy adults: a systematic review with meta-analysis. Br J Sports Med. 2009, 43, 556-68.

[10] E. Kellis, and V. Baltzopoulos. Isokinetic eccentric exercise. Sports Med. 1995, 19, 202-22.

[11] M. C. Kostek, Y. W. Chen, D. J. Cuthbertson, R. Shi, M. J. Fedele, K. A. Esser, and M. J. Rennie. Gene expression responses over 24 h to lengthening and shortening contractions in human muscle: major changes in CSRP3, MUSTN1, SIX1, and FBXO32. Physiol Genomics. 2007, 31, 42-52.

[12] S. Hody, P. Leprince, K. Sergeant, J. Renaut, J. L. Croisier, F. Wang, and B. Rogister. Human muscle proteome modifications after acute or repeated eccentric exercises. Med Sci Sports Exerc. 2011, 43, 2281-96.

[13] H. Langberg, H. Ellingsgaard, T. Madsen, J. Jansson, S. P. Magnusson, P. Aagaard, and M. Kjaer. Eccentric rehabilitation exercise increases peritendinous type I collagen synthesis in humans with Achilles tendinosis. Scand J Med Sci Sports. 2007, 17, 61-6.

[14] K. Falconer, and D. A. Winter. Quantitative assessment of co-contraction at the ankle joint in walking. Electromyogr Clin Neurophysiol. 1985, 25, 135-49.

[15] M. Solomonow, R. Baratta, B. H. Zhou, and R. D'Ambrosia. Electromyogram coactivation patterns of the elbow antagonist muscles during slow isokinetic movement. Exp Neurol. 1988, 100, 470-7.

[16] G. Guilhem, C. Cornu, and A. Guevel. Neuromuscular and muscle-tendon system adaptations to isotonic and isokinetic eccentric exercise. Ann Phys Rehabil Med. 2010, 53, 319-41.

[17] M. Pensini, A. Martin, and N. A. Maffiuletti. Central versus peripheral adaptations following eccentric resistance training. Int J Sports Med. 2002, 23, 567-74.

[18] S. Colson, M. Pousson, A. Martin, and J. Van Hoecke. Isokinetic elbow flexion and coactivation following eccentric training. J Electromyogr Kinesiol. 1999, 9, 13-20.

[19] C. A. Moore, L. W. Weiss, B. K. Schilling, A. C. Fry, and Y. Li. Acute effects of augmented eccentric loading on jump squat performance. J Strength Cond Res. 2007, 21, 372-7.

[20] D. Paddon-Jones, M. Leveritt, A. Lonergan, and P. Abernethy. Adaptation to chronic eccentric exercise in humans: the influence of contraction velocity. Eur J Appl Physiol. 2001, 85, 466-71.

[21] M. F. Bobbert, and G. J. van Ingen Schenau. Coordination in vertical jumping. J Biomech. 1988, 21, 249-62.

[22] A. J. Van Soest, A. L. Schvab, M. F. Bobbert, and G. L. van Ingen Schenau. The influence of bi-articularity of the gastrocnemius muscle on vertical jumping achievement. J Biomech. 1993, 26, 1-8.

[23] H. J. Hermens, B. Frerics, C. Disselhorst-Klug, and G. Rau. Development of recommendations for SEMG sensors and sensor placement procedures. J Electromyogr Kinesiol. 2000, 10, 361-74.

[24] C. J. De Luca. The use of surface electromyography in Biomechanics. Journal of Applied Biomechanics. 1997, 13, 135-63.

[25] T. Horita, P. V. Komi, C. Nicol, and H. Kyrolainen. Interaction between pre-landing activities and stiffness regulation of the knee joint musculoskeletal system in the drop jump: implications to performance. Eur J Appl Physiol. 2002, 88, 76-84.

[26] C. D. Marsden, J. A. Obeso, and J. C. Rothwell. The function of the antagonist muscle during fast limb movements in man. J Physiol. 1983, 335, 1-13.

[27] S. H. Westing, A. G. Cresswell, and A. Thorstensson. Muscle activation during maximal voluntary eccentric and concentric knee extension. Eur J Appl Physiol Occup Physiol. 1991, 62, 104-8.

[28] T. Hortobagyi, J. Barrier, D. Beard, J. Braspennincx, P. Koens, P. Devita, L. Dempsey, and J. Lambert. Greater initial adaptations to submaximal muscle lengthening than maximal shortening. J Appl Physiol. 1996, 81, 1677-82.

[29] V. Paschalis, M. G. Nikolaidis, A. A. Theodorou, G. Panayiotou, I. G. Fatouros, Y. Koutedakis, and A. Z. Jamurtas. A weekly bout of eccentric exercise is sufficient to induce health-promoting effects. Med Sci Sports Exerc. 2011, 43, 64-73.

[30] G. A. Dudley, P. A. Tesch, B. J. Miller, and P. Buchanan. Importance of eccentric actions in performance adaptations to resistance training. Aviat Space Environ Med. 1991, 62, 543-50.

[31] R. M. Enoka. Eccentric contractions require unique activation strategies by the nervous system. J Appl Physiol. 1996, 81, 2339-46.

[32] P. Aagaard, E. B. Simonsen, J. L. Andersen, S. P. Magnusson, J. Halkjaer-Kristensen, and P. Dyhre-Poulsen. Neural inhibition during maximal eccentric and concentric quadriceps contraction: effects of resistance training. J Appl Physiol. 2000, 89, 2249-57.

[33] P. V. Komi, and E. R. Buskirk. Effect of eccentric and concentric muscle conditioning on tension and electrical activity of human muscle. Ergonomics. 1972, 15, 417-34.

[34] V. Linnamo, T. Moritani, C. Nicol, and P. V. Komi. Motor unit activation patterns during isometric, concentric and eccentric actions at different force levels. J Electromyogr Kinesiol. 2003, 13, 93-101.

[35] T. Hortobagyi, J. P. Hill, J. A. Houmard, D. D. Fraser, N. J. Lambert, and R. G. Israel. Adaptive responses to muscle lengthening and shortening in humans. J Appl Physiol. 1996, 80, 765-72.

[36] N. N. Mahieu, P. McNair, A. Cools, C. D'Haen, K. Vandermeulen, and E. Witvrouw. Effect of eccentric training on the plantar flexor muscle-tendon tissue properties. Med Sci Sports Exerc. 2008, 40, 117-23.

[37] C. Bosco, J. T. Viitasalo, P. V. Komi, and P. Luhtanen. Combined effect of elastic energy and myoelectrical potentiation during stretch-shortening cycle exercise. Acta Physiol Scand. 1982, 114, 557-65.

[38] V. Linnamo, R. Bottas, and P. V. Komi. Force and EMG power spectrum during and after eccentric and concentric fatigue. J Electromyogr Kinesiol. 2000, 10, 293-300.

[39] T. W. Kaminski, C. V. Wabbersen, and R. M. Murphy. Concentric versus enhanced eccentric hamstring strength training: clinical implications. J Athl Train. 1998, 33, 216-21.

17

Employee performance appraisal in health clubs and sport organizations

Kaprinis Stylianos[1], Kipreos George[1], Vrondou Ourania[1], Kakkos Vasilios[2]

[1]Department of Sport Management, University of Peloponnese, Greece
[2]General Director at Olympic Athletic Center of Athens, Greece

Email address:
skaprinis@yahoo.gr(K. Stylianos), Kipreos@uop.gr(K. George)

Abstract: Human Resources evaluation constitutes a useful management tool which can help prosperity, rivalry and the achievements of organizational goals. The company's ability to evaluate executive performance, using valid, reliable and objective processes to identify actual employee's performance discrepancies to the ones desired contributes to long-term success, growth, profitability and organizational improvement. Especially, in the highly competitive health and fitness club industry, which are recorded as 133.000 fitness centers worldwide with profits of 72.7 billion dollars, an organization in order to be viable requires from the employees maximum work performance. Job performance is overall a complex meaning, from which its definition and measurement depends on various factors that should be encoded through a scientific documented effort, rather than arbitrary, spasmodic or informally. This review highlights the importance of a valid and reliable human resources assessment where as organizations prosperity competitiveness and effectiveness is increased as well as a strategic planning is developed.

Keywords: Performance Evaluation, Fitness Trainer, Health Clubs, Sport Organizations

1. Introduction

In today's era of intense and tough competition, and in a rapidly changing environment, human resources are recognized as an important source and competitive advantage to companies and organizations. (Barney, 1995; Newstrom & Davis, 2002; Prahaland & Hamel, 1990; Storey, 1989; Thomas, 1997). An organization's prosperity, effectiveness and rivalry relies mostly on the knowledge, talents, ideas and abilities of people who staff these organizations. (Chelladurai, 2006; Collins & Porras, 2001). Especially, in places that provide services, such as gymnasiums and sport organizations, where the quality of services is considered a prerequisite for their success, if not for their survival, the organizations recognize that apart from the facilities, programs and their reliability, the human factor is pivotal.

Additionally, according to the International Health Racquet & Sports Club Association's (IHRSA, 2012) report, the health and fitness club industry recorded dramatic growth globally; in 2011, over 133.000 gymnasiums worldwide provided services to 129.000.000 members and their revenues reached up to 72.7 billion dollars. In Europe, despite that many countries face a difficult economic climate, there are 48.000 gymnasiums recorded with 43.500.000 members and their revenues surpass 31 billion dollars. In Greece, there are 975 gymnasiums active with 385.000 members and their revenues reach up to 257.000.000 dollars (IHRSA, 2012). These facts prove that fitness industry is highly competitive and therefore, in order to survive, an organization needs the maximum efficiency from its staff. The management of staff performance, the assessment process of how well an employee executes his duties against a constant standard, contributes to this and offers companies a competitive advantage (Mathis & Jackson, 2000; Strebler, Robinson & Heron, 1997).

Despite the apparent usefulness of the staff appraisals, European studies (Papalexandris, 1997; Papalexandris, Chalikias, Panagyotopoulou, 2001) shows that in countries such as Greece, Spain, Germany, Norway and Finland only half of the companies adopt an evaluation system. This is in contrast to France, Great Britain, Sweden and Holland where the organizations have implemented appraisal methods for their employees.

Aim of this study was to review the published literature on the concept and philosophy of human resource evaluation.

Furthermore, to briefly record the evaluation systems objectives and targets and lastly to imprint the performance assessment criteria's the fitness instructors' assessments and the evaluation system design and process. This review highlights the importance of a valid and reliable human resources assessment where as organizations prosperity competitiveness and effectiveness is increased as well as a strategic planning is developed.

Method section of narrative literature: This present study, aims to a critical review of the research conducted during the last three decades (1983-2013, concerning the human resources evaluation performance and in particular fitness trainers and aerobics instructors evaluation performance. Some articles from earlier specified periods, with significant importance were accepted. Firstly, the research question was formulated; the criteria were identified and were recorded into an electronic base. For example, articles referring to employee's evaluation working in the sports industry were accepted, as well as the articles referring generally to service sectors since in this category sports organizations and gymnasiums are included. The main terms that were searched were: "personnel assessment", "fitness trainer performance appraisal", "aerobics instructor", "performance evaluation", "performance appraisal criteria for fitness instructors". From this study "grey literature" (e.g. Ph.D Thesis, Master Thesis, etc.) was excluded. As the numbers of publications were too large, the methodology that was used was "preview, question, read, summarize" (PQRS). Following, research classification into a Leader board was held, based on the work content of the evaluated (fitness trainers, personal trainers, sports coaches, PE teachers and out of the sports industry employees). Concerning the theoretical approach of the evaluation performance, secondary sources were sought (handbooks, journals, etc.) aiming to provide to the reader a comprehensive background in order to fully understand this particular study.

2. Evaluation History

Although employee performance appraisal is a distinct management process, it has become the subject of scientific research only in the past century; whereas the concept of evaluation in its broader sense is encountered for millennia. Information which establishes the existence of procedures and assessment tools can be found as far back as at least the third millennium BC (Dubois, 1970; Guba & Linkoln, 1983). According to Dulewicz (1989) there is a human tendency for everyone to judge themselves and the people with whom they work. Usually though, these approaches are informal, unofficial, erratic and mostly arbitrary. The first official attempt to evaluate was found during the 16th century at the Dublin Evening Post, in which attempts were made to define criteria's for employees evaluation based on their individual characteristics. (Huber & Fuller, 1998)

In Europe, the first staff evaluations were implemented, in the early 1800s, in the northern industrial countries. At the cotton factories in New Lanark of Scotland, Robert Owens, classified the employee's profitability levels by placing different colored cubes on their workstation, therefore indicating their value based on their contribution to the company. The evaluation attempts that were used in industry, where mostly used as a method of establishing salaries based on merit rating logic and performance pay philosophy.

The first official organized workforce assessment in the USA, began in 1813 in the US armies ranks (Randell, 1994; Wiese & Buckley, 1998). In the written reports of General Lewis Cass, the soldier's evaluations were conducted under the terms of « Good Character» or « Contemptible». Later in the First World War, when the need for the proper allocation of millions of men in the armed forces arose, Carnegie – Mellon University developed the first structured evaluation method based on physiological characteristics, known as *«Officer with Officer Comparison»* (Peters & Pierre, 2011). The encouraging results of the army's evaluation methods, primarily based on psychometric criteria adaptation, led to the dissemination of the evaluation methods into the world of business.

The Industrial Revolution (1815-1870) gave an enormous impetus to management thinking and practice. Pioneering studies by Frederic Taylor (1911) in the USA and Henry Fayol (1976) in France helped develop the «Classical Theory» in management thinking in which specific factors were highlighted as critical, i.e. careful employee selection, specialization, analysis and job description and productive results evaluation (Warr & Wall, 1975). Later, new classical approaches, which complemented the conclusions of the classical theorists, turned their interest towards the employees' behaviors and their motives as organizational growth factors. However, McGregor considers that developing the employees without perfecting working methods to be the cause of low productivity in organizations. (Bennis, 1966)

After the Second World War, modern approaches prevailed in human resource management; the performance appraisal is differentiated from staff behaviors. The work of Drucker (1954) focused predominantly on the organization's productivity in relation to employees' performance assessed against objective targets (Management by Objectives). Later on, the researchers' attention becomes focused on customer's satisfaction and quality services that are meet the customer's needs and desires. So, the Total Quality Management model is introduced. Today, as Campbell and Garfinkel (1996) support, large companies in Europe and in the United States aim to evaluate employees as objectively as possible. As such, they simultaneously use multiple personnel evaluator sources (superiors, peers and subordinates), applying a cyclic evaluation model *(360 Degree Feedback)*. Huber and Fuller (1998) support that today 80%-90% of the organizations in the United States use a personnel performance evaluation method.

3. Personnel Performance Evaluation Concept

The Performance evaluation is a formal, scientifically structured process for measuring and assessing performance against the relevant job description, the behavior and the results of the employee, aiming at the measurement and the valuing of his productivity, in order to determine if the employee engages effectively or can improve his productivity in the near future. (Kanobear 2002; Field & Holley, 1982). It is a process that provides relevant and valid information regarding the overall capabilities and abilities of the individual (Bratton & Gold, 2003), an assessment process of how well an employee perform his job tasks in relation to his/her job description. (Mathis & Jackson, 2000). The evaluation is an administrative function that contributes to the exercise of effective management. (Papalexandris & Mpourantas, 2003).

Through the procurement of reliable information about an individual,, the process of evaluation enables a team, a company or an organization manage to proceed to valid and updated decisions in order to solve any issues they are experiencing (Randell, 1994; Guion, 1998). Through this advanced process of decision making, the organization is empowered to place the most appropriate employees in the right job post at the right time (Golec & Kahya, 2007). The evaluative ordinances do not only concern the organization's prosperity, rivalry and effectiveness, but also constitute an employee's feedback process which helps him/her to realize and fully exploit his/her skills. Result of this feedback is the stimulation, evolution and improvement of the employee (Cascio, 1998).

According to Moulder (2001) and Maddux (1987), the appraisal of work produced offers a communication opportunity between the organization and the employee to discuss what is expected from each other and to find out whether each other's expectations are fulfilled. In medium and large organizations, the personnel performance evaluation constitutes distinct, demarcated and separated Human Resources Management functions, which assesses the extent to which an employee completes his job tasks efficiently. (Judge T. & Ilies R, 2002).

Nowadays, most researchers (Mescon, Bovee & Thill, 1999; Cascio, 1995; French, 1994) support that evaluation constitutes a new prominent scientific area related to the management, employee selection, education and development. It also focuses on the strategic processes and practices in business and to the changes and improvement of the organizations people.

4. Aims and Objectives of an Employee's Performance Evaluation

Osborne & Gaebler (1992) stress that if outputs results are not evaluated and if the outcome of a project is not appraised, then it is not possible to distinguish between success and failure. MacLean (2001) supports that it is important and necessary to evaluate the human resources of a sport organization for three mainly reasons: a) an organization's success relies on the quality of the human resource performance, b) it is impossible to manage efficiently without reliable information on employees' performance, c) so as to determine the customers' orientation and satisfaction.

A Human Resource's evaluation system firstly aims to identify the gaps between the real employees performance to the one desired, to identify the weaknesses and take corrective measures to continuously improve employees performance and to increase the organization's efficiency (Boone & Kurtz, 2005; Wilson & Western, 2000). The evaluative procedures aim to identify whether a person responds effectively in work, according to certain predefined criteria standards (Byars & Rue, 2003). However, an organization's and company's primary importance is finding and highlighting employees' strong side and exploiting their strengths without being occupied with their weaknesses (Mondy & Noe, 2005; Drucker, 1954). Jackson & Schuler (2003) report that main objectives of evaluation are employees' motivation, productivity enhancements and the facilitation of strategic planning. Therefore, for organizations, the evaluation performance is mainly directed towards the future as they encourage employees' development whilst contributing positively to the entire organization. (Soltani, Gernnard, Van der Meer & Williams, 2005). The traditional approach of Human Resources Management, where evaluation is characterized by the orientation in control based on past performance, is considered obsolete. The most important has a formative character and aims at identifying actions for improvement. The actions concern the identification of educational needs, staff training needs, targeted training activities programs to support the individual to achieve maximum efficiency. (Werther & Davis, 1996; Levin, 1986; Campell, Dunnette, Lawler & Weick, 1970).

One of the most cited evaluation goals are wage management and the determination of the remuneration system. The valuation of work produced by each employee provides the basis for reward efficiency (bonus) and determines the new wage levels. (Cole, 2004; Werther & Davis, 1996; Levin, 1986). Gomez-Mejia & Welbourne (1991) support that connection between wage and efficiency has a positive impact in effectiveness and in human resources efficiency, assuming that promotions and salary increases affect positively employees' motivation. Of course, some researchers support that it is wrong to connect wages with efficiency. They stress that high efficiency has to remain stable and permanent, while wage increases cannot be given continuously by the organization. They consider that evaluation has to be disconnected from salary increase, bonus provision, and to be associated with education and lifelong learning. (Papanis & Rontos, 2007; Van Yperen & Hagedoorn, 2003). However, evaluation is also concerned with the non-official benefits distribution (Sashkin, 1986), the decision making for promotions, internal movements and redundancies.

The evaluation performance is mostly useful in providing information for the employees profile, especially when he is a newcomer to the organization. So through this evaluation system the candidate selection can be validated -a general assessment of the operation system for attracting and selecting new staff and determination if through these procedure's suitable partners are chosen for the staffing of the organization. (Deadrick & Gardener, 1999). Furthermore, potential deficiencies of shortage in human resources or processes related to staff are identified (Werther & Davis, 1996).

Many researchers (Baruch, 1996; Bratton & Gold 2003; Campell, 1993; Cole 2004; Rendero, 1980) conclude that perhaps the most sufficient assessment role concerns the employee's performance feedback, which in return helps the stimulation, activation and maintenance of a high performance level. The purpose of feedback is the provision of encouragement, strengthening and correction. Furthermore, according to Moulder (2001), evaluations are useful because they help employees to set goals, and performance goals and directly regulate their effort and action.

Researchers (Babakus, Cravens, Johnston & Moncrief, 1996; Cotton & Tuttle 1986; Jaworski & Kohli, 1993) show that an important assessment objective relates to doubt reduction both from the side of the employee and from the side of the organization. This means that the employee has the chance to be informed any time about the quality of his performance. His comparative performance against that of his colleagues enables him to feel stability, justice and meritocracy within the organization and also re-enforces his professional and evolutionary development. From the organizations perspective the verification for the suitability of an employee to a job certifies its expectations, for the proper use of employee's talents and skills for maximum efficiency. The evaluation system can also help exploit hidden resources.

Especially in the area of fitness centers, where physical education instructors have to fulfill various roles, including those of a teacher, an instructor, a nutrition advisor and an active lifestyle councilor (Chen, 2006), it is important for an organization to design an efficient appraisal performance system for instructors in order to ensure that they provide the best possible services. (Penman & Adams, 1980). Additionally the quality of fitness trainers' services may significantly affect the fitness centers reputation. (Tai & Chiu, 2007). Quality fitness instructors are the cornerstone of an established and profitable exercise program. Their classes are innovative that motivate trainees and promote them to an active lifestyle; they are safe, effective and popular amongst gymnasiums' members. Through organized efficiency assessments, recognition, reward and professional development opportunities, fitness center managers can ensure that physical educators continue to bring quality, prestige and energy to a fitness center (Chiu, Lee & Lin, 2010).

5. Evaluation System Design and Process

The evaluation process according to Hansen (2002) consists of a systematic and scientific substantiated effort, which includes a definition of a clear and commonly accepted framework on how performance is estimated, the ongoing assessment of the employee's performance and progress, formal discussions and interactive communication regarding efficiency. The structural elements that constitute a well-designed evaluation system, according to many researchers (Cascio, 1998; Hansen, 2002; Werther & Davis, 1996) are:

Defining criteria performance, on which the evaluation will be performed

Defining the performance standings.

Designing (Method) of the Evaluation System.

Feedback of the assessed.

DeNisi & Griffin (2001); Longenecker & Fink (1999) suggest that after completing the evaluation process, the criteria performance definition and performance standards, communication with the employee should be followed up, in order to clarify the performance standards, advice and training.

Furthermore, according to Joinson (2001) an evaluation system in order to be sustainable and effective it must be valid, reliable, unbiased, easily implemented and accepted by all. Critical factor in the validity and reliability are the assessment criteria.

6. Performance Assessment Criteria's

Job Performance is a multidimensional concept, the definition and measurement of which depends on a variety of factors (Bates & Holton, 1995). Therefore, performance assessment cannot be carried out using a single criterion, but a set of criteria need to be established, a multidimensional tool. Today, multilevel and multiform assessment systems have been designed. Commonest assessment criteria, without these being contradictory and mutually exclusive are the features of traits, behavior, competencies, achievement of objectives and opportunities for improvement (Latham & Latham, 2000; Mondy & Noe, 2005). Mathis and Jackson (2000) add to the above work, quantity and quality, time management, work time completion, constant work presence and required performance skills. Jenks (1996) supports that in an objective assessment system, criteria must focus on efficiency and not on an employee's character, and neither on their past performance, but criteria should be oriented to employee's stimulation and improvement.

Smith (1976) suggests that skills, abilities, knowledge, behaviors and motivation, are a general evaluation field for human resources. MacLean (2001) supports that a fitness instructor's evaluation field should include knowledge of the subject, teaching efficiency, classroom management, trainee's activity levels, use of voice, a variety of activities and exercise, communication and administrative skills. Penman & Adams (1980) counted the essential professional possibilities and assessment fields of a fitness trainer as follows: a) Financial management regarding budgets, equipment and employees b) communication skills c) public relations d) knowledge e) quality service f) personality g) organizational management skills h) activities management i) equipment management j) knowledge and corporate culture management. According to Stiff (1993) the important skills that a physical education instructor must hold are: high module level, professionalism, excellent customer management, communications skills, first aid basic skills, computer knowledge skills, marketing skills, skills of setting personal targets and appropriate dress code. Chen (1989) specifies the area of expertise of a successful physical education teacher as: principle knowledge and sport diagnostics technique, teaching results, principles of a suitable sports environment, leadership skills, personality and understanding of corporate philosophy. According to Eickhoff- Shemek (2004) assessment criteria may include: a) quality indicators regarding the warming up of the trainee, the gradual increase of intensity, adaptability at the trainee level b) Instructions, feedback, interest for the trainee and c) issues, such as selecting and adjusting exercises, charisma, energy, a variety of intensity control, security, use of music, etc. Campell, (1993) and Chelladurai, (2006) add the following to the above: written and oral communication, leadership, effective trainee management, customer management and administrative skills.

Literature reviews have produced a wide range of criteria, which make the assessment process vague and difficult. Chiu, Lee & Lin (2010) tried to explore the assessment criteria for a physical education instructor through the Analytic Hierarchy Process [AHP] model of Saaty (1980). The AHP method has been widely used in different diagnostic areas and scientific fields in order to examine the problems that occur from numerous evaluation criteria where the researcher can select the most relevant criteria. The assessment in the study of Chiu, Lee & Lin, (2010) include a total of three dimensions and fifteen factors. The three dimensions are: *teaching, achievement* and *service*. The teaching dimension includes the quality of lessons, their innovation, the training and interaction with the client, etc. The dimension of achievement refers to lesson sales, customer attraction, communication skills, marketing, etc. The service dimension includes administration management, image improvement of fitness center, interaction with others, participation in relevant activities, customer information provision. The results of the research showed that priority to assessment efficiency of a personal physical instructor are the achievements (0,637), teaching (0,258) and services (0,105). Within these dimensions the most important factors were: in the «training» section appropriate criterion is considered *quality of lessons*, in the « achievement» sector the factor that dominates is the *course sale*, while in the «services» section the factor that emerges is the *administration management.* However, researchers underline that, despite the emergence of the « achievement» sector as the main evaluation index, gymnasiums cannot ignore service quality and are required to adjust appropriately to meet the needs of trainees and generally develop a customer-oriented strategy (Chiu, Lee & Lin, 2010).

On the coaching field MacLean & Chelladurai (1995) created a multidimensional assessment model, *the Scale of Coaching Performance (SCP)*. The assessment criteria are classified into two categories, those that refer to the product / results (behavioral product factors) and those that refer to the process (behavioral process factors). The two categories are structured into six factors. The factors that refer to the product are described as example win-loss record, number of blue-ship athletes, improvement from season to season, etc. The factors that refer to the process are analyzed as effecting teaching methodology; communicate effectively with athletes, understanding of appropriate age-group skills, motivation of athletes, etc. The following figure analyzes the evaluation criteria's per factor.

But whatever is chosen as evaluation criteria in an organization, according to many researcher's (Chelladurai, 2006; MacLean, 2001; Campbell, 1993) these have to be specific to the job, relevant, valid, comprehensive and measurable. In order for these criteria identified a job analysis must be undertaken (Noe et all, 2007; Jackson & Schuler, 2003; Mathis & Jackson, 2000; Murphy & Cleveland, 1991; Ilene & Barnes – Farrell, 1984; Sashkin, 1981). According to research by Eickhoff – Shemek (2004) while the 88% of the fitness center managers implemented an evaluation system, few explicitly declared the significant criteria or the performance standards. As such, while many of them provided written feedback to the assessed, significant errors occurred in the evaluation system.

7. Evaluation Systems Errors

Verma, DeNisi & Peters (1996) stress that evaluators inevitably judge based on their values, ideas, knowledge and prejudice, but also the emotional attachment they might have with the assessed and all these factors positively or negatively affect their judgment. As such, the evaluator's suitability and a wrong choice of an evaluation method are included in lists of frequent errors in relation to evaluating staff. Avoiding evaluation mistakes is not easy, for this reason Mathis & Jackson (2000) support that educating evaluators is essential for the objectivity and reliability of the evaluation system. From the bibliography (Byars & Rue, 2003; Mathis & Jackson, 2000; Mondy et al. 1999) the common error types are:

7.1. Halo and Horn Effect

This error type occurs when the evaluator marks low (horn) or high (halo) in all factors, focusing on an intense characteristic of the individual. The halo effect is the evaluator's natural tendency to have the whole evaluation based on the general picture he has for the assessed (Kanellopoulos, 1991). This specific mistake type is usually found in the grading of the employee's personality, where the evaluator expresses in a subjective way his sympathy or antipathy towards the assessed Nathan & Tippins (1992). For the limitation of the halo effect, employees should be evaluated in only one factor or characteristic each time before the evaluator proceeds to the next factor Mathis & Jackson (2000).

7.2. Leniency Errors

This error type is observed when personal preferences are located in the highest points of the grading scale. According to Hitiris (2001) this occurs from a conscious error where the evaluator biases and grades his employee higher than his real value. This happens because the evaluator may want to avoid tension and friction from the employees side. As such, they tend to evaluate them with leniency and not according to what they really deserve (Mathis & Jackson, 2000). The leniency errors are mainly found when the evaluation criteria are vague, indefinite and when they are not quantified (Kane, Bernardin, Villanova & Peyrefitte, 1995).

7.3. Strictness Errors

This specific error type is observed when the value judgments are identified in the lower points of the grading scale. And, here, biased and stereotypical evaluators attitudes are intervening. Lenient or austerity phenomena are found in organizations where vague and indefinite optimum performance levels are found. (Kantas, 1998). According to Kanellopoulos (1991) the evaluator's education helps the limitation of this specific error.

7.4. Central Tendency

The evaluator commits central tendency errors when he does not wish to consider the assessed as ineffective neither wants to estimate them as excellent employees, so he evaluates them within a limited range, which is consisted in the same context of the grading scale (Mathis & Jackson, 2000). This error is committed from the evaluator in order to avoid the justification of higher or lower grading. (Hitiris, 2001). For the limitation of central tendency error, a detail recording of each criteria is required and a clarification of the differences in work performance, so the evaluator has a clear knowledge of the grade he submits. (Byars & Rue, 2003).

7.5. Regency Effect

This error is committed when the evaluator is influenced from recent incidents and strongly emphasizes the events and behaviors during the last years (Byars & Rue, 2003). The evaluator commits this error especially when the evaluation period has a long time gap (e.g. yearly) and it is possible for him not to remember the previous employee's contribution (Hitiris, 2001). The most recent method for eliminating this error is the constant behavior recording, all year round (Mathis & Jackson, 2000).

7.6. Stereotyping and Prejudice

The evaluators grading, often deviates from objectivity due to prejudices such as employees' gender, age, nationality or religion. (Byars & Rue, 2003). For example, it is has been found that men receive better assessments than woman, even if the evaluator is a woman (Kanellopoulos, 1991). A way of eliminating this type of error is the evaluation should be carried out from more than one evaluator (Byars & Rue, 2003).

7.7. Similar to Me Effect

Common characteristics between the evaluator and the assessed (e.g. origin, education, political beliefs, etc.) create sympathies that lead to an error of similarity or intimacy, as a result of the favorable evaluation rating of the evaluator towards the assessed. (Papanis & Rontos, 2007; Hitiris, 2001).

7.8. Mathew Effect

One of the main errors in the evaluation procedure according to Gabris & Mitchell (1989) occurs when the employee receives the same evaluation results every year regardless of the efforts he makes. According to the Mathew effect, previous evaluations prejudge any future attempt.

Many researchers have studied the evaluation errors, in an effort to identify and clarify them so as to reduce or eliminate them, referring to the type and the frequency of their occurrence. Lefkowitz (2000) observes an employee's leniency grading from the evaluators, which is due to the low desire they have for low performance punishment or due to good interpersonal relations. Heneman, Greenberger & Anonyou (1989) support that evaluators frequently classify their employees into teams "in" or "out" categories. The first ones are rated in favor and are consistent to reap fees and promotions, and the second ones often stagnate in their development. Te existence of social relationships between evaluators and the assessed constitutes, according to Stredwick (2005) an objective difficulty in negative rating. Antonioni (1994) states that when the evaluator knows in advance that the evaluation results will be notified to the employee, an attitude of lenient and favorable rating is observed. Longenecker, Sims & Gioia (1987) consider that the reasons that one evaluator may discriminate and view favorable towards an employee, is to avoid a possible confrontation and conflict, to avoid a written justification for low efficiency, to submit a bonus to someone he likes, while negative evaluation is given to employees in order to render wise, the evaluator to validate power trends or to present written data upon employees dismissal.

In order to avoid error assessments, above all, education of the managers who conduct the evaluations is required. Keeping a logbook of each employee's performance and conducting an evaluation based on data from many sources also assists in error avoidance (Mathis & Jackson, 2000).

8. Human Resources Assessors

One of the basic, but controversial, issues of the evaluation process is assigning the appropriate evaluator, i.e. who will conduct the performance evaluation. In the traditional approach this task is undertaken from the direct supervisor. In the last few years, however, a turn to new sources is observed, which include self-appraisal, evaluation from external consultants, evaluation from colleagues, employees, customers or evaluation from many other sources simultaneously (Byars & Rue, 2003; Jackson & Schuler, 2003; Latham & Wexley, 1981; Mathis & Jackson, 2000; Mondy et al. 1999). In large organizations, the function designing and development of the evaluation system is executed by the Human Resources department (Mondy et al. 1999). Below, the various people responsible for conducting the evaluation process are presented:

8.1. Direct supervisor

Although the supervisor was the main source of information for the majority of organizations until the late '70s (Lazer & Wilkstrom, 1977), in many organizations, the supervisor, still remains the key evaluation personnel (Soltani, 2003). Theoretically he might be the most appropriate, as he has a clear picture for each employee, he is aware of behavior aspects, abilities and potentials of the assessed, and his opinion should be significant (Ghorpade & Chen, 1195). Additionally, he is the person who will recommend for the employees changes (promotion, training, relocation, benefits, etc) and therefore his judgment is significant. In order to avoid partiality errors, favorable or unfavorable treatment, his judgment is usually subjected to approval by the Senior Manager.

8.2. Self-Appraisal

In this process, each employee is asked to evaluate their own efficiency. In this way the employee has the opportunity to identify by himself his abilities and weaknesses. As a process, it usually encounters a positive response and acceptance from the employees, and it is a unique technique to increase the employees' simulation and improvement. It increases the employees' commitment towards the objective target (Mathis & Jackson, 2000). However, several researchers (Byars & Rue, 2003; Jackson & Shuler, 2003; Fox et al. 1994) support that the self-appraisal method often subjects to lenient errors, to discriminatory ordinances and is not always objective, therefore, self-appraisal should be combined with other assessment sources. Research from Eichener & Lombardo (2003) supports that employees self–appraisal rarely has similarities with the opinions of the direct supervisors, and therefore they suggest having combined models from evaluators.

8.3. Evaluation Performed by Colleagues

It is an essential source of valuable information because employees spend the whole of their working time with their colleagues, and are aware of the assessed weaknesses and strengths, which makes their opinion particularly significant (Atwater, Roush & Fichthal, 1995). Additionally, several researchers (Maurer, Raju, & Collins 1998; Zingheim & Schuster, 1995) support that colleagues evaluations can offer reliable information to identify the assessed educational needs. However, friendly and hostile interpersonal relationships may threaten the objectivity of this specific technique (Mathis & Jackson, 2000), in contrast with groups that have basic features cooperation, mutual respect and understanding, the results may be particularly significant (Scott & Einstein, 2001).

8.4. Evaluation Performed by Subordinates

It is also named as Reverse or Upward Appraisal. It is a technique that gives the chance to subordinates to express their opinion and judgments concerning their superiors' performance. It is an essential information source for the employee's evolution and development rather than their provision of rewards or incentives (Taylor & Morgan, 1995). Several researchers (Antonioni, 1994; Fox, Caspy & Reiser, 1994) support that anonymity is essential for the technique's objectivity because subordinates usually are afraid to express their opinion freely, for fear of dismissal. The subordinate's assessment according to Shaw et al. (1995), encounters great acceptance in government agencies in the USA (State Patrol) and in large private companies (IBM, Syntex). One of the positives of this specific assessment source, is that the information concerning an employee's positive or negative behavior is transferred to the higher administrative levels and effectively employees' relationships improve.

8.5. Evaluation from Customers

Chellandurai, (2006) supports that services organizations, such as gymnasiums, customers are a particularly interesting source of evaluation data regarding employees efficiency and behavior. It is particularly important for organizations to know what customers believe concerning the service level they are offered. Customer satisfaction ratings provide a reliable indicator for quality and services (MacLean, 2001; Milliman, Zawacki, Schulz, Wiggins, & Norman, 1995; Yakovac, 1996).

8.6. Evaluation from External Consultants

Many organizations use the services of external consultants to perform the assessment process with the assistance of the supervisors. The consultant, in co-operation with the supervisor, initially uses the interview method to collect job data and information concerning the employee's efficiency. Following that, another interview is performed with the employee discussing, about the outcomes of the first interview. (Byars & Rue, 2003; Mathis & Jackson, 2000)

8.7. 360 Degree Feedback – Cyclic Evaluation

The main characteristic of 360 degree feedback is the combination of all the above assessment sources. Supervisors, equivalent grade colleagues, subordinates, customers and the assessed themselves express their appreciation and judgments concerning an employee's efficiency (Carson, 2006; Mondy et al. 1999; Vinson, 1996). The multiple information sources offer quality, reliable and valid results (Bratton & Gold, 1999). Engaging a group of people, instead of an individual, reduces the evaluation errors and the biased judgments (Jackson & Shuler, 2003). Additionally it tends to supplement the total quality management principles as emphasis is given to the customer (Sherman, Bohlandern & Snell, 1998). The cyclical evaluation method enjoys great acceptance and tends to replace traditional evaluation methods in modern organizations (Toegel & Conger, 2003). For many though, it constitutes an expensive, time-consuming process and a bureaucratic method (Newstrom & Davis, 2002; Mathis & Jackson, 2000). It requires the managing of complexity since all answers have to be combined, and many of them are often conflicting (Sherman et al. 1998). However, because it is a multifaceted creative process, which encounters the employees' consent and acceptance (Huet, Nielsen, Sundsrton, 1999), a large number of companies (General Electric, Mobil Oil, Disney, Nabisco, Lockheed, Warner, Lambert, etc.) use the cyclical evaluation method widely.

In conclusion, someone could support that all assessment sources have advantages and disadvantages. A combination of sources, according to Ghorpade & Chen (1995),

throughout the assessment process, lends credibility, validity and objectivity.

9. Human Resources Evaluation Frequency

An important decision that an organization has to make is how often an assessment process should take place. A formal and organized procedure takes place in regular and specific periods. Mondy and Noe (2005), support that in a modern and constantly changing environment it is desired that organizations should often perform assessment systems. The majority of organizations perform the *Focal – Point system*, evaluating their employees on a yearly of even on an every six months basis. Possibly yet, the yearly evaluation might be considered insufficient (Mondy & Noe, 2005). Additionally Cascio (1998) considers the yearly based evaluations, have fundamental disadvantages, due to the workload in a short period of time, and the evaluator's influence from recent events and employees behaviors. Schuler & Jackson (2000) consider that an assessment process should be performed only when the evaluator has full knowledge of the employees' job performance level, without being influenced from time restrictions and commitments. This philosophy has been imprinted by the term *Natural Time Span of the Job*. Several organizations adopt evaluation processes every time that a project finishes. So, on the firsthand, they expect to convert the operational targets into employee's personal targets, and on the other hand to ensure objective and impartial judgments (Mondy & Noe, 2005). In cases of a new recruited employee evaluation, the first assessment takes place in the first 30-90 days, following the employee is assessed again in six months, and the last phase takes place after the completion of the first year (Mathis & Jackson, 2000).

What has a particular importance is that organizations should understand that the evaluation performance is not a static process that is performed every year, they should realize that it is a dynamic, substantial and sustained process to achieve human resource development, consequently improving the organization's rivalry and prosperity.

10. Relations between Evaluators and Assessed

The performance evaluation process is according to Bratton and Gold (2003) the most controversial and less popular operation of Human Resources Management. Spence & Keeping (2010) support that evaluation procedures are often a painful experience for the assessed and for the assessors. For employees there is distrust, a dissatisfaction and even fear (MacLean, 2001). Evaluation processes amongst employees, are recorded as low trust and acceptance, sense of efficiency and often lead to rivalries and conflicts between evaluators – employees (Smither, 1998).

According to several researchers (Hitiris, 2001; Deming, 1998, Longenecker & Goof, 1992; Sherman, 1998) evaluation processes have received overwhelming critics and arguments from those who are negatively disposed to the evaluation philosophy, and refer that the evaluation function creates fear to the employees, it makes the employees feel that their personality is being reduced, it creates injustices and inequalities, it promotes competition between colleagues and it does not develop the team spirit. Additionally they stress that efforts have temporary short-term results and most importantly that employees are being discouraged instead of being motivated. Deming (1986), considers the evaluation function as one of the "seven deadly diseases" and that it is opposed to the Total Quality Management principles. According to Ghorpade and Chen (1995), supporters of the Total Quality Management, evaluation systems are considered unfair, as that they promote behaviors which endanger quality, and quality is sacrificed for the sake of the numbers. Lastly, evaluation systems discourage employees considering them responsible for issues that the organization is to blame. However, the problem is not exactly the evaluation itself, but the way it is performed. The strongest reason of employees' dissatisfaction is due to management's inability to cultivate a supportive culture for the human resources evaluation system. The modern understanding of a performance evaluation system is that it cannot have a punitive character, but it has to focus on improving and developing employees' skills and consolidating performance with the organizations strategic targets (Longenecker & Goof, 1992).

Perquisite for the success of a performance evaluation system, according to Terzidis (2004) is the acceptance of the assessed. Incomplete acceptance of the system, from the side of the assessed, leads to negativism, resistance and hostility towards the evaluation system. However, acceptance is not easily achieved. Employees need to be persuaded and possibly involved/consulted during the development of such a system, especially during the selection of performance criteria in order to ensure acceptable of an evaluation system. It is particularly important for employees to understand that even when they receive a negative assessment, if it is accompanied by constructive and creative intention; it helps them overcome their present difficulties and improve their performance. (Fedor, Eder & Buckley, 1989).

But managers, who are invited to conduct assessments, often find themselves in an uncomfortable position and experience feelings of guilt because they tend to view assessments as an aggressive act towards their employees (Levinson, 1970). Either because there is no evaluation culture within the organization or there is no experience or training in evaluation systems, or there is a lack of trust in the workplace, assessment remains even nowadays an uncertain and a controversial issue. It is an intense emotional process and without a developmental direction is impossible to succeed (Cascio, 1998).

11. Traditional and Contemporary Approaches to Evaluation Performance

In the traditional approach of management human resources evaluation performance is characterized by the element of control. The appraisal of work that is produced mainly focuses on past performance, while productivity improvement is based on a «reward» and «punishment» system as a result of employee's comparison and ranking. Consequently, the assessed role remains passive, without any involvement in the evaluation process. The aftereffect of the above, is the non – acceptance of such system by the assessed and a defensive and reactive attitude (Papalexandris & Mpourantas, 2003).

Evaluation only makes sense when it is future oriented, with a formative character and aims at identifying actions for improvement. Thus, in the modern conception of human resource evaluation, the assessment systems are characterized by a developmental nature giving emphasis to employees possibilities for future progression and performance. Performance improvement is attempted through education, motivation and the empowering of human recourses. Improved performance is attempted through targeted, continuous feedback, the analysis strengths and weakness and through guidance. The role of the assessed is substantial as he is participating in the process (Papalexandris & Mpourantas, 2003). In the modern concept of assessment, firstly the assessed has to be convinced about the assessments' necessity and importance. If this is achieved, then employees acquire an enhanced understanding for the needs and requirements of their job, they build up relationships based on trust and maintain positive feelings towards their organization (Fletcher & Williams, 1996). On the contrary, it is observed that organizations that do not the incorporate regular performance assessments suffer reduced performance, increased frustration and withdrawal (Longenecker & Fink, 2001).

12. Discussion

In a challenging business environment, the continuous development of human resources is essential for the company's effectiveness and competitiveness. For this reason, companies seek to develop means for evaluating and further developing their human resources. According to Jackson & Schuler (2000) the function of evaluation aims to activate staff's talents and behaviors of an organization, in ways which will contribute to the creation and completion of the organization's mission, vision and goals.

However, the evaluation function constitutes a controversial issue and with differing opinions being expressed. Supporters of performance measurement, consider that the evaluation process to be a critical aspect of the organizational life (Lawrie, 1990), whereas researchers who are skeptical and do not see the evaluation process as a panacea, believe that it is inherently wrong and impossible to be perfected (Derven, 1990). Indeed, Deming (1986) considers that the evaluation process is one of "the seven deadly diseases" which are opposed to the Total Quality Management-TQM principles.

Although evaluation is used as useful tool for increasing staff's stimulation and improving their efficiency, even more controversial issues and many differing opinions are expressed in relation to how the evaluation processes should be implemented, how often it should take place and who the evaluators should be. Intense concerns are being expressed with regard to whose goals are being served by the evaluation process. There are many researchers who believe in the benefits of performance valuation and evaluation, and as it has the potential to contribute to staff's development and improvement. However, they condemn every effort made to link these assessments to rewards and recognition schemes which results in salary increase, productivity premium or promotions. On the other hand, there are supporters who believe that benefits should be distributed fairly to the most deserving employee's according to their qualifications, to their efforts and their results.

Even critics of evaluation's systems believe that negative

evaluation results usually occur due to the application of the wrong evaluation system/method. As such, they express their skepticism in relation to the inadequacy of methods and usability of systems rather that the philosophy of evaluation. (Hitiris, 2001).

Evaluation contributes to improved administration and the normal operation of an organization as capable, highly trained and skilled personnel constitute a necessity for an organization. The science of human resources management, through the means of evaluation, attempts to identify the best personnel. This study aims to highlight that the evaluation of human resources is not a luxury for an organization, but a necessity which should be incorporated as an integral part of any organization's culture. It should not be treated by companies as a cost to be avoided, but as an opportunity to invest in people with the ultimate goal of an organization's prosperity.

During the last decade, the rapid growth of sports industry and the large profits from sports organizations, created the need for educating the organization leaders – sport managers, aiming to maintain the competitiveness with other industries. In order to meet the needs of the specific profession, according to N.A.S.P.E. – N.A.S.S.M, more than 250 Universities in the United States educate their human resources executives derived from physical studies. Sport Managers, endeavor through the functions of developing human resources, soliciting, managing and evaluating, to fulfill the needs of the trainees and to gain the consumers loyalty. Their target is human resources empowerment improvement. Researches indicate that on average gymnasiums lose 40% of their customers each year (Sawyer & Smith, 1999) and the 50% of the consumers that begin to participate in athletic programs, drop out at the first six months (Gerson, 1999). In conclusion, quality determination as a strategic and human resources evaluation performance are identified as a significant source of a competitive advantage since high-level of customer satisfaction leads to a higher level of loyalty and devotion towards the organization and is linked to the behavioral intention of reusing the specific services (Bloemer, Ko de Ruyter & Wetzels, 1999, Zeithaml & Bitner, 2000, Roest & Verhallen, 1995).

References

[1] Alexandris, K, Zahariadis, P., Tsorbatzoudis, C. & Grouios, G. (2004). An empirical investigation of the relationships among service quality, satisfaction and psychological commitment in a health club context. *European Sport Management Quarterly,* 4: 36-52.

[2] Antonioni, D., (1994). The effects of feedback accountability on upward appraisal ratings, *Personnel Psychology,* Vol. 47, 349-360.

[3] Atwater, L.E., Roush, P., & Fichthal, A. (1995) The influence of upward feedback on self and follower rating of leadership, *Personnel Psychology, Vol. 48 (1), 35-60.*

[4] Babakus, E. D., Cravens, W., Johnston M., & Moncrief W. C., (1996), Examining the Role of Organizational Variables in The Salesperson Job Satisfaction Model, Journal *of Personal Selling & Sales Management*, 16 (3), 33-46.

[5] Barney J. (1995), Looking Inside for Competitive Advantage. *Academy of Management Executive,* Vol. 9, 49-81.

[6] Baruch, Y., (1996) Self performance appraisal vs. direct-manager appraisal: A case of congruence, *Journal of Managerial Psychology,* Vol. 11 Iss: 6, pp.50 - 65

[7] Bates, R & Holton, E., (1995) Computerized performance monitoring: a review of human resource issues. *Human resource management review, Winter 1995, 267-288.*

[8] Beer, M. (1987). *Performance appraisal.* In J.W. Lorsch (Ed). Handbook of organizational behavior (pp 286-290). Englewood Cliffs, NJ: Prentice Hall.

[9] Bennis, W. G. (1966). *Changing Organizations.* New York: Mc Craw Hill.

[10] Boone L., Kurtz D., (2005), *Contemporary Business*, South-Western Thomson, Mason

[11] Bratton J. & Gold J. (2003), *Human Resource Management: Theory and Practice,* New York: Palgrave Macmillan.

[12] Bratton, J. and Gold, J. (1999), *Human Resource Management*, Macmillan, Hampshire.

[13] Byars, L., & Rue, L., (2003) *Human Resource Management.* McGraw - Hill. U.S.A

[14] Campbell, J, P., (1993). *A theory of performance.* In N. Schmitt, W. C. Borman and associate (Eds). Personnel selection in organizations (pp35-70). San Francisco: Jossey Bass.

[15] Campbell, J., Dunnette, M., Lawler E., & Weick K., (1970) "*Managerial behavior performance and effectiveness*" New York, McGraw – Hill.

[16] Campbell, R.B., & Garfinkel, L.M., (1996) Strategies for Success, *HR Magazine,* 98-104.

[17] Carson M, (2006), Saying it like it isn't: The pros and cons of 360-degree feedback. *Business Horizons, 49, 395-402.*

[18] Cascio, W.F. (1995). *Managing human resources, productivity, quality of work life, profits*, New York, McGraw-Hill.

[19] Cascio W., F., (1998): *Managing Human Resources,* Boston, McGraw Hill Publishing Company.

[20] Chellandurai, P., (2006). *Human Resource Management in Sport and Recreation,* second edition, Human Kinetics.

[21] Chen, C. C. (1989). *The development of fitness instructors.* Taipei, Taiwan, ROC: Aerobic Fitness and Health Association of Taiwan.

[22] Chen, C. C. (2006). Discussion of the market of fitness centers and personal trainers in Taiwan. *Sport Management*, 11, 35-44.

[23] Chiu, W.-Y., Lee, Y.-D., & Lin, T.-Y. (2010). Performance Evaluation Criteria for Personal Trainers: An Analytical Hierarchy Process Approach. *Social Behavior and*

Personality: an international journal, *38*(7), 895–905.

[24] Cole G., (2004), *Management Theory and Practice*, 6th ed., Thomson, London

[25] Collins J. C. & Porras, J.I., (2001) *Built to Last. Successful Habits of Visionary Companies,* Harper Business, NY.

[26] Cotton, J and Tuttle, J (1986). Employee turnover: A meta-analysis and review with implication for research. *Academy of Management Review*, 11 (1), 55-70.

[27] Deadrick, D. & Gardner, D. (1999). Performance distributions: Measuring employee performance using total quality management principles. *Journal of Quality Management, 4*(2) 225-242.

[28] Deming W, (1986). *Out of Crisis*, Centre of Advanced Engineering Study Massachusetts Institute of Technology. Cambridge.

[29] DeNisi A. S. & Griffin R. W., (2001) *Human Resources Management,* 2nd ed. Houghton Mifflin Co., Boston.

[30] Dubois, P., H., (1970). *"A History of Psychological Testing"*, Allyn & Bacon, Boston.

[31] Dulewicz, V., (1989) *"Performance appraisal and counseling",* in Herriot, P., *Assessment and selection in organizations: methods and practices for recruitment and appraisal",* New York, John Wiley & Sons, pp645-649.

[32] Drucker P. (1954) *The practice of Management.* Harper and Row, New York.

[33] Eichiner, R. W. & Lombardo, M. M. (2003). *Knowledge Summary Series: 360-degree assessment.* Human Resource Planning Magazine.

[34] Eickhoff-Shemek, J. (2004). Conducting performance appraisals of group exercise leaders. Lecture presented at the American College of Sports Medicine Health and Fitness Summit, Orlando.

[35] Fedor, D.B., Eder, R.W. & Buckley, M.R. (1989) The contributory effects of supervisor intentions on subordinate feedback responses, *Organizational Behavior and Human Decision Processes*, Vol 44, 396-414.

[36] Field, H. S., & Holley, W. H. (1982). The relationship of performance appraisal system characteristics to verdicts in selected employment discrimination cases. *Academy of Management Journal*, 25, 392-406.

[37] Fletcher C. & Williams R. (1996), Performance Management, Job Satisfaction and Organizational Commitment, *British Journal of Management,* Vol. 7, 169-179.

[38] Fox, S., Caspy T., Reiser A, (1994), Variables, Affecting Leniency, Hallo and Validity of Self Appraisal, Journal of Occupational and Organizational Psychology, Vol. 67, (1) 45-46.

[39] French, W., (1994). *Human Resources Management*, 3rd Edition Boston: Houghton Miffin.

[40] Gabris G.T., Mitchell k., (1989), The impact of merit raise scores on employee attitudes; the Matthew Effect of performance appraisal, *Public Personnel Management,* Vol 17, No 4 (Special Issue).

[41] Ghorpade, J. & Chen, M. M. (1995). Creating quality-driven performance appraisal systems, *Academy of Management Executive*, Vo. 9, 32-35.

[42] Golec, A., & Kahya, E. (2007): A fuzzy model for competency-based employee evaluation and selection. *Computer & Industrial Engineering* 52, 143-161.

[43] Gomez-Mejia, L. R. & Welbourne, T. M. (1991). Compensation strategy in a global context. *Human Resource Planning,* 14(1), 29-42.

[44] Guion, R., (1998). *"Assessment, Measurement, and Prediction for Personnel Decisions",* Mahwah, NJ, Lawrence Erlbaum and Associates.

[45] Guba, E., & Linkoln, N., Y., (1983): Effective Evaluation, Jossey-Bass, Washington.

[46] Hansen, D., *(2002) Performance Appraisal. Tips Help Page, http://iso9k1.home.att.net/pa/performance-appraisal. html* , Retrieved 3/12/2012.

[47] Heneman, R.L., Greenberger, D.B. & Anonyou C., (1989) Attributions and exchanges: the effects of interpersonal factors on the diagnosis of employee performance, *Academy of Management Review*, Vol 32, No 2.

[48] Hitiris S.L. (2001) Administration of Human Resources, Interbooks Publications, Athens.

[49] Hoffman, R., (1995), Ten Reasons You Should Be Using 360-Degree Feedback, *HR Magazine, 40, 82.*

[50] Huber, V. L., & Fuller, S. R. (1998). *Performance appraisal and compensation.* In M. Poole, & M. Warner (Eds.), The IEBM Handbook of Human Resource Management. London: International Thomson Business Press.

[51] Huet-Cox, G., Nielsen, T., Sundstron, E., (1999) Get the Most from 360- Degree Feedback: Put it on the Internet, *HR Magazine,* May 1999*, 99-103*

[52] IHRSA (2010). `European Health Club Report: International Health Racquet & Sports Club Association. http://www.ihrsa.org/cbi/2010/12/21/the-2010-european-health-club-report-paints-a-detailed-port.html Retrieved 11-3-2013

[53] IHRSA (2012). The 2012 IHRSA Global Report: The State of the Health Club Industry. International Health Racquet & Sports Club Association. http://www.ihrsa.org/media-center/2012/5/23/the-2012-ihrsa-global-report-analyzes-industry-performance-a.html, Retrieved 11-3-2013

[54] Ilgen, D. R., & Barnes-Farrell, J. B. (1984). *Performance planning and evaluation.* Booklet in *Modules in management* edited by F. Kast & J. Rosensweig. Chicago: Science Research Associates.

[55] Jackson E. S. & Schuler, R. (2003): «Managing Human Resources through Strategic Partnerships» 8th Edition, Thomson South – Western Publishing.

[56] Jackson E. S., & Schuler R. (2000) *Managing Human Resources*, South Western College, Ohio.

[57] Jaworski, B. J., & Kohli, A. K., (1993) Market Orientation Antecedents and Consequences *Journal of Marketing*, Vol. 57: 53-70.

[58] Jenks M. J., (1996): The personnel Management Source

Book, Alexander Hamilton Institute, Kritirio, Athens.

[59] Joinson, C., (2001), Performance appraisal effectiveness *HR Magazine,* March, pp 38-41.

[60] Judge T. & Ilies R. (2002): Relationship of personality to performance motivation: A meta-analytic review. *Journal of Applied Psychology, Vol. 87(4), 797-807.*

[61] Kanellopoulos H, (1991) *Effective Human Resources Management Theory – Practice,* Stamoulis Publication, Athens.

[62] Kanobear, Inc. (2002). *Performance Appraisal,* Retrieved 17/6/2011 http://www.geocities.com/Athens/Forum/3126/htmlperfapp.html.

[63] Kantas A. (1998) Organizational - Industrial Psychology. Part 2nd Athens, Ellinika Grammata.

[64] Latham G., & Latham S.D., (2000). *Overlooking theory and research in performance appraisal at one's peril: Much done, more to do.* In C. L, Cooper & E. A. Locke (Eds) Industrial and Organizational Psychology: Linking theory with practice (pp199-215). Massachusetts, U.S.A: Blackwell Publishers Inc.

[65] Latham, G. P., and Wexley, K. N. (1981). Increasing Productivity Through Performance Appraisal. Reading, MA: Addison-Wesley.

[66] Lazer, R. I., & Wikstrom, W. S., (1977). *Appraising managerial performance: Current practices and future directions. New York:* Conference Board.

[67] Levin H. Z., (1986), "Performance appraisal at work" *Personnel,* Vol 63 (6) pp63-71.

[68] Levinson, H. 1970. Management by whose objectives? *Harvard Business Review* 44:4 July–August: 125–34.

[69] Lefkowitz J. (2000), The Role of Interpersonal Affective Regard in Supervisory Performance Ratings: A Literature Review and Proposed Casual Model. *Journal of Occupational and Organizational Psychology,* 73, 67-85.

[70] Liu, C. C. (1991). The human resources management of professional fitness instructors. *National Sports Quarterly,* 20 (4), 46-57.

[71] Longenecker, C.O., & Fink, L.S., (1999), Creating Effective Performance Appraisals, *Industrial Management,* Vol (5), 18-23.

[72] Longenecker C.O. & Fink L.S. (2001), Improving Management Performance in Rapidly Changing Organizations. *Journal of Management Development,* Vol.20 No.1, 7-18.

[73] Longenecker C.O., & Goof S.J., (1992) *"Performance Appraisal Effectiveness: A matter of perspective"* SAM Advanced Management Journal 57(2).

[74] Longenecker C. O., Sims, H. P., & Gioia D. A., (1987), Behind the Mask: The politics of Employee Appraisal, *The Academy of Management Executive,* Vol, 1, 183-193.

[75] MacLean, J. C., (2001), *Performance Appraisal for Sport and Recreation Managers.* Human Kinetics

[76] MacLean, J. C., & Chelladurai, P. (1995). Dimensions of coaching performance: Development of a scale. *Journal of Sport Management, 2, 194-207.*

[77] Maddux, R. B., (1987), *Effective Performance Appraisals,* Los Altos, CA: Crisp Publications.

[78] Mathis, R., & Jackson, J., (2000). *Human Resource Management.* South – Western Thompson Learning, U.S.A

[79] Maurer, T. J, Raju, N. S. & Collins, W. C., (1998), Peer and Subordinate Appraisal Measurement Equivalence, *Journal of Applied Psychology, Vol. 83, No 4, 693-702.*

[80] Mescon M., Bovee C., Thill J., (1999), *Business Today,* Prentice Hall, New Jersey.

[81] Milliman, J., Zawacki, R., Schulz, B., Wiggins, S., & Norman, C., (1995), Customer Service Drives 360-Degree Goal Setting, *Personnel Journal, Vol. 74, 136-142.*

[82] Mondy R., W., Noe R., M., & Premeaux S. (1999), *Human Resources Management,* Prentice Hall.

[83] Mondy R., W., & Noe R., M., (2005), *Human Resources Management,* ninth edition, Pearson Prentice Hall.

[84] Mondy R.W., & Noe R., M., (1996), *Human Resources Management,* 6th edition, Prentice Hall International Inc. N.J.

[85] Moulder, E., (2001), *"Performance Appraisal for Local Government Employees: Programs and Practices" Special Data Issue,* Washington DC, International City Managers Association.

[86] Murphy, K. R. & Cleveland, J. N. (1991). *Performance appraisal: An organizational perspective.* Boston, MA: Allyn & Bacon.

[87] Nathan B.R & Tippins N., (1992). The Consequences of Hallo Error in Performance Ratings, *Journal of Applied Psychology,* Vol. 77, 975-985.

[88] Newstrom, J.W., Davis, K. (2002). *«Organizational Behavior – Human Behavior at Work».* McGraw- Hill. London.

[89] Noe, R., Hollenbeck, J., Gerhart, B., & Wright, P., (2006) *Houman resource management: Gaining a competitive advantage, Vol. A,* Translation Athens, Publications Papazisi.

[90] Noe, R., Hollenbeck, J., Gerhart, B., & Wright, P., (2007) *Houman resource management: Gaining a competitive advantage, Volume B,* Translation Athens, Publications Papazisi.

[91] Osborne D., Gaebler T., (1992). *Reinventing Government.* Reading, MA: Addison – Wesley.

[92] Papalexandris N (1997) *Comparative Research in Human Resource Practices in Greece and Europe,* AUEB - Cranfield University, Athens.

[93] Papalexandris N., Chalikias J., Panagyotopoulou L., (2001) *Comparative Research in Human Resource Practices in Greece and Europe,* 1st Edition, Benos Publications, Athens (2001).

[94] Papalexandris N., & Mpourantas D., (2003) *Human Recourses Management,* Athens, Benou Eds.

[95] Papanis, E., & Rontos, K., (2007) *Performance Evaluation Employees,* Retrieved 17/2/2012 http://epapanis.blogspot.com/2007/09/blog-post_285.html

[96] Parasuraman, A., Berry, L., & Zeithaml, V. (1996). The behavioral consequences of service quality. *Journal of Marketing, 6(2),* 31-46.

[97] Penman, K. A., & Adams, S. H. (1980). *Assessing athletic and physical education programs: A manual with reproducible forms.* Boston: Allyn & Bacon.

[98] Peters B. G, & Pierre, J., (2011): The SAGE Handbook of Public Administration. Los Angeles, SAGE.

[99] Prahaland C. K. & Hamel G. (1990), The Core Competencies of the Corporation. *Harvard Business Review, Vol.68, 79-91.*

[100] Randell, G. (1994), *Employee appraisal,* in Sisson, K. (Ed.), Personnel Management: A Comprehensive Guide to Theory and Practice in Britain, Blackwell, Oxford, pp. 221-52.

[101] Redman, Snape & McElwee (1993). Appraising employee performance: A vital organizational activity? *Education & Training 35,* 3 – 13.

[102] Rendero, T., (1980), "Performance appraisal practices", *Personnel* Vol 57 (6) pp 4-12.

[103] Saaty, T. L. (1980). *The analytic hierarchy process.* New York: McGraw Hill.

[104] Sashkin, M., (1986), *"Becoming a visionary leader: A guide for understanding and developing visionary leadership",* Bryn Mawr, PA: Organization Design and Development.

[105] Sashkin, M. (1981), *Assessing Performance Appraisal,* San Diego, California.

[106] Scott, S, G., & Einstein W.O., (2001) Strategic Performance Appraisal in team-based organizations: One side does not fit all. *Academy of Management Executive, Vol. 15 No.2, 107-116.*

[107] Sherman, A., (1998) Managing Human Resources, South-Western, Ohio.

[108] Sherman A. W, Bohlander, G. W., Snell, S. A., (1998), *Managing Human Resources,* 11th ed., Thomson Publishing, Pennsylvania.

[109] Shaw, C. Schneier, R. Beatty & Baird L., (1995). *Performance measurement, management and appraisal sourcebook.* HRD Press: Amherst, Massachusetts.

[110] Smith, P.C., (1976). *Behaviors, results and organizational effectiveness.* In M. Dunnette (Ed.), Handbook of industrial and organizational psychology. Chicago: Rand-McNaly.

[111] Smither, R. D., (1998) *The psychology of work and human performance,* 3rd edition, New York: Longman.

[112] Soltani, E., (2003). Towards a TQM-driven HR performance evaluation: en empirical study. *Employee Relations,* Vol. 25, Issue 4.

[113] Soltani E., Gernnard J., Van der Meer R. & Williams T. (2005), *An Empirical Study of Performance Management Systems in Quality – Oriented Organizations.* Paper, Glasgow: University of Strathclyde.

[114] Stiff, M. C. (1993). The personal trainer. *Fitness and Sport Review International,* 28, 83-88.

[115] Stredwick J. (2005). *An Introduction to Human Resource Management,* Oxford: Elsevier Butterworth Heinemann.

[116] Strebler M, Robinson D and Heron P. (1997) Getting the Best Out of Your Competencies, Institute of Employment Studies, University of Sussex, Brighton.

[117] Storey J., (1989). New perspectives on H.R.M. London: Routledge & Kegan Paul.

[118] Tai, L. S., & Chiu, W. Y. (2007). The case study of management in world gym. *Journal of Physical Education,* 14, 77-81.

[119] Taylor G. L., & Morgan, M. N., (1995), The Reverse Appraisal: A Tool for Leadership Development. *Quality Progress, Vol. 28 (12) 81-87.*

[120] Terzidis, K. (2004). Management. A Strategic Approach, Athens, Edition: Modern Editions

[121] Thomas S. L. (1997), Performance Appraisals: Any Use for Training? *Business Forum,* Vol.22, 29-33.

[122] Toegel, G., Conger, J., A., (2003). 360-degree assessment: Time for reinvention, *Academy of Management Learning & Education,* Vol, 2, pp 297-311.

[123] Torrington, D & Hall, L., (1998) *Human Resource Management,* 4th ed. Prentice- Hall International Inc, U.K.

[124] Yakovac M. A., (1996), Paying for Satisfaction, *HR Focus, Vol. 63, No 6, 10-11.*

[125] Van Yperen N., & Hagedoorn M., (2003). Do high job demands increase intrinsic motivation or job strain or both? The role of job control and social support, *Academy of Management Journal,* Vol 46, No 3.

[126] Verma, A., DeNisi A. S., & Peters L. H., (1996), "Interpersonal Affect and Performance Appraisal: A Field Study," *Personnel Psychology,* 49, 341-360.

[127] Vinson, M., (1996) The Pros and Cons of 360-Degree Feedback: Making it Work. *Training and Development, April 1996, 11-12.*

[128] Warr, P. B, & Wall, J. D., (1975). *Work and Well-being.* HarmondsWorth: Penguin.

[129] Werther W., B. & Davis J., K., (1996), *Human Resources and Personnel Management,* fifth edition, Irwin Mc Graw – Hill.

[130] Wiese, D. S., & Buckley, R. M., (1998). The evolution of performance appraisal process, *Journal of Management History, 4, 233.*

[131] Wilson J. P. & Western S. (2000), Performance Appraisal: an Obstacle to Training and Development? *Journal of European Industrial Training, 24/7, 384-390.*

[132] Zingheim P. K., & Schuster J. R., (1995) Supporting Teams with Multi-Rater Performance Reviews, *Compensation and Benefits Management,* Vol, 11 (3) 41-45.

[133] Sawyer, S. & Smith, O. (1999).The management of clubs, recreation and sport: concepts and applications. Champaign, IL: Sagamore.

[134] Gerson, R. (1999). Members for life: proven service and retention strategies for health - fitness and sports clubs. Champaign, IL: Human Kinetics Publishers.

[135] Bloemer J, Ko de Ruyter, Wetzels M, (1999) "Linking perceived service quality and service loyalty: a

multi-dimensional perspective", European Journal of Marketing, Vol. 33 Iss: 11/12, pp.1082 – 1106

[136] Roest H., Verhallen T, (1995), "Quality Marks: Prospective Tools in Managing Service Quality Perceptions", in: Managing Service Quality, QMS Series Volume 1, Chapter 5, P. Kunst and J. Lemmink (eds.), SAGE (Paul Chapman) Publications, London, 65-78

[137] Zeithaml V., Bitner M., (2000) *Services Marketing: Integrating customer focus across the firm*, 2nd ed., Irwin/ McGraw-Hill, Boston, M.A

18

Slow recovery of the right and left ventricular deformation after conversion from atrial fibrillation

Roman Leischik, Henning Littwitz

Dept. Prevention and Sports Medicine, University Witten-Herdecke, Chair Cardiology, Prof. M. Seyfarth, Hagen, Germany

Email address:
info@dr-leischik.de (R. Leischik)

Abstract: Atrial fibrillation (AF) is a possible complication of sport in middle-aged athletes. When sinus rhythm has been restored, at what time is deformation restored too? This question has never been answered. We studied an one 47-year old cyclist and runner with acute lone atrial fibrillation. A day before, he trained hard intervals and felt at the next day an irregular rhythm, training was not possible. He told this would occure 2 times a year , but after the light training the irregular puls will disappear. At the chest-pain unit we performed echocardiography inclusive strain measurements of the right and left ventricle during atrial fibrillation and immediately after the recovery of the sinus rhythm. He recovered to sinus rhythm during the exercise test. Global strain was at the moment of atrial fibrillation – 11.8%, direct after the recovery of the sinus rhythm -17,2%, and -20.5% at the next day, even though the normalized diastolic function directly after conversion from AF. It seems to be that the heterogenity of the deformation need time to recovery after the conversion to the sinus rhythm, even though the diastolic function seems to be normalized. The further endurance training should be continued only after normalization of deformation values.

Keywords: Atrial Fibrillation, Endurance Sport, Deformation, Strain-Echocardiography, Cardiac Fatique

1. Introduction

Atrial fibriallation (AF) related to sport is known phenomenon since the 60-ties [1]. The recurrent atrial fibrillation in athletes has a variety of reasons: individual disposition, underlying atrial or conductional disease. Other reasons are speculative too: atrial ectopic beats, inflammatory changes, changes in electrolytes, atrial enlargement with dilatation, increased vagal tone [2]. There are different reports about the risk of AF in endurance athletes. The most of them refer an increased risk of AF in endurance athletes in comparison to general population [2] , in contrast only Pelicca at al. [3] reported about low incidence of AF among competitive athletes (0.2%) similar to that general populations of comparable age or sex.

In the ongoing search for possibilities to overcome the subjectivity of echocardiography as a diagnostic tool for the assessment of LV function [4], novel quantitative technique for deformation analysis has been introduced. Strain is defined as the speed at which deformation occurs, shortening is often expressed as negative strain and as percentage [5]. Besides the advantages that strain imaging offer, there is still a number of challenges that limit their clinical utility such as challenging image acquisition and a lack of consensus regarding optimal parameters and methods. Global Strain measurement seems to be easy and practicable in clinical setting [6] to assess the left [6] and right ventricular function [7].

2. Case Report

One 47-year old cyclist and runner (172cm /72kg), (1x Trans-Alp, Half-Marathon time 1.30h) has since 8 years 2x year AF-events. He train 6 days a week (4xtimes bike for 3-5 hours) and runs 50 km weekly since 6 years. He lost 5 years before 50 kg weight, because he was extremely obese. Endurance sport was for him a part of the lifestyle change. Underlying illness is not known. Arterial hypertension is not known. He developed AF suddenly, one day after hard training with intervalls up to 150 to 280/Watts over 2 hours. Training in this day was not possible, he took 100 mg flecainid, but nothing happened, so he came to the cardiologic chest pain unit. He reported, in cases of AF, he would obtain sinus rhythm after light bike-training.

3. Methods and Results

The echocardiographic exam [8] was performed with the commercially available ultrasound device VIVID 9 by General Electrics (GE) Medical Systems GmbH, Germany. The ultrasound probe that was used is a “Matrix Array”; Sector 3.5 – 4.3 MHz. The recorded data were transferred by a local network and saved on a storage device. For the exercise test an Ergoline stressecho-chair was used. Strain-Echocardiography was performed in the AFI-Mode [6]. For the right ventricle analysis we used only the 4 apical-view and the P-Lax option in the AFI-program.

In 12-canal ECG a typical atrial fibrillation could be noted. 2-D Echocardiography showed normal left atrial dimensions (3,6cm/38ml volume) and normal left ventricular size (4,7cm /100ml enddiastolic volume). Myocardial thickness was with 11mm normal (septum and posterior wall). Right ventricular volume was 38ml without enlargement. We decided to perform stress-echocardiography to assess a possible cardiac dysfunction during exercise and to obtain a conversion to the sinus rhythm regarding the successfully recovery in the patients history. We used the Bruce-protocol with 50 Watts and increased each 2 minutes 25 watts. At 125 Watts level and 140heart rate, sinus rhythm occurred. There were no signs of ischemia during the exercise in regarding the stress-echocardiography, during AF, ECG was not interpretable in cause of false-positive ST-depression due to the AF. Strain echocardiography was performed at rest 5 minutes after the peak exercise. Strain values of the different time points are visualized for all left ventricular views (Table 1).

It is shown in the Figure 2, that the deformation of the right ventricle after 24 hours is not homogenous in comparison to the left ventricle. It could be caused by the “exercised induced cardiac fatique” of the right ventricle. This issue is already under discussion [9, 10]. LaGerche et al. [9] described right ventricular “overload” after vigorous exercise.

Table 1.*Strain Values*

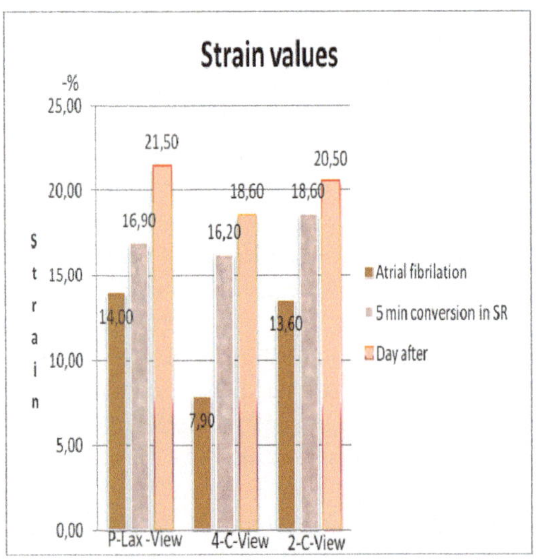

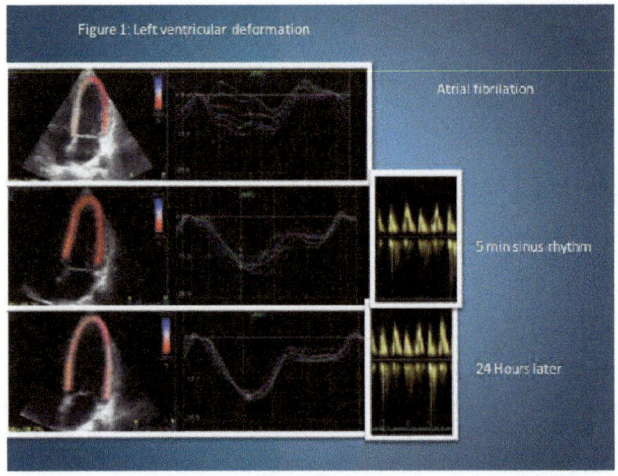

Figure 1. *Left ventricular deformation during atrial fibrillation, 5 Min after conversion to sinus rhythm and 24 hours later*

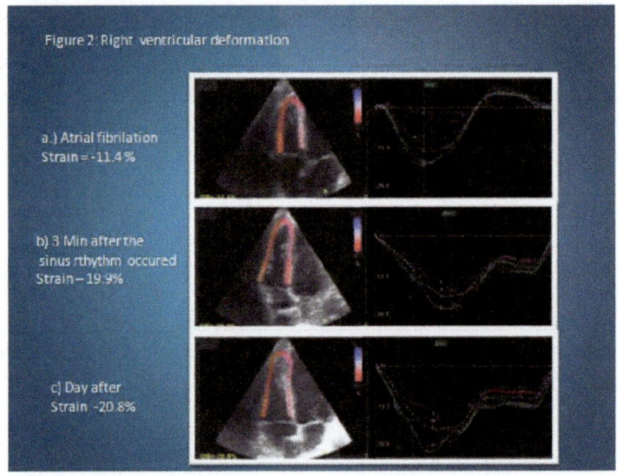

Figure 2. *Right ventricular deformation during atrial fibrillation, 3Min after conversion to sinus rhythm and 24 hours later*

4. Discussion

Atrial fibrillation in middle aged athletes is one common phenomenon. The athletes have higher risk for AF than controls (OR 5.29 (CI 3.57–7.85). For therapy we have the option of the intermittent drug therapy or the better option of circumferential pulmonary vein ablation [11]. Long term drug therapy introduces a lot of problems with decreased performance of the athletes or pro-arrhythmogenic effects caused by changes of electrolytes. In cases of occurred AF in endurance athletes we have to try to find the possible reason of the arryththmia. The problem is there are e a lot of possibilities [2, 12]. Gallagher at al. [13] discussed a broad field of underlying diseases from myocarditis to myocardial degeneration. The last problem is under scientific discussion. The degeneration and fibrosis of the atrial tissue is one possible mechanisms [14].

It is not known how much physical activity is good for health [15, 16]. One of the recommendations is to use 490/kcal/day regarding to Late Paeolithic times (50000-10000 BP) [17]. The further proposal is to be active up to 41/Mets-hrs/day [18]. For all “joggers” or ambitious middle aged triathletes it is not enough. They have to train and suffer from arrhythmias, but they live longer [19-21]. The study by Marijon et al. [22] reports positive effects professional endurance sport. Professional cyclists presented a 41 % percent lower all-cause mortality than the general population. Also the current meta-analysis by Teramoto and Bungum [23] reports a lower mortality (especially cardiovascular) and a longer life span of elite athletes. Of course, the results have to be interpreted with caution. Lifestyle and genetic predisposition may be more advantageous than the variables in the general population. The investigation of 2612 male elite athletes of Sarna et al. [24] also showed an increase in life-expectancy of endurance athletes compared with the control group (75.6 vs. 69.0 years).

There is no doubt, that athletes have a higher incidence of atrial fibrillation an bradyarrhythmia in old age [2, 19]. The relevance of possible fibrosis of the left atrium remains open [14]. In the case of 52.755 cross-country skyers of the Vasa-race [19] atrial fibrillation and bradyarrhythmia occurs more frequently (14.3/10000/patients/years and 1.9-2.8/10000/ patients/years). However frequent occurrence of supraventricular/ventricular tachycardia and cardiac arrest compared with the general population was not seen.

The general discussion of arrhythmias and sport remains controversial, because the causes and effects are still not clear at present (underlying disease, predisposition, training situation, circumstances). Sport itself is not arrhythmogenic. It needs perhaps a "triggerpoint": an inflammation or genetic disposition [13].

The recent general reviews on the potential side effects of ambitious endurance sport have partly different views. Scharhag et al. [25] thesis is that ambitious endurance sport will not lead to a myocardial damage or negative effects. O'Keefe et al. [26] agree with the statement that ambitious endurance athletes have lower mortality ratios, however, they also suggest the hypothesis that excessive endurance training may lead to negative cardiovascular remodeling. To verify this hypothesis endurance athletes should be identified. The latest publication of the Nixdorf-Recoll study revealed that for older athletes >50 years not the increase in troponin during marathon, but the individual risk of cardiovascular disease is of prognostic significance [27]. These studies indicate that endurance sport per se does not present a risk, but that "individual burden of disease" determines the risk for mortality.

5. Critical View

We introduced strain measurements for the situation of AF. We are using only one cardiac cycle (from R-wave to R-wave), so we can obtain one strain-value for a practical assess of the left or right ventricular deformation. In our opinion this assess of deformation can be used, even though AF occurred. Otherwise we have only the conventional assessment [8]. We observed that in cases of advanced heart failure with AF, the strain values decreased further until -8%. We considered, it might be possible to use this method and we have to develop further studies in similar issues.

6. Summary

Atrial fibrillation (AF) in the endurance athletes >45 years endurance sport is common phenomenon [2]. The prevention of frequency of arrhythmias or atrial fibrillation in athletes is unknown. It is possibly, that aerobic training [28] and consequent treatment of arterial hypertension [29] have the impact to avoid the frequency of occurrence of AF. The treatment with ACE inhibitors or AT1-receptor antagonists is seems to be one option [30, 31]. Further studies on this issue are necessary.

References

[1] Zehender, M., T. Meinertz, J. Keul and H. Just (1990) *ECG variants and cardiac arrhythmias in athletes: clinical relevance and prognostic importance.* Am Heart J. 119, 1378-1391.

[2] Calvo, N., J. Brugada, M. Sitges and L. Mont (2012) *Atrial fibrillation and atrial flutter in athletes.* Br J Sports Med. 46 Suppl 1, i37-43.

[3] Pelliccia, A., B.J. Maron, F.M. Di Paolo, A. Biffi, F.M. Quattrini, C. Pisicchio, A. Roselli, S. Caselli and F. Culasso (2005) *Prevalence and clinical significance of left atrial remodeling in competitive athletes.* J Am Coll Cardiol. 46, 690-696.

[4] Voigt, J.-U., B. Exner, K. Schmiedehausen, C. Huchzermeyer, U. Reulbach, U. Nixdorff, G. Platsch, T. Kuwert, W.G. Daniel and F.A. Flachskampf (2003) *Strain-rate imaging during dobutamine stress echocardiography provides objective evidence of inducible ischemia.* Circulation. 107, 2120-2126.

[5] Heimdal, A., A. Støylen, H. Torp and T. Skjærpe (1998) *Real-time strain rate imaging of the left ventricle by ultrasound.* Journal of the American Society of Echocardiography. 11, 1013-1019.

[6] Feigenbaum, H., R. Mastouri and S. Sawada (2012) *A practical approach to using strain echocardiography to evaluate the left ventricle.* Circ J. 76, 1550-1555.

[7] Simsek, Z., M.H. Tas, E. Gunay and H. Degirmenci (2013) *Speckle-tracking echocardiographic imaging of the right ventricular systolic and diastolic parameters in chronic exercise.* Int J Cardiovasc Imaging. 29, 1265-1271.

[8] Lang, R.M., M. Bierig, R.B. Devereux, F.A. Flachskampf, E. Foster, P.A. Pellikka, M.H. Picard, M.J. Roman, J. Seward and J. Shanewise (2006) *Recommendations for chamber quantification.* European Journal of Echocardiography. 7, 79-108.

[9] La Gerche, A., A.T. Burns, D.J. Mooney, W.J. Inder, A.J. Taylor, J. Bogaert, A.I. MacIsaac, H. Heidbüchel and D.L. Prior (2012) *Exercise-induced right ventricular dysfunction and structural remodelling in endurance athletes.* European heart journal. 33, 998-1006.

[10] Oxborough, D., K. Birch, R. Shave and K. George (2010) *"Exercise-induced cardiac fatigue"--a review of the echocardiographic literature.* Echocardiography. 27, 1130-1140.

[11] Calvo, N., L. Mont, D. Tamborero, A. Berruezo, G. Viola, E. Guasch, M. Nadal, D. Andreu, B. Vidal and M. Sitges (2010) *Efficacy of circumferential pulmonary vein ablation of atrial fibrillation in endurance athletes.* Europace. 12, 30-36.

[12] Lubitz, S.A., E.J. Benjamin, J.N. Ruskin, V. Fuster and P.T. Ellinor (2010) *Challenges in the classification of atrial fibrillation.* Nat Rev Cardiol. 7, 451-460.

[13] Gallagher, M.M. and J. Camm (1998) *Classification of atrial fibrillation.* Am J Cardiol. 82, 18n-28n.

[14] Burstein, B. and S. Nattel (2008) *Atrial Fibrosis: Mechanisms and Clinical Relevance in Atrial Fibrillation.* Journal of the American College of Cardiology. 51, 802-809.

[15] Blair, S.N., H.W. Kohl, N.F. Gordon and R.S. Paffenbarger, Jr. (1992) *How much physical activity is good for health?* Annu Rev Public Health. 13, 99-126.

[16] Lee, I.M. and P.J. Skerrett (2001) *Physical activity and all-cause mortality: what is the dose-response relation?* Med Sci Sports Exerc. 33, S459-471; discussion S493-454.

[17] Eaton, S.B., L. Cordain and S. Lindeberg (2002) *Evolutionary Health Promotion: A Consideration of Common Counterarguments.* Preventive Medicine. 34, 119-123.

[18] Bellavia, A., M. Bottai, A. Wolk and N. Orsini (2013) *Physical activity and mortality in a prospective cohort of middle-aged and elderly men - a time perspective.* Int J Behav Nutr Phys Act. 10, 94.

[19] Andersen, K., B. Farahmand, A. Ahlbom, C. Held, S. Ljunghall, K. Michaelsson and J. Sundstrom (2013) *Risk of arrhythmias in 52 755 long-distance cross-country skiers: a cohort study.* Eur Heart J. .

[20] Farahmand, B.Y., A. Ahlbom, O. Ekblom, B. Ekblom, U. Hallmarker, D. Aronson and G.P. Brobert (2003) *Mortality amongst participants in Vasaloppet: a classical long-distance ski race in Sweden.* J Intern Med. 253, 276-283.

[21] Gajewski, A.K. and A. Poznanska (2008) *Mortality of top athletes, actors and clergy in Poland: 1924-2000 follow-up study of the long term effect of physical activity.* Eur J Epidemiol. 23, 335-340.

[22] Marijon, E., M. Tafflet, J. Antero-Jacquemin, N. El Helou, G. Berthelot, D.S. Celermajer, W. Bougouin, N. Combes, O. Hermine and J.-P. Empana (2013) *Mortality of French participants in the Tour de France (1947–2012).* European heart journal. 34, 3145-3150.

[23] Teramoto, M. and T.J. Bungum (2010) *Mortality and longevity of elite athletes.* J Sci Med Sport. 13, 410-416.

[24] Sarna, S., T. Sahi, M. Koskenvuo and J. Kaprio (1993) *Increased life expectancy of world class male athletes.* Med Sci Sports Exerc. 25, 237-244.

[25] Scharhag, J., H. Lollgen and W. Kindermann (2013) *Competitive sports and the heart: benefit or risk?* Dtsch Arztebl Int. 110, 14-23; quiz 24; e11-12.

[26] O'Keefe, J.H., R.P. Harshal, C.J. Lavie, A. Magalski, R.A. Vogel and P.A. McCiiough (2012) *Potential Adverse Cardiovascular Effects From Excessive Endurance Exercise.* Mayo Clin Proc. 87, 587-595.

[27] Mohlenkamp, S., K. Leineweber, N. Lehmann, S. Braun, U. Roggenbuck, M. Perrey, M. Broecker-Preuss, T. Budde, M. Halle, K. Mann, K.H. Jockel, R. Erbel, and G. Heusch (2014) *Coronary atherosclerosis burden, but not transient troponin elevation, predicts long-term outcome in recreational marathon runners.* Basic Res Cardiol. 109, 391.

[28] Whelton, S.P., A. Chin, X. Xin and J. He (2002) *Effect of aerobic exercise on blood pressure: a meta-analysis of randomized, controlled trials.* Ann Intern Med. 136, 493-503.

[29] Kaplan, N.M., R.B. Deveraux and H.S. Miller, Jr. (1994) *26th Bethesda conference: recommendations for determining eligibility for competition in athletes with cardiovascular abnormalities. Task Force 4: systemic hypertension.* J Am Coll Cardiol. 24, 885-888.

[30] Ehrlich, J.R., S.H. Hohnloser and S. Nattel (2006) *Role of angiotensin system and effects of its inhibition in atrial fibrillation: clinical and experimental evidence.* Eur Heart J. 27, 512-518.

[31] Brilla, C.G., R.C. Funck and H. Rupp (2000) *Lisinopril-mediated regression of myocardial fibrosis in patients with hypertensive heart disease.* Circulation. 102, 1388-1393.

[32]

19

Macronutrient consumption prior to, and during, a mountain marathon

Elizabeth Mahon[1], Allan Hackett[1], Timothy Stott[1], Keith George[2], Ian Davies[1]

[1]Faculty of Education, Health and Community, Liverpool John Moores University, Liverpool, United Kingdom
[2]Research Institute for Sport and Exercise Sciences, Liverpool John Moores University, Liverpool, United Kingdom

Email address:
E.Haywood@ljmu.ac.uk (E. Mahon)

Abstract: Participation in ultra-endurance events such as mountain marathons is increasing, yet analysis of the nutritional intake and requirements of this group of athletes have received relatively little attention. This field study examined athletes' food intake prior to, and during a mountain marathon event to assess compliance with recommendations and to identify associations with performance. Nineteen male athletes competing in the Longmynd Hike (LH) completed a 7-day food diary in the week prior to the event and a weighed food inventory of all items consumed during the event. Despite reported intentions to increase carbohydrate (CHO) consumption in the week prior to the event, there was no significant change in consumption across the week. The mean daily CHO intake of 4.5 g/kg/d was below that recommended to effectively enhance glycogen stores. CHO and energy consumption prior to the event were positively associated with performance [energy (kJ/kg/d): $r = .56$, $p = 0.03$; CHO (g/kg/d): $r = .54$, $p = 0.04$]. Energy and CHO consumption during the event were also positively correlated with performance [energy (kJ/kg/h): $r = .80$, $p < 0.001$; CHO (g/kg/h): $r = .75$, $p = 0.001$)], despite most participants again failing to meet recommendations for intake. Further research is needed to determine reasons for non-compliance with nutritional guidelines and to investigate to what extent type and timing of macronutrient intake during such events impacts on performance.

Keywords: Ultra-Endurance, Exercise, Carbohydrate, Fat, Running, Hill-Walking

1. Introduction

The popularity of ultra-endurance sport, both as a leisure time activity and in competitive events, is rising [1]. Popular ultra-endurance races in the United Kingdom (UK) include mountain marathons, which are typically either two-day (with a mid-camp) or continuous races combining fell-running and orienteering over steep, uneven terrain [2]. They can either be supported, where food and drink is provided at aid stations, or unsupported in which participants must carry their own provisions. The prolonged duration of such events and additional factors; such as weather conditions, backpack weight and severity of terrain can result in exceptional physiological and metabolic demands being placed on the competitors [3]. Consequently, the nutritional requirements of these athletes are likely very important to health and performance but have received little attention.

Maintaining an energy supply to meet the physiological demands of prolonged exercise is paramount to performance [4-5], and several strategies exist to accomplish this. Supercompensating muscle glycogen levels by carbohydrate (CHO) loading in the days prior to an endurance event can improve performance by 2-3% [6]. Secondly, convincing evidence from numerous studies now indicates that CHO ingestion during exercise of one hour or more can improve work capacity and performance [7-10]. The American College of Sports Medicine (ACSM) recommends intakes of 30 – 60 g/h of CHO during endurance exercise [11], whilst the latest International Olympic Committee (IOC) consensus statement on sports nutrition 2010 [12] advises that athletes participating in events lasting > 2.5 h may benefit from higher intakes up to 90 g/h. Other strategies include utilizing fat as an alternative fuel to attempt to enhance rates of fat oxidation during exercise and reduce rates of muscle glycogen use [13-14]. Studies on prolonged low-moderate intensity exercise have shown an enhanced fat oxidation to be the major energy source [15-16].

It is evident that nutritional strategies are very dependent on the format of the race to be completed and in particular the intensities of exercise involved. An important feature of the mountain marathon is the varying intensity at which athletes must work. Whilst no study has measured percentages of maximal oxygen uptake (VO_2 max) during mountain marathon events, studies performed on hill walkers have shown that they typically work at a range of 25-70% VO_2 max [17]. Mountain marathoners are likely to reach higher intensities due to the competitive nature of the sport, and so such events are examples of where a mix of nutritional strategies may be required.

To date very few studies have investigated the dietary practices of mountain marathon competitors [2,18-19]. Kruesman *et al.* observed the fluid and fuel intake of 42 amateur runners in a 44 km Swiss mountain marathon [18]. Mean hourly intakes of energy, CHO, fat and protein were 590 kJ, 31 g, 2 g and 0.8 g, respectively. Whilst the mean CHO intake was within the recommended range provided by the ACSM [11], more than half the runners were unable to meet energy balance and accumulated a deficit of between 7,908 – 10,341 kJ during the race. It is hypothesized in an unsupported race, where runners must carry their own food; even greater energy deficits would be observed. Clarke *et al.* recorded the nutrient intakes of 90 athletes competing across four different two-day unsupported mountain marathon events in the UK [2]. Nutrient data are not provided on a g/h basis and so cannot be compared to current guidelines, but g/kg/h of athletic effort for energy, CHO, fat and protein were 20.67 kJ, 0.89 g, 0.11 g and 0.10 g, respectively. It is clear that CHO consumption was below that required to reach maximal oxidation rates. Energy expenditure was not calculated and as no indication of distance or time taken to complete the course was provided, it is difficult to estimate energy balance. Performance was positively associated with energy, CHO and protein intake. Stuempfle *et al.* analyzed the race diet of competitors in the Western States Endurance Run; a 161 km supported mountain footrace [19]. They compared the nutrient intakes of those who finished compared to the non-finishers and found significantly higher intakes of overall energy (4.6 ± 1.7 vs. 2.5 ± 1.3 kcal/kg/h), CHO (0.9 ± 0.43 vs. 0.56 ± 0.32 g/kg/h) and fat (0.06 ± 0.03 vs. 0.02 ± 0.02 g/kg/h), respectively. However, the sample sizes were very small; only six participants finished the race and there was large variation in the nutrient intakes.

It is evident that there are few detailed reports of nutrient intakes in mountain marathoners. Whilst CHO appears to be beneficial to performance during such events, there are no existing accounts of nutrient consumption prior to events with regard to whether high-CHO or high-fat diets are optimal. Further research is therefore warranted in this area to determine optimal strategies. The main objective of this study was to provide descriptive information on the food intakes of athletes prior to, and during, a continuous unsupported mountain marathon event to assess compliance with recommendations and to identify associations with performance. Secondary objectives were to record athletes' intended race-diet strategies in order to explore whether these led to appropriate nutrient intakes; determine whether nutrient intake differed depending on age and experience; and to measure blood β-ketones to provide an objective measure of energy metabolism and macronutrient utilization during the event.

2. Method

2.1. Setting

The event used for this study was the Longmynd Hike (LH), held in October 2009. The LH is an 80.5 km continuous, competitive mountain marathon set in the countryside of South Shropshire and the Welsh Marches UK, with approximately 2,400 m of climbing over eight summits. The course profile is displayed in Fig. 1. No food was provided and so competitors were required to carry sufficient food for the duration of the event. The event attracts a wide spectrum of competitors ranging from elite fell-runners to recreational athletes. This event was chosen, as previous studies on mountain marathons have either used two-day events [2], which make interpretation of dietary intake and association with performance difficult, or supported events [18-19]. An unsupported event was used as larger differences in food selection and energy consumption are likely to be seen. Weight of food carried is a concern for competitors and as a result food intake might be restricted [2].

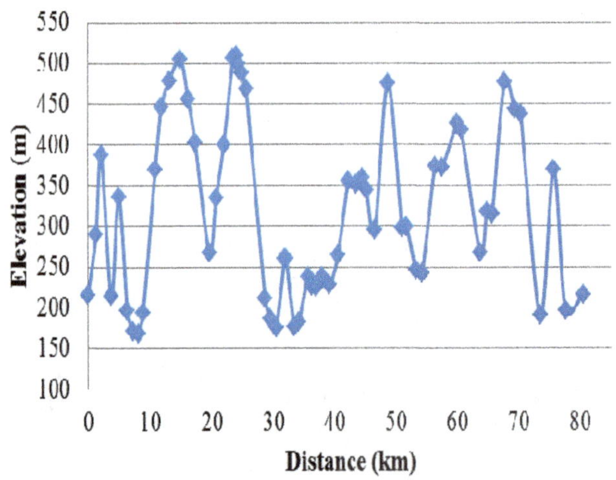

Figure 1. *Longmynd Hike course profile (plotted from course data available on the event website [20]).*

2.2. Participants

Ethical approval was granted by Liverpool (Adult) Research Ethics Committee and Liverpool John Moores University Ethics Committee. Competitor participants were recruited through links on the event website and flyers sent out with entry packs. Volunteers registered their intent to participate via email and consent to take part in the different elements of the study was obtained in writing.

2.3. Protocol and Procedures

Self-administered questionnaires were sent to all participants prior to the event to collect data on participant characteristics; dietary habits prior to and during previous ultra-endurance events; and level of experience in mountainous environments and in ultra-endurance racing.

2.3.1. Food Intake and Analysis

Dietary intake was assessed with a seven-day weighed food diary in the week prior to the event. To record consumption during the event participants were asked to compile an inventory (at home prior to the event) of all the food (including sports drinks) which they had packed to take with them. They were provided with a proforma to complete which asked them to provide a detailed description of the foods and the weight (in grams) of each food item. On arrival at the event headquarters on the day of the race, participants were asked to present their paperwork to a researcher who checked that it was complete, questioned any ambiguities and added detail where necessary on the food diary and food inventory forms. After the event, any leftover food was weighed by the researchers on site and net consumption was calculated and inputted onto the food inventory forms. Leftover food was weighed using digital scales accurate to 1 g.

Food data and macronutrient intakes were analyzed using dietary software (MicroDiet, version 1.2). The macronutrient content was taken from standard food tables [21], available datasets on the MicroDiet software programme, or specialist items were inputted manually using information collected from food labels provided by participants or product websites.

2.3.2. Anthropometrics

The body mass (BM) and pack weight of each participant was recorded using calibrated scales accurate to 0.1 kg. Height was measured using a stadiometer to the nearest 1 mm. Measurements were performed to standard protocol on the morning of the event.

2.3.3. Blood Analyses

Blood β-ketones were measured as an indicator of energy metabolism and macronutrient utilization. Levels of β-ketones below 0.6 mmol/L are considered normal and those over 1.5 mmol/L elevated. In this study β-ketones were measured from a fresh capillary whole blood sample taken from the fingertip and analyzed using the MediSense (Optium™) instrument. Precision and accuracy testing shows that results typically vary by no more than 3.1 – 3.8% coefficient of variation [22]. Measurements were taken pre- and post-event. Participants were asked to report to the testing area, a room at the event headquarters, as soon as they had completed the event.

2.3.4. Performance

Performance was calculated as a reciprocal percentage of the winning time [2], times were age-adjusted:

$$200 - (\text{Individual time} / \text{winning time} \times 100)$$

2.4. Statistical Procedures

Statistical analyses were performed with SPSS (version 17.0). Descriptive statistics (mean, standard deviation (SD), minimum, maximum) were calculated for completion time, participant characteristics, nutrient intakes and blood ketones. Frequencies were reported for questionnaire responses and number of participants meeting dietary recommendations. All data were tested for normality and non-parametric tests were used where appropriate.

A one-way repeated measures ANOVA explored the differences in CHO consumption during the week prior to the event and the Wilcoxon Signed Rank Test was used to detect significant changes in blood ketone levels. Associations between various aspects of dietary intake, participant characteristics and performance were tested with Pearson's and Spearman's rank correlation coefficients and a standard multiple linear regression model, with factors statistically associated with performance, was employed to determine the best predictor of performance. All tests were two-tailed, with alpha < 0.05.

3. Results

3.1. Participant Characteristics

Nineteen male participants volunteered from the 550 registered for the LH. The sample was split into the following age categories to reflect the classes that athletes compete in: 'male' 18 – 39 y; 'male senior' 40 – 49 y; and 'male veteran' 50+ y. Sample characteristics were as follows: n = 19; age (18 – 39 y: n = 5, 40 – 49 y: n = 7, 50+ y: n = 7); BM: 76.3 (10.3) kg; body mass index (BMI); 24.3 (3.3) kgm^{-2}; and course completion time 16 (±3) h.

The majority of participants (18/19) had previously taken part in the same event before. Experience can be important to performance in such events and so was classified as the number of times participants have previously taken part in the event. The sample was split as follows: 'never or once' (n = 7); '2 to 5 times' (n = 8); and 'more than 5' (n = 4).

3.2. Food Intake in the Week Prior to the Event

On the pre-event questionnaire 95% of all participants commented that food consumed in the week prior to an event can impact on performance, with 78% claiming to have changed their diet in the past to aid performance. The main dietary change reported was an increase in CHO consumption (86%). Regarding the targeted event, 74% of participants reported planning to change their diet with 86% of these planning to increase their CHO intake. Only one participant planned to increase their fat consumption.

Macronutrient intakes are presented in Table 1. There was no difference in nutrient consumption with respect to age, and no noteworthy differences with respect to experience when taking BM into account. There was however, considerable between-participant variation.

Consequently all further analyses represent the entire cohort (with age and experience groups collapsed). Despite reported intentions to increase CHO consumption, there was no significant change in CHO consumption throughout the week (Table 2).

Table 1. *Mean macronutrient consumption prior to the event*

Nutrient	Mean (SD)	Range
Energy (kJ/kg/d)	145 (39)	77 - 238
CHO (g/kg/d)	4.5 (1.1)	2.3 – 6.8
Protein (g/kg/d)	1.3 (0.4)	0.7 – 1.9
Fat (g/kg/d)	1.3 (0.4)	0.7 – 2.3

Table 2. *CHO intake in the week prior to the event*

Day of food diary	CHO (g/kg/d)	
	Mean (SD)	Range
1	4.6 (1.5)	2.2 – 7.5
2	4.7 (1.6)	2.8 – 8.7
3	3.9 (1.6)	1.6 – 7.5
4	4.4 (1.8)	2.0 – 9.9
5	4.5 (1.6)	1.8 – 8.4
6	4.6 (1.7)	2.5 – 8.0
7	4.9 (1.4)	2.3 – 7.7

3.3. Food Intake During the Event

All participants reported that food consumed during the event has some influence on performance. A wide range of food stuffs were consumed, both specialized sports products and traditional foods (see table 3 for full details). Sports products included: sports drinks; energy gels; energy bars; and energy tablets. Such products were used by 74% of competitors contributing from 0 to 97% of total energy. Popular traditional snack products included: cereal bars; chocolate; dried fruit; nuts and jelly babies.

Table 3. *Popular food items consumed during the event*

Food item	Number of participants who consumed
Chocolate	13
Sandwich	12
Energy gel	11
Dried fruit	11
Energy/sports bar	10
Banana	10
Energy/sports drink	10
Nuts	10
Cereal/muesli bar	9
Energy tablets	9
Sweets (jelly babies)	9
Malt loaf	7
Pasta	4

Energy and macronutrient intake is shown in table 4. Total nutrient intake data was divided by the number of hours on the course to give hourly estimates. Nutrient intake data did not vary with age or experience. The mean hourly CHO consumption was 28 (± 17) g/h.

Table 4. *Mean macronutrient consumption during the event*

Nutrient	Mean (SD)	Range
Total Energy (kJ)	9827 (3458)	5396 - 15975
Total CHO (g)	413 (195)	197 - 932
Total Protein (g)	57 (43)	13 - 186
Total Fat (g)	61 (31)	11 - 125
Energy (kJ/kg/h)	8.7 (4.4)	2.5 – 16.7
CHO (g/kg/h)	0.4 (0.3)	0.08 – 1.0
Protein (g/kg/h)	0.05 (0.04)	0.02 – 0.19
Fat (g/kg/h)	0.05 (0.03)	0.01 – 0.13
Energy density (kJ/g)	12 (3)	9 - 20
Total food carried (g)	854 (405)	282 - 1780

3.4. Blood β-Ketone Levels

Blood β-ketones significantly increased during the event (Fig. 2). There was a significant increase from pre [*Md* = 0.00 (0.00 – 0.00) mmol/L] to post [*Md* = 0.90 (0.35 – 1.15) mmol/L] event (z = -3.63, p < 0.001, n = 17). Those consuming less CHO tended to have higher post-ketone levels (CHO < 30 g/h: n = 11, mean post β-ketones = 1.24 (± 1.0) mmol/L; CHO 30-60 g/h: n = 3, mean post β-ketones = 0.63 (± 0.4) mmol/L; CHO > 60 g/h: n = 1, post β-ketones = 0.30 mmol/L). Correlation analysis showed a significant negative relationship between post-ketones and performance (Table 5).

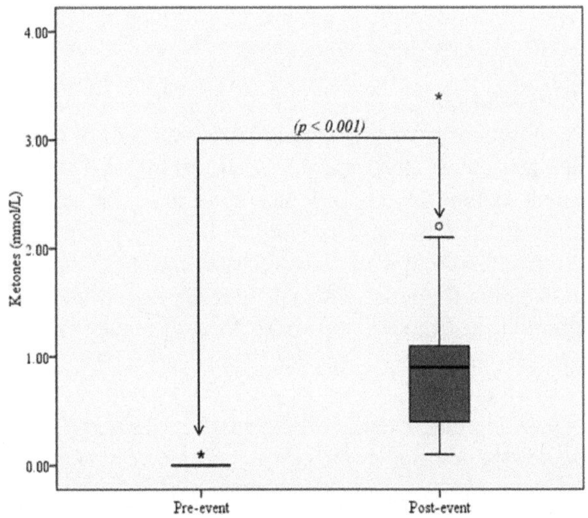

Figure 2. *Change in blood β-ketone levels during the event (o indicates outliers, * indicates outliers that are more than three box-lengths from the edge of the box).*

*Table 5. Correlation coefficients showing association with performance (*p < 0.05, **p < 0.01, *** p < 0.001)*

	Nutrient	Performance
Nutrient intake in the week prior	Energy (kJ/kg/d)	0.56*
	CHO (g/kg/d)	0.54*
	Protein (g/kg/d)	0.38
	Fat (g/kg/d)	0.43
Nutrient intake during the event	Energy (kJ/kg/h)	0.80***
	CHO (g/kg/h)	0.75**
	Protein (g/kg/h)	0.39
	Fat (g/kg/h)	0.46
	Energy density (kJ/g)	0.07
Other predictors	Post-event β-ketones (mmol/L)	- 0.60*
	BM (kg)	- 0.65**
	BMI (kgm^{-2})	- 0.55*
	Pack weight (kg)	- 0.46

3.5. Predictors of Performance

Both total energy and CHO consumed in the week prior to the LH were positively associated with performance when adjusted for BM (Table 5, Fig. 3). No such associations were seen with the other macronutrients. CHO consumption (g/kg/d) on days 4, 6 and 7 was also significantly associated with performance (Day 4: $r = .57, p = 0.03$; Day 6: $r = .59, p = 0.02$; Day 7: $r = .61, p = 0.02, n = 16$).

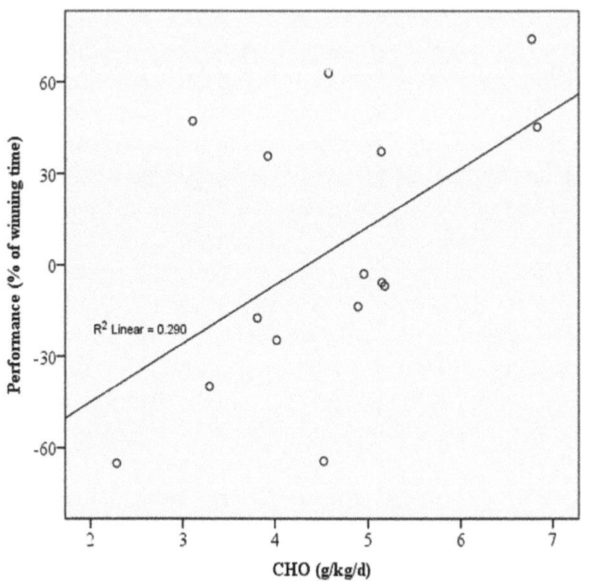

Figure 3. *Relationship between CHO consumed in the week prior and performance*

Energy and CHO consumed during the event also showed significant positive correlations with performance (Table 5, Fig. 4). No significant correlations were observed between fat, protein or energy density and performance. Asides from nutrient intake, lower BM and BMI were also associated with better performance.

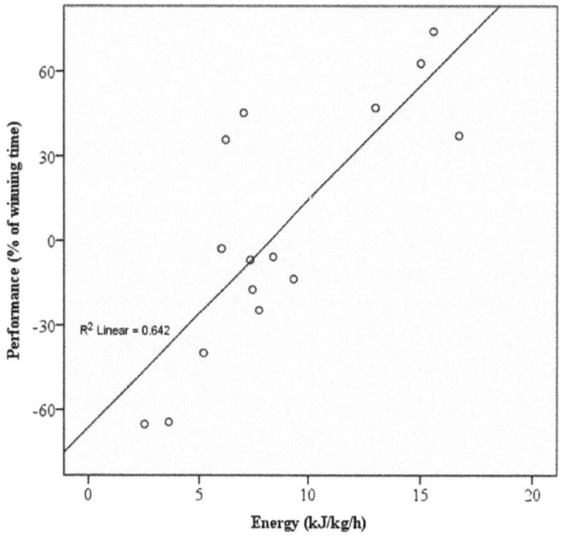

Figure 4. *Relationship between energy consumed during the event and performance*

Table 6 shows results from the multiple regression analysis that was performed for those variables that were associated with performance. The model performed suggests that together these variables explain 69% ($R^2 = .693$) of the variance in performance, with energy consumed during the event (kJ/kg/h) making a statistically significant unique contribution to performance (*beta* = 1.10, $p = 0.037$).

*Table 6. Linear regression model for performance (*p < 0.05)*

Model Summary: $R^2 = .693$, Adjusted $R^2 = .522$			
Variable	Regression coefficient (*beta*)	*t*	*p*
Energy prior (kJ/kg/d)	- .128	- .302	.770
CHO prior (g/kg/d)	.428	.965	.360
Energy during (kJ/kg/h)	1.096	2.452	.037*
CHO during (g/kg/h)	- .735	- 1.619	.140
BMI (kgm^{-2})	- .301	- 1.085	.306

4. Discussion

4.1. Nutrient Intake in the Week Prior to the Event

Energy consumption in the week prior to the event (145 kJ/kg/d, Table 1) was lower than that observed in other studies measuring energy intake from 7-day food diaries in male endurance athletes. Intakes of 280 kJ/kg/d have been previously reported for self-reported adequate eaters and 180 kJ/kg/d for small eaters [23], and intakes of 230 kJ/kg/d for Australian marathon runners [24]. However, the athletes in these studies were highly-trained and presumably undertaking larger quantities of training than the recreational athletes in the present study. In order to determine the extent of under-reporting, energy expenditure would need to be measured. It is important to note though that the athletes in the present study were volunteers and are therefore likely to be highly motivated and want to receive valuable feedback, which should limit conscious under-reporting.

Mean CHO intakes for the week were below the recommended 5-7 g/kg/d to meet the daily fuel needs of an athlete with a moderate training programme [25]. Despite over 65% of athletes reporting that they intended to increase their CHO intake in the week prior to the event, no participants came close to the CHO-loading recommendations of 10-12 g/kg/d in the 48 hours leading up to the event [25]. This is in line with findings from a previous study which reported that whilst CHO-loading is a well-known term, athletes in real-life often fail to reach daily CHO targets needed to maximize glycogen storage [26]. Similar findings were reported in a study observing the dietary intakes of cyclists prior to, and during, a 210 km cycle race [27]. They noted that the mean self-reported CHO intake of forty-five cyclists in the three days leading up to the race was just 5.6 ± 1.7 g/kg/d. Regarding alternative strategies, there was no indication in the present study of chronic high-fat diets with no participants meeting high-fat protocols published in previous research (2.6 g/kg/d) [28].

Both energy and CHO were positively associated with performance. These findings support those from controlled, intervention studies that have shown CHO loading can improve performance [6], and provides evidence that higher intakes of CHO can be beneficial in a 'real-life' setting. Results indicated that CHO consumption, particularly in the latter half of the week was more important to performance than earlier in the week. This supports the guidelines that shorter CHO loading protocols should be sufficient [29-30]. This is an important message for athletes since they appear to struggle to consume the amounts recommended.

4.2. Nutrient Intake During the Event

The mean overall energy consumption during the event (9,827 kJ) appears low. Energy expenditure was not calculated during this study, due to financial constraints and the difficulties in accurately measuring this in the field. However, a study carried out measuring energy expenditure by the doubly labelled water technique over ten consecutive days of hill-walking reported values of approximately 21,000 kJ/day [31]. Given the distances covered in the hill-walking study ranged from 10-35 km per day, and the distances in the present study were substantially higher, it is likely that the participants in the present study were in significant negative energy balance. This appears to be the case in many ultra-endurance studies; during an ironman triathlon endogenous fuel stores contributed to half or more of the total energy requirements of the athletes [5].

Energy intake was positively associated with performance during the event. This finding is similar to those reported by others observing similar races [2,18]. This suggests that negative energy balance is detrimental, but further evidence is warranted.

Endurance athletes are advised to consume at least 30-60 g/h of CHO during exercise [11], and up to 90 g/h for exercise lasting longer than 2.5 hours [12]. The average intake in this sample was just 28 g/h. On an individual basis eleven participants consumed < 30 – 60 g/h, four within the range and one participant higher. Adjusting for BM, only three participants met the 0.5 – 1 g/kg/h recommendation for CHO consumption during prolonged moderate-intensity exercise [32]. A similar mean intake of 31 g/h was reported in a Swiss mountain marathon, with over half the runners not meeting the minimal recommendation [18]. Other studies involving ultra-marathon running have reported slightly higher intakes; a mean figure of 43 g/h was published from seven subjects during a 100 km road running race [33]. Literature available on ultra-endurance exercise suggests that athletes struggle to meet these requirements unless other disciplines are included, for example: intakes of 69 g/h have been observed during an ironman triathlon [5], with the majority being consumed during the cycle leg; 63 g/h in male cyclists during a 210 km race [27]; and 52 g/h during a 384 km cycling event [34]. In order to meet the CHO demand during running events, the form of foods consumed and their mode of consumption requires further investigation.

As reported by Clark *et al.* [2], countless other studies performed on endurance exercise of shorter duration [10], and several cycling ultra-endurance events [27,34], CHO intake was positively associated with performance. This suggests that despite the potentially lower exercise intensity in such an event, CHO is the most important substrate to fuel the activity. In addition, those consuming sub-optimal amounts of CHO had higher levels of blood β-ketones post-event and post-blood β-ketone levels were negatively associated with performance, this further supports the need for CHO intake during prolonged events, given that ketones are an indicator of fat metabolism. During periods of glucose deficiency, such as fasting or prolonged exercise, ketone bodies can play a key role in sparing glucose utilization [35]. In a study performed on post-exercise ketosis it was found that whilst training status had no effect on post exercise ketone levels, diet prior to exercise did [36]. High-CHO diets were shown to prevent the onset of post-exercise ketonaemia whilst low-CHO diets enhanced it. The highest post-exercise ketone levels (3.88 mmol/L) were recorded in marathon runners following a glycogen-stripping regimen [36].

Other predictors of performance included BMI and BM. A key factor in performance may be leanness; however estimating body composition in the field is problematic. Conversely, lower BMI may reflect training status. Linear multiple regression analysis suggested that overall energy intake during the event was the best predictor of performance, stronger than physical characteristics, such as BMI, and nutrition in the week prior to the event. This suggests that advice should focus on increasing energy intake during such events, and in particular energy from CHO. Further research is needed regarding the type of CHO consumed and timing of intake.

4.3. Limitations

There are several limitations to this study. Having no measures of physical activity in the week prior to the event makes it difficult to measure the accuracy of the food diaries. It is likely that a certain degree of underreporting of dietary intake exists. Nutrient intake data during the event from the food inventory form, however, is likely to be more accurate. Food items consumed were known prior to the race and participants had time to note down details of the products they were taking with them. Food items listed on the inventory were checked by a researcher prior to the event and all leftover food was weighed on completion. It would have been useful to have a measure of energy expenditure though, so that the energy balance status of athletes could have been accurately assessed.

The sample size was small, given the total number of runners in the event, but is comparable to those in other field studies of similar design [5,33-34]. Finally, being a cross-sectional, observational study, no causal relationship can be drawn between intake and performance and various factors that could be contributing to performance are missing, such as measures of fitness, body composition and hydration status.

5. Conclusions

The present study shows that a range of foods, both specialized sports products and traditional whole-foods are consumed by athletes taking part in mountain marathons. Whilst CHO and energy intakes both prior, and in particular during the event, appear to be beneficial to performance, the intakes of athletes in this sample were below current recommendations for endurance athletes. Whilst the possibility of under-reporting exists regarding the pre-event food diaries, nutrient intake data obtained during the event is likely to have good accuracy. It can therefore be concluded with some certainty that participants were consuming suboptimal amounts of energy and CHO during the race. Reasons for this could be: lack of knowledge of recommendations; inadequate practical nutrition skills or food composition knowledge [32]; the weight burden of carrying sufficient food during events; or purposefully limiting intake due to potential gastro-intestinal discomfort associated with high intakes.

It is apparent that athletes need more guidance in order to meet the current recommendations and further research is needed to identify the best way to do this. Additional research is warranted to take into account the type and timing of macronutrient intake, fluid consumption, and the effects of other dietary constituents such as caffeine which have also been shown to improve endurance performance.

Acknowledgments

We would like to thank the event organizer: Simon Lumley, for his help and support with this study; the participants of the event who kindly gave up much of their time and made this research possible; and John and Sarah Haywood, Lee Mahon, Jackie Richards, Leo Stevenson, Nicola Davies, Ruth Hackett, Ian Lovegrove, Genevieve and Anthony Warburton and Rebecca Gobbi for their assistance with data collection.

References

[1] A. La Gerche, D.L. Prior, and H. Heidbuchel, "Strenuous endurance exercise: is more better for everyone? Our genes won't tell us." British Journal of Sports Medicine, vol. 45, pp. 412-426, 2011.

[2] H.R. Clark, M.E. Barker, and B,M. Corfe, "Nutritional Strategies of Mountain Marathon Competitors – An Observational Study." International Journal of Sport Nutrition and Exercise Metabolism, vol. 15, pp. 160-172, 2005.

[3] P.N. Ainslie, I.T. Campbell, J.P. Lambert, D.P.M. MacLaren, and T. Reilly, "Physiological and Metabolic Aspects of very Prolonged Exercise with Particular Reference to Hill Walking." Sports Medicine, vol. 35, pp. 619-647, 2005.

[4] R.B. Kreider, "Physiological considerations of ultraendurance performance." International Journal of Sport Nutrition, vol. 1, pp. 3-27, 1991.

[5] N.E. Kimber, J.J. Ross, S.L. Mason, and D.B. Speedy, "Energy balance during an ironman triathlon in male and female triathletes." International Journal of Sport Nutrition and Exercise Metabolism, vol. 12, pp. 47-62, 2002.

[6] J.A. Hawley, E.J. Schabort, T.D. Noakes, and S.C. Dennis, "Carbohydrate-loading and exercise performance: an update." Sports Medicine, vol. 24, pp. 73-81, 1997.

[7] C.J. Hulston, and A.E. Jeukendrup, A.E. "No placebo effect from carbohydrate intake during prolonged exercise." International Journal of Sport Nutrition and Exercise Metabolism, vol. 19, pp. 275-284, 2009.

[8] J.W. Smith, J.J. Zachweija, F. Peronnet, D.H. Passe, D. Massicotte, C. Lavoie, and D.D. Pascoe, "Fuel selection and cycling endurance performance with ingestion of [^{13}C] glucose: evidence for a carbohydrate dose response." Journal of Applied Physiology, vol. 108, pp. 1520-1529, 2010.

[9] K.L. Osterberg, J.J. Zachwieja, and J.W. Smith, "Carbohydrate and carbohydrate + protein for cycling time-trail performance." Journal of Sports Science, vol. 26, pp. 227-33, 2008.

[10] J. Temesi, N.A. Johnson, J. Raymond, C.A. Burdon, and H.T. O'Connor, "Carbohydrate ingestion during endurance exercise improves performance in adults." The Journal of Nutrition, vol. 141, pp. 890-897, 2011.

[11] American College of Sports Medicine (ACSM), American Dietetic Association & Dieticians of Canada. "Nutrition and Athletic Performance." Medicine and Science in Sports and Exercise, vol. 41, pp. 709-731, 2009.

[12] International Olympic Committee (IOC). "IOC consensus statement on sports nutrition 2010." Journal of Sports Sciences, vol. 29:sup1, pp. S3-S4, 2011.

[13] L.M. Burke, and J.A. Hawley, "Effects of short term fat-adaptation on metabolism and performance of prolonged exercise." Medicine and Science in Sports and Exercise, vol. 34, pp. 1492-1498, 2002.

[14] J.A. Hawley, F. Brouns, and A.E. Jeukendrup, A. "Strategies to enhance fat utilisation during exercise." Sports Medicine, vol. 25, pp. 241-257, 1998.

[15] R.J. Maughan, P.L. Greenhaff, M. Gleeson, C.E. Fenn, and J.B. Leiper, "The effect of dietary carbohydrate intake on the metabolic response to prolonged walking on consecutive days." European Journal of Applied Physiology, vol. 56, pp. 583-591, 1987.

[16] P.N. Ainslie, I.T. Campbell, K.N. Frayn, S.M. Humphreys, D.P.M. MacLaren, and T. Reilly, "Physiological and metabolic responses to a hill walk." Journal of Applied Physiology, vol. 92, pp. 179-187, 2002.

[17] L.G.C.E. Pugh, "Accidental hypothermia in walkers, climbers, and campers: report to the Medical Commission on Accident Prevention." British Medical Journal, vol.1, pp. 123-129, 1966.

[18] M. Kruesman, S. Bucher, M. Bovard, B. Kayser, and p.A. Bovier, "Nutrient intake and performance during a mountain marathon: an observational study." European Journal of Applied Physiology, vol. 94, pp. 151-157, 2005.

[19] K.J. Stuempfle, M.D. Hoffman, L.B. Weschler, I.R. Rogers, and T. Hew-Butler, "Race diet of finishers and non-finishers in a 100 mile (161 km) mountain footrace." Journal of the American College of Nutrition, vol. 30, pp. 529-535, 2011.

[20] The Longmynd Hike. "The Hike Route." Available at: http://www.longmyndhike.org.uk/hikeroute (Accessed on: 29.11.09).

[21] R.A. McCance, and E.M. Widdowson, "The Composition of Foods", 6th Edition. Food Standards Agency and the Institute of Food Research. Cambridge: Royal Society of Chemistry, 2002.

[22] Abbott. "Optium Blood Glucose Monitoring System: User's Guide." Abbott Laboratories Ltd: Abbott Diabetes Care, 2009.

[23] J.L. Thompson, M.M. Manore, and J.S. Skinner, J.S. "Daily energy expenditure in male endurance athletes with differing energy intakes." Medicine and Science in Sports and Exercise, vol. 27, pp. 347-354, 1995.

[24] L.M. Burke, R.A. Gollan, and R.S.D. Read, "Dietary intakes and food use of groups of elite Australian male athletes." International Journal of Sports Nutrition, vol. 1, pp. 378-394, 1991.

[25] L.M. Burke, J.A. Hawley, S.H.S. Wong, and A.E. Jeukendrup, "Carbohydrates for training and competition." Journal of Sports Sciences, vol. 29:sup1, pp. S17-S27, 2011.

[26] L.M. Burke, and R.S.D. Read, "A study of carbohydrate loading techniques used by marathon runners." Canadian Journal of Sports Science, vol. 12, pp. 6-10, 1987.

[27] L. Havemann, and J.H. Goedecke, "Nutritional practises of male cyclists before and during an ultraendurance event." International Journal of Sport Nutrition and Exercise Metabolism, vol. 18, pp. 551-566, 2008.

[28] A.L. Carey, H.M. Staudacher, N.K. Cummings, N.K. Stepto, V. Nikolopoulos, L.M. Burke, and J.A. Hawley, "Effects of fat adaptation and carbohydrate restoration on prolonged endurance exercise." *Journal of Applied Physiology, vol. 91*, pp. 115-122, 2001.

[29] W.M. Sherman, D.L. Costill, W.J. Fink, and J.M. Miller, "Effect of exercise-diet manipulation on muscle glycogen and its subsequent utilisation during performance." International Journal of Sports Medicine, vol. 2, pp. 114-118, 1981.

[30] V.A. Bussau, T.J. Fairchild, A. Rao, P. Steele, and P.A. Fournier, "Carbohydrate loading in human muscle: an improved 1 day protocol." European Journal of Applied Physiology, vol. 87, pp. 290-295, 2002.

[31] P.N. Ainslie, I.T. Campbell, K.N. Frayn, S.M. Humphreys, D.P.M. MacLaren, T. Reilly, and K.R. Weserterp, "Energy balance, metabolism, hydration and performance during strenuous hill walking: the effect of age." Journal of Applied Physiology, vol. 93, pp. 714-723, 2002.

[32] L.M. Burke, G.R. Cox, N.K. Cummings, and B. Desbrow, "Guidelines for daily carbohydrate intake: do athletes achieve them?" Sports Medicine, vol. 31, pp. 267-299, 2001.

[33] K.E. Fallon, E. Broad, M.W. Thompson, and P.A. Reull, "Nutritional and fluid intake in a 100-km ultramarathon." International Journal of Sports Nutrition, vol. 8, pp. 24-35, 1998.

[34] K.E. Black, P.M.L. Skidmore, and R.C. Brown, "Energy intakes of ultraendurance cyclists during competition, an observational study." International Journal of Sport Nutrition and Exercise Metabolism, vol. 22, pp. 19-23, 2012.

[35] L. Laffel, "Ketone bodies: a review of physiology, pathophysiology and application of monitoring to diabetes." Diabetes, Metabolism Research and Reviews, vol. 15, pp. 412-426, 1999.

[36] J.H. Koeshlag, T.D. Noakes, and A.W. Sloan, "Post-exercise ketosis." Journal of Physiology, vol. 301, pp. 79-90, 1980.

20

An assessment of the hydration status of recreational endurance athletes during mountain marathon events

Elizabeth Mahon[1], Allan Hackett[1], Timothy Stott[1], Keith George[2], Ian Davies[1]

[1]Faculty of Education, Health and Community, Liverpool John Moores University, Liverpool, United Kingdom
[2]Research Institute for Sport and Exercise Sciences, Liverpool John Moores University, Liverpool, United Kingdom

Email address:
E.Haywood@ljmu.ac.uk (E. Mahon)

Abstract: Changes in hydration status have been shown to have deleterious effects on physiological functioning, physical performance, mental decision making, and subjective sensation of effort. This exploratory study assessed the hydration status of athletes taking part in mountain marathon events and the implications on performance, cognition and well-being markers. Twenty-nine male recreational athletes from the Original Mountain Marathon (OMM) and nineteen from the Longmynd Hike (LH) provided urine samples before, at mid-point (in the OMM) and after the events. Body mass; reaction time tests; and subjective ratings of well-being and effort were also collected/performed at these time points. Post-urine specific gravity (U_{sg}) values [(OMM: 1.023 (range: 1.008 – 1.038) g/ml; LH: 1.024 (range: 1.014 – 1.035) g/ml] were significantly higher than pre-values [(OMM: 1.013 (range: 1.002 – 1.026) g/ml; LH: 1.013 (range: 1.002 – 1.026) g/ml] in both events ($p < 0.01$), but there was no significant change from mid- to post-event in the OMM ($p > 0.05$). There was no association between hydration status and overall performance in the LH, whilst change in U_{sg} from pre- to mid-event was positively associated with performance in the OMM (r = .561, $p = 0.004$). Whilst no associations were observed between hydration status and reaction time, rate of perceived exertion and subjective ratings of nausea showed positive associations with U_{sg}. These findings suggest that although changes in hydration status of this level may not significantly affect performance, they can impact on participant sensations of effort and well-being.

Keywords: Fluid, Exercise, Cognition, Running, Hill-Walking

1. Introduction

Prolonged exercise increases the requirement for water intake in order to maintain hydration. Even modest changes in hydration status (equivalent to 2% loss in body mass) can have deleterious effects on physical performance [1-2], mental decision making, physiological functioning and temperature regulation [3], all important safety considerations in a mountainous environment. Previous research has shown that during a two-day mountain marathon, only 13% of subjects finished well hydrated and 27% reported symptoms of dehydration such as headaches, cramps, and feeling faint [4]. Consuming fluid at regular intervals during exercise is therefore important to optimize performance and safeguard health and well-being.

Guidelines for fluid consumption during exercise have changed over the years; an ultra-distance runner in the 1940s – 1960s was cited in Noakes (2003, p.199) [5]: *"To run a complete marathon without any fluid replacement was regarded as the ultimate aim of most runners and a test of their fitness"*. In the 1970s, athletes were advised to stay ahead of thirst and maximising rehydration during events was of primary concern [6]. However, following several cases of hyponatremia as a result of over-hydration in endurance events [7], it has since been realised that taking on too much fluid can be as serious as taking on too little and therefore fluid replacement guidelines need to take into account a myriad of factors, such as: exercise intensity; duration; environmental conditions; and individual sweat rates. The International Olympic Committee (IOC) [8] state that the goal of drinking during exercise should be to limit dehydration to less than about 2% of body mass (BM), but not to drink so much that weight is gained during exercise.

Although it is commonly believed that dehydration equal to 2% BM loss can have a detrimental effect on endurance performance [9], the data regarding the effects in temperate conditions remains equivocal. Whilst several studies have observed detriments to performance [10-11], others have shown improvements in performance with markers of dehydration [4,12]. Therefore, more research is needed to resolve the impact of fluid balance on endurance performance. This is particularly important in prolonged exercise, as the longer the exercise duration the greater the cumulative effects of any differences between fluid needs and fluid replacement. As a result one would expect that dehydration or over-hydration in prolonged events would have the potential to have greater negative effects on performance and health.

The main objective of the present study was to assess the hydration status of athletes competing in mountain marathon events and to study the association between levels of hydration and performance. As a secondary objective, the associations between hydration status and cognitive performance and well-being were also investigated as these may be important to athletes whilst in mountain environments. The majority of research studying the effects of dehydration on cognitive function have used heat and exercise to induce rapid dehydration in laboratory settings [13], which may yield very different results to progressive and slower development of dehydration in temperate conditions out in the field. In addition, given the wide range of ages of the competitors that take part in mountain marathons, hydration status was compared with respect to age to determine whether, as published elsewhere [14-15]; older athletes are more prone to dehydration.

2. Method

2.1. Study Design

This cross-sectional study was designed to assess the hydration status of recreational athletes competing in two UK mountain marathon events in the autumn of 2009. Hydration status was then related to measures of overall performance, cognition, rate of perceived exertion (RPE) and subjective ratings of well-being.

2.2. Setting

The events used were the Original Mountain Marathon (OMM) and the Longmynd Hike (LH). The OMM is an unsupported (no food or drink is provided) two-day race combining fell-running and orienteering over mountainous terrain, held in a different region of the UK each year. The 2009 event was held at the end of October in the Elan Valley, Wales. Participants compete in teams of two and it is designed to test fitness and orienteering skills in extreme circumstances. Each team must carry all their equipment including that needed for an overnight camp. Participants are grouped into classes, dependent on fitness and experience: Long (approximately 65 km over the two days), Medium (approximately 50 km) or Short (approximately 45 km).

The LH is an 80.5 km continuous, individual competitive mountain marathon set in the countryside of South Shropshire and the Welsh Marches UK, during the first weekend of October each year. The course includes approximately 2,400 m of climbing covering eight summits. No food is provided during the event; however water is available at the checkpoints on route.

2.3. Participants

Recreational athletes were targeted for entry into the study as a growing number of such athletes are taking up ultra-endurance racing [16]. Once ethical approval was granted for the study by the Liverpool (Adult) Research Ethics Committee, event organizers were approached via email for permission to recruit participants. Competitors were encouraged to participate through links on the event websites and flyers sent out with entry packs. In total 48 male participants were recruited to this study; sample characteristics were as follows: OMM [$n = 29$; age (18-39 y: $n = 16$, 40-49 y: $n = 7$, 50+ y: $n = 6$); class (long: $n = 6$, medium: $n = 12$, short: $n = 11$)], LH [$n = 19$; age (18-39 y: $n = 5$, 40-49 y: $n = 7$, 50+ y: $n = 7$); course completion time 16 (± 3) h]. There were various levels of participation in the study; this is reflected in the results.

2.4. Protocol and Procedures

All procedures described below were performed immediately prior to the start of the mountain marathons at the event headquarters, at the mid-point campsite at the end of day one (for the OMM only), and at the end of the events.

2.4.1. Body Mass

The BM of each participant was recorded using calibrated scales accurate to 0.1 kg. Participants were weighed with their clothes on, but without shoes and accessories (caps, bottles, bags, wallets, keys etc). Total BM change was used as an indicator of fluid loss/gain.

2.4.2. Estimation of Fluid Intake

Fluid consumption was estimated by participants retrospectively (at mid-camp and post-event) to the nearest half-litre per hour by questionnaire [4].

2.4.3. Urine Sampling and Analysis

Urine specific gravity (U_{sg}) was used to assess hydration status as the validity and reliability has been tested and it is considered one of the most appropriate methods for use in the field [17]. Percentage BM loss over the events was used as a second measure, however these data must be considered with caution as athletes were not weighed naked, and it is generally only considered accurate over relatively short time periods of 1 to 4 hours. When measurements are taken over intervals larger than this water exchange due to substrate oxidation and respiratory water loss become significant factors [18].

U_{sg} was measured using a visual hand held refractometer (Model: Index Instruments Ref: 301). Liquid reference standards with an accuracy of ± 0.0005 refractive index were used prior to each testing period to check for precision of the instrument. Participants were provided with a sample pot and were asked to provide a midstream urine sample as close as possible to the start, mid-point and the end of the events. U_{sg} was assessed immediately on receipt of the sample in a well-lit area. During each testing period 10% of the samples were tested twice to test the reliability of the refractometer. Pre-event samples were considered euhydrated with values ≤ 1.020 g/ml. The ACSM's position on Exercise and Fluid Replacement (2007, p.385) [19] state that *"a person with a first morning U_{sg} ≤ 1.020 can be considered as euhydrated"*. Post-event samples were considered in the normal range with values between 1.013 and 1.029 g/ml; samples with values of 1.030 g/ml or higher being considered to be significantly dehydrated; and values below 1.012 g/ml were considered hyperhydrated. These values are based on what is typically seen during dehydration, exercise and rehydration [20].

2.4.4. Cognitive Performance

As mountain marathons involve competitors making quick navigational decisions, a choice reaction time test (CRT), considered a decision task, was the most suitable cognitive test to mimic the tasks involved in the 'real-life' setting. Diet and exercise interventions have shown that CRTs show greater sensitivity than simple reaction time tests [21]. A unique laptop-based CRT was designed, programmed and tested (r = 0.91) for this study. Participants completed a familiarisation trial prior to their first recorded attempt as prior testing (unpublished) showed it to be subject to learning effects which may affect the test-retest reliability.

2.4.5. Subjective Measurements

A questionnaire was designed to allow participants to rate their feelings of "thirst", "nausea", "tiredness", "physical fatigue" and "mental fatigue". These ratings were assessed by a 100-mm visual analogue rating scale labelled from "not at all" to "extremely". Participants were advised to mark a line through the scale at a point between the two extremes of the symptom being rated, which they considered to indicate the degree of the subjective feeling they were experiencing. The nature of these rating scales and their validity in relation to fluid and food consumption have been previously described [22], and have been used in studies of similar design [23].

To determine perception of fatigue during the event, participants were asked to provide a score using the Borg 15-point rating of perceived exertion (RPE) scale [24]. Ratings were taken at mid-point and at the end of the events. This scale has been adopted as the standard instrument for evaluating the perception of whole-body exertion during exercise and has been used by countless studies in the sports and exercise field in laboratory settings [21,25], in mountainous environments [26], and during ultra-endurance events [27].

Finally, mid- and post-event questionnaires were used to gather information on the occurrence of symptoms during the marathons that may be linked to dehydration (e.g. headaches), where fluid was obtained from during the events, and whether participants felt they had drank sufficient amounts.

2.4.6. Overall Performance

Overall performance was calculated as a reciprocal percentage of the winning time [4], times were age-adjusted and class-specific for the OMM:

200 – (individual time / winning time x 100)

2.5. Statistical Procedures

Statistical analyses were performed with SPSS (version 17.0). Descriptive statistics (mean, standard deviation (SD), minimum, maximum) were calculated for pre, mid and post BM, percentage BM loss, U_{sg} and cognitive test scores. The change in measurement from pre-, to mid-, to post-event was also calculated for these variables. Frequencies were reported for hourly estimates of fluid consumption, reported symptoms and number of participants meeting hydration cut-offs.

A one-way ANOVA was used to investigate differences in U_{sg} values between participants of different age or class, and to determine whether there were any statistically significant differences in cognitive performance depending on hydration status. Paired sample t-tests were used to detect for significant differences between BM, U_{sg} and cognitive test scores at different time points. Independent sample t-tests were employed to identify any differences in U_{sg} values between those reporting having experienced a symptom and those not. Pearson's and Spearman's rank correlation coefficients were performed to examine associations between U_{sg} values and overall performance, and subjective ratings. All tests were two-tailed, with alpha < 0.05.

3. Results

3.1. Fluid Intake and Hydration Status

Table 1. *Hourly fluid consumption estimates*

Fluid consumption (L/h)	LH (n = 19)	OMM Day 1 (n = 29)	OMM Day 2 (n = 28)
< 0.25	5	10	9
0.25 – 0.5	12	19	13
> 0.5 - 1	2	0	2
> 1 – 1.5	0	0	2
> 1.5	0	0	2

Information from questionnaires revealed that the majority of participants in both events estimated their fluid consumption whilst running to be between 0.25 – 0.5 L/hour (Table 1). In the LH, water was available at the checkpoints on route; responses from questionnaires indicated that all runners made use of this. In addition, 74% of participants carried their own drinks. In the OMM, no drinks were provided (with the exception of water at mid-camp) and so fluid was either obtained from that carried or from natural sources. On day one, 57% of participants carried their own drinks, whilst on day two this dropped to 32%. A considerable percentage of both samples felt that they drank insufficient fluids: 37% of the LH and 64% of the OMM on day one and 52% on day two. Timing of intake and type of fluid consumed was not recorded.

Data regarding hydration status is presented in Tables 2 and 3. U_{sg} significantly increased from pre- to mid-event (OMM: $t = -6.03$, $p < 0.001$, $n = 27$) and pre- to post-event (OMM: $t = -5.65$, $p < 0.001$, $n = 27$; LH: $t = -4.13$, $p = 0.001$, $n = 17$). There was no further significant increase from mid- to post-event in the OMM. For both samples the mean pre-event U_{sg} was considered euhydrated (≤ 1.020 g/ml). Only two participants in each sample started the event with an U_{sg} > 1.020 g/ml. In the LH, the mean post-event U_{sg} was > 1.020 g/ml but below that considered significantly dehydrated in sportsmen (> 1.029 g/ml) [20]. Using this higher figure, just four participants in the LH sample were considered significantly dehydrated at the end of the event. In the OMM, only one participant was considered significantly dehydrated at the end of day one, but eight by the end of day two. There were no significant differences in U_{sg} values between participants of different age or class.

BM significantly decreased from pre- to mid-event ($t = 5.83$, $p < 0.001$, $n = 27$) and pre- to post-event (OMM: $t = 4.94$, $p < 0.001$, $n = 27$; LH: $t = 6.83$, $p < 0.001$, $n = 18$). There was no further significant decrease from mid- to post-event in the OMM. The mean percentage BM losses (LH: 1.4%; OMM: 1.3% day one, 1.4% overall) were within the 0 – 2% range considered acceptable during endurance exercise [19]. In the LH, four of the seventeen participants lost more than 2% of their BM during the event and no participants gained weight. In the OMM, three lost greater than 2% of their BM on day one and seven throughout the event as a whole. One individual lost more than 5% of their total BM. Conversely, two participants gained weight. However, there was no relationship between percentage BM loss and U_{sg} in either sample.

In the LH there were no associations with U_{sg} and overall performance in the event. In the OMM change in U_{sg} from pre- to mid-event (day one) was positively associated with performance ($r = .561$, $p = 0.004$, $n = 24$) (Fig.1).

Table 2. *Hydration measures of OMM participants (**Significant difference in values between pre and post (p < 0.01), †† Significant difference in values between pre and mid (p < 0.01))*

Measurement	Time point	OMM ($n = 27$)	
		Mean (SD)	**Range**
Specific gravity of urine (U_{sg}) (g/ml)	Pre	1.013 (0.006)	1.002 - 1.026
	Mid	1.021 (0.007)††	1.010 - 1.033
	Post	1.023 (0.008)**	1.008 - 1.038
Body mass (kg)	Pre	81.0 (10.0)	60.9 - 104.8
	Mid	80.0 (10.2)††	60.3 - 104.5
	Post	79.9 (10.0)**	60.7 - 103.0
Body mass loss (%)	Day One	1.3 (0.7)	-0.41 - 4.29
	Overall	1.4 (1.5)	-0.85 - 5.36

Table 3. *Hydration measures of LH participants (**Significant difference in values between pre and post (p < 0.01))*

Measurement	Time point	LH ($n = 18$)	
		Mean (SD)	**Range**
Specific gravity of urine (U_{sg}) (g/ml)	Pre	1.013 (0.009)	1.002 - 1.026
	Post	1.024 (0.007)**	1.014 - 1.035
Body mass (kg)	Pre	76.3 (10.3)	63.7 - 109.2
	Post	75.2 (10.4)**	63.0 - 108.7
Body mass loss (%)	Overall	1.4 (0.9)	0.07 - 2.99

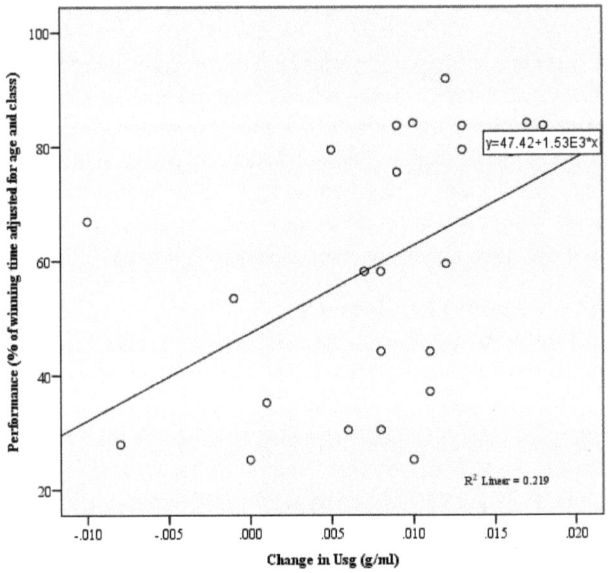

Figure 1. *Change in Usg and performance during day one of the OMM*

3.2. Hydration Status and Cognitive Performance

Reaction time tests were performed pre-, mid- and post-event to determine the effects of hydration status on cognitive function. The results are displayed in Table 4. In the LH, mean time taken to respond to the reaction time test significantly increased from pre- to post-event. In contrast, there were no significant differences in reaction times between the three time points in the OMM. When grouped according to hydration status (< 1.013 g/ml; 1.013 – 1.029 g/ml; and > 1.029 g/ml) there were no significant differences between groups in either absolute reaction times or changes in reaction times across the events (Fig.2).

Table 4. *Choice reaction time test scores: pre, mid and post event (**Significant difference in values between pre and post (p < 0.01))*

Event	Time point	CRT (time taken to respond (ms))	
		Mean (SD)	**Range**
OMM ($n = 25$)	Pre	3248 (644)	1970 – 4593
	Mid	3314 (624)	2348 – 4840
	Post	3251 (590)	2461 – 4610
LH ($n = 17$)	Pre	3121 (629)	2457 – 4615
	Post	3788 (872)**	2512 – 6328

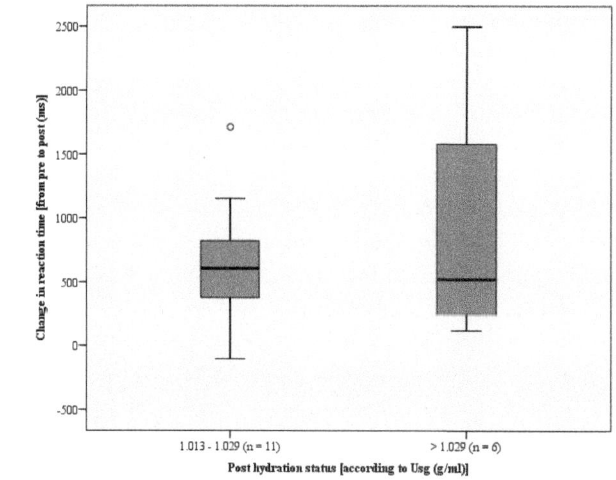

Figure 2. *Change in choice reaction time with hydration status in LH participants (*^{O} *Indicates outliers)*

3.3. Hydration Status and Subjective Measures of Well-Being

Correlation analyses were performed to identify associations between hydration status (according to absolute, and changes in, U_{sg} values) and subjective sensations, such as those reported on the visual analogue scales and RPE scores. In both samples there were strong positive correlations between U_{sg} values and self-reported ratings of nausea; in the LH post U_{sg} was positively associated with ratings of nausea on the post subjective-measures questionnaire ($r = .534$, $p = .027$, $n = 17$), and in the OMM mid-event U_{sg} values were positively associated with day one ratings of nausea ($r = .513$, $p = .007$, $n = 26$). In addition, in the OMM sample, mid-point RPE scores showed positive correlation with change in U_{sg} values over day one ($r = .566$, $p = .005$, $n = 23$).

On the mid- and post-event questionnaires participants were asked to report whether they suffered from any symptoms characteristic of dehydration. In the LH, mean post-event U_{sg} values were higher in those suffering from headache, cramp, stomach discomfort and nausea, compared to those who did not report these symptoms. However, there were only significant differences in post U_{sg} values between those experiencing headaches [1.029 (± 0.004) g/ml; $n = 6$] and those not [1.022 (± 0.008) g/ml; $n = 11$; $p = 0.044$] (Fig.3) and those suffering from stomach discomfort [1.031 (± 0.004) g/ml; $n = 4$] and those not [1.022 (± 0.007) g/ml; $n = 13$; $p = 0.025$].

In the OMM, mean mid-event U_{sg} values were significantly higher in those suffering from headaches [1.029 (± 0.003) g/ml; $n = 4$] than those not [1.019 (± 0.006) g/ml; $n = 22$; $p = 0.007$] (Fig.4); in those experiencing cramp [1.025 (± 0.005) g/ml; $n = 12$] than those not [1.017 (± 0.006) g/ml; $n = 14$; $p = 0.001$]; in those who reported stomach discomfort [1.027 (± 0.004) g/ml; $n = 6$] compared to those who did not [1.019 (± 0.006) g/ml; $n = 20$; $p = 0.003$]; and in those who expressed having felt nauseous [1.028 (± 0.002) g/ml; $n = 7$] in comparison to those who did not [1.018 (± 0.005) g/ml; $n = 19$; $p < 0.001$], during day one. No significant differences were observed with post-event U_{sg} values and day two symptoms.

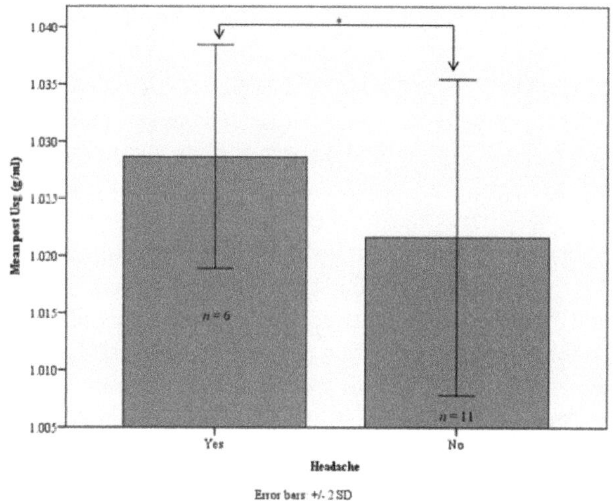

Figure 3. *A comparison of post urine specific gravity and occurrence of headaches in LH participants (*Significant difference between groups (p < 0.05))*

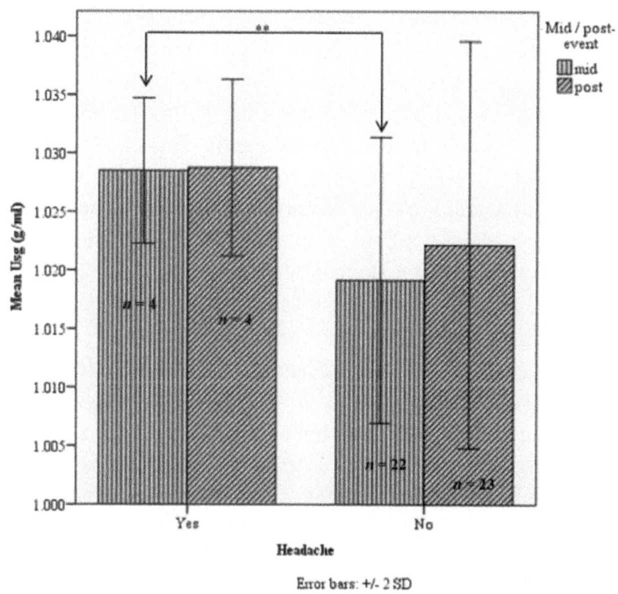

Figure 4. *A comparison of urine specific gravity and occurrence of headaches mid and post-event in OMM participants (**Significant difference between groups (p < 0.01))*

4. Discussion

4.1. Fluid Intake and Hydration Status

Hourly fluid intake could not be determined exactly but estimates are similar to those in other mountain races. A study on mountain marathon athletes using the same method reported that over three-quarters of athletes estimated their fluid consumption to be ≤ 500 ml/h [4]. In studies where fluid intake was more precisely measured: intakes of 545 ml/h have been published during a 44 km Swiss mountain marathon [28]; and 422 ml/h in runners during an 80 km mountain trail race [29]. Studies investigating different types of ultra-endurance events have found higher intakes when other disciplines apart from running are involved; intakes of 716 ml/h have been reported during an ironman triathlon [30]. The differences seen in fluid intake will not only be due to the format of the event, but also due to the environmental temperature and whether aid stations are available. In the present study, those competing in the OMM often had to rely on finding water from natural sources, whereas in the LH it was available at checkpoints. In those studies described above where fluid was measured, these values were all recorded from fluids taken from aid stations.

Due to different race conditions, comparing fluid intake is not the most useful measure, as requirements will differ, therefore it is more important to monitor the hydration status of athletes. In this study the specific gravity of urine samples was measured to assess hydration status. In the LH, the post-event range in U_{sg} values was 1.014 – 1.035 g/ml, representing wide variation in the hydration status of athletes completing the event (Table 3). Whilst the mean value (1.024 g/ml) was within the range considered normal 1.013 – 1.029 g/ml after exercise [20], four out of the 18 participants had values considered significantly dehydrated (> 1.029 g/ml). In the OMM, the mean U_{sg} values were similar at the end of each day (Day 1 (mid): 1.021 g/ml; day 2 (post): 1.023 g/ml) (Table 2), although the range was larger at the end of day two and more participants were significantly dehydrated; eight post-event versus just one at mid-camp. This could suggest that some participants failed to sufficiently re-hydrate at mid-camp and started day two in an already dehydrated state. This agrees with findings from Clark *et al.* [4] who took a measure of hydration status at the start of day two across a range of mountain marathon events. They found that whilst some participants had managed to rehydrate over the mid-camp rest, others remained severely dehydrated. Conversely, four participants in the OMM had U_{sg} values < 1.013 g/ml at the end of both days, suggesting potential over-drinking, which is generally associated with inexperienced runners. In studies where athletes have had to qualify for entry into the mountain race, and thus include possibly more experienced runners, there have been no reports of athletes drinking to excess [29].

A surprising finding of the present study, given the wide range of ages represented, was that no significant differences were found in hydration status with age. Several studies have reported that older athletes are more likely to become dehydrated [14,15]. Whilst older adults have been shown to consume adequate volumes of fluid on a daily basis under normal conditions, an age-related blunting of thirst response to water deprivation or exercise exists, making them more susceptible to dehydration [31,32]. One suggestion for this is that older adults tend to have an increased resting plasma osmolality, which may lead to a higher osmotic operating point for thirst sensation [33]. As a result older adults are often slower to restore body fluid homeostasis. It is possible that in the present study there were not large enough numbers of older athletes to detect significant differences in hydration status.

The majority of field studies that have estimated hydration status have used percentage BM loss as an indicator. Mean BM loss in the present study was considerably lower (approximately 1.4%) than that reported in other ultra-endurance studies of around 3-5% [28-29,34]. As BM loss was not associated with U_{sg} values in either sample it is likely that there is considerable error associated with the percentage BM loss data in this study. Firstly, it is important to establish euhydrated BM in participants in order to use BM change as an indicator of dehydration; secondly, over prolonged exercise substrate oxidation may contribute to changes in BM; for example, fat oxidation actually results in a net gain in BM as the mass of the carbon dioxide generated is less than the mass of the oxygen consumed [35-36]. The latter, however, is unlikely to result in profound changes and will result in similar errors in the other studies mentioned. It is likely that the main reason BM losses in the current study were less than those previously reported is that the participants in this study were weighed with their clothes on, which were likely heavier at the end due to wet weather conditions during both events.

4.2. Hydration Status with Performance

In the LH there was no association with U_{sg} values and overall performance; however, in the OMM day one U_{sg} values were positively associated with overall performance (Fig.1). This finding supports those of Clark *et al.* [4]; who reported that dehydration at the end of day two was positively associated with performance and Kao *et al.* [12]; who showed a significant relationship between percentage BM loss in a 24 hour ultra-marathon and performance. These findings contradict those of McConell *et al.* [10] and Fallowfield *et al.* [11], who previously reported negative effects of dehydration on endurance exercise performance in temperate climes. These conflicting results suggest that the relationship between hydration status and performance is complex and is not only likely due to temperature, exercise intensity, duration, and protocol, but also individual fitness and the physiological characteristics of the study participants. The different findings between the OMM and the LH could be due to the type of athletes the events attract. Whilst the LH is a smaller event comprising predominantly of local recreational athletes, the OMM is an international event attracting more experienced athletes. It has been proposed that top-level athletes may be better able to sustain performance, despite becoming dehydrated and it may be that the improvement in performance observed is due to them carrying less weight as fluid [4].

The possible physiological mechanisms for an increase in performance with dehydration are unclear, however the author hypothesises that dehydrated blood would lead to elevated blood glucose concentrations, which could result in increased transport of glucose into cells. In addition, blood concentration of haematocrit would also increase consequently enhancing blood oxygen levels. As glucose and oxygen are rate limiting in exercise performance, higher concentrations of these could be the reason for the improvement in performance seen.

This is therefore another study that challenges the well-established belief that euhydration is necessary to maintain performance during endurance exercise. Marino *et al.* [37] also did this when they reported participants performed as well when exercising for 60 minutes at 20°C when fully hydrated, as at 33°C without hydration. They investigated neuromuscular responses to hydration status and found adjustments were made allowing the attainment of similar core body temperatures, heart rates and performance times. It has been suggested [38] that these adjustments could be made as the exercise was self-paced, not of fixed-intensity like many of the exercise protocols used [10-11], which have led to the current recommendations. Whereas fixed intensity exercise to exhaustion only allows an all-or-nothing response, self-paced exercise of a set distance, like that performed in mountain marathons, allows continual behavioural adjustments that may affect performance [38].

Another theory is rather than dehydration itself negatively impacting on performance, it may be that not drinking to the satisfaction of thirst is responsible for the decrement in exercise performance found in many studies [39]. A meta-analysis of two research articles and eight individual studies reported drinking according to the dictate of thirst was associated with an increase in TT performance compared with a rate of drinking below (+5.2 ± 4.6%, p = 0.01), or above (+2.4 ± 5.0%, p = 0.40), thirst [39]. This could account for why dehydration has not been found to negatively affect performance in many observational studies on "real-life" events when participants are free to drink as they desire [4,12], providing fluids are available.

Therefore, whilst laboratory-based studies are useful to determine physiological responses to exercise, field-based research is crucial to determine the effects in 'real-life' competition. Whilst this present study cannot conclude that dehydration improves performance, it suggests that moderate levels of dehydration in cool climates do not significantly reduce overall performance.

4.3. Hydration Status and Cognitive Performance

A greater decline was seen in performance in the reaction time tests in the LH sample than the OMM (Table 4). This is likely to be due to the continuous nature of the LH event allowing no time for rest and recovery. Improvements in performance were seen in the mean post-event scores of OMM competitors compared to mid-event scores, suggesting that the previously discussed learning effect associated with such tests outweighed any effects of fatigue. This indicates that perhaps further familiarisation is required with such tests before their use in the main study.

No significant differences were observed in either event between hydration status and cognitive performance in the CRT test (Fig.2). These findings were surprising; as it might be expected that dehydration would impair cognitive performance as adequate hydration is required for homeostasis and maintaining brain function [13]. Whilst the effects of dehydration on cognitive performance and brain function are not entirely known, there are several hormonal and cellular theories [40]. Dehydration leads to the activation of the hypothalamic-pituitary-adrenocortical axis and to increased production of the stress hormones i.e. cortisol. Studies have shown that hyercortisolaemia tends to worsen various cognitive functions such as perception, spatial ability and memory [41-42]. Other work has shown that changes in electrolyte concentrations during dehydration can alter brain activity [40]. However, it is likely that the reason no negative effect of dehydration on cognitive performance was seen in the present study, was that dehydration was not severe enough among these participants. A recent review of the literature has reported that the performance of simple attention tasks, such as reaction time, is not usually impaired at dehydration levels of 1-2% in cold environmental conditions [43]. There are however some studies that have found a deterioration, for example; a negative effect of dehydration on cognitive processing time has been reported in hill-walkers [14]. It is therefore possible that individuals respond differently to dehydration and some are better able to cope than others. The large range of results displayed in Figure 2 support this hypothesis and consequently a larger sample size would be needed to make any firm conclusions. Another possible factor in the response to dehydration may be age. In the hill-walking study [14] where dehydration did affect cognition, the mean age of the sample was 56 ± 3 years, older than the present study sample.

4.4. Hydration Status and Well-Being

Whilst the findings from this study suggest that the level of dehydration reported here does not significantly affect measures of performance, it does appear to have an impact on the athletes' well-being. In the OMM, RPE at the end of day one was associated with higher changes in U_{sg} values, which agrees with a laboratory-based study that reported an increased rating of fatigue with 2.8% dehydration versus euhydration [44]. Moran *et al.* [45] showed that perception of effort, using the Borg scale, was closely related to level of dehydration. They reported that an exercise intensity rated at 13.4 ± 0.5 ("somewhat hard") when participants were dehydrated to 1.1% of BM was rated at 17.6 ± 0.3 ("very hard") when dehydration was at 4.2% of BM. These findings suggest an association between the development of dehydration and subjective sensation of effort, which could ultimately impact on performance and also enjoyment of the event, the latter perhaps of particular importance to recreational athletes.

Incidence of headaches, cramps, stomach discomfort and nausea was also associated with higher U_{sg} values. It is not surprising that those who were more dehydrated tended to suffer from headaches as this is a common symptom associated with dehydration and has been regularly reported by others [46]. Cramps were reported by a considerable proportion of subjects in both events (44% in the OMM and

35% in the LH), again this is as expected as cramps have been cited by many as one of the most common complaints, particularly during endurance events such as triathlons and marathons, to be reported to medical staff [1,47]. Whilst dehydration alone may not be the sole cause of muscle cramps, studies have shown that remaining well hydrated could help delay the onset [48]. The findings that stomach discomfort and nausea were more common in those dehydrated is supported by the positive association observed in both studies between self-reported ratings of nausea and U_{sg} values. However, athletes should be careful not to drink large volumes of fluid during exercise as that too can cause gastrointestinal discomfort [49]. The temperature of fluids should also be taken into account and may have varied greatly in this study; cold water from natural sources in comparison to warmer fluids carried in backpacks could have impacted upon levels consumed and symptoms experienced. This area warrants further investigation.

4.5. Limitations

It is evident from this study and from comparison with existing research that the effects of hydration status on exercise are complex. There is not only likely to be considerable individual variation, but the exercise protocols used, the level of dehydration, the environmental conditions and the method used to determine hydration status will all influence the outcome. As a result, the findings must take into account these factors and the limitations of the study.

Several limitations have been discussed such as the errors associated with using BM loss as a hydration marker, but it is important to note that urine values such as U_{sg} can also provide misleading results in certain cases. Levels of dehydration may have been under-reported in this study as ideally U_{sg} values should be taken after several hours of stable hydration status. If a dehydrated individual consumes a substantial volume of hypotonic fluid prior to testing they will have large amounts of urine production long before euhydration is re-established and U_{sg} values may indicate euhydration when the individual is still dehydrated [19]. It is also best practise to establish both BM and U_{sg}, and the relationship between them, in euhydrated participants before exercise commences so that individual results can be interpreted more accurately. As access to participants in a controlled environment, prior to the events, was not possible this could not be done and as a result the findings must be taken with caution.

The type and timing of fluid ingestion was not investigated which can significantly affect the ability of an individual to remain hydrated or to effectively re-hydrate. Several authors have written about the importance of electrolyte consumption during exercise. Coyle [2] stated that sodium should be included in fluids consumed during exercise lasting more than two hours, and Shirreffs and Sawka [50] explained that if rapid recovery is desired, such as during mid-camp events like the OMM, aggressive drinking of fluids and consumption of electrolytes is necessary to facilitate recovery for subsequent competition. Further research is therefore needed in this area, which takes into account not only quantity, but also quality of fluid consumption, in order to investigate whether mountain marathon athletes are currently meeting such recommendations.

5. Conclusions

A wide range of hydration levels were observed in these athletes; with some remaining well-hydrated, others finishing significantly dehydrated and others perhaps over drinking. Dehydration was not negatively associated with performance; however it was related to an increased incidence of various well-being measures such as headaches, cramps and nausea. Whilst the majority of elite athletes are primarily concerned with performance measures, recreational athletes are likely to be as concerned with factors that affect their enjoyment and so hydration strategies that could help to improve this are likely to be well-received.

Due to the wide variation in hydration levels observed it is likely that athletes would benefit from more individualised hydration strategies rather than blanket recommendations. Whilst it is difficult for recreational athletes to get individualised advice, it is possible to provide simple suggestions for athletes participating in particular events that take into account the nature and the environment of the event. Athletes competing in the OMM should be made aware of situations where availability of water from natural sources may be limiting and that greater effort should be put into rehydration at mid-camp where water is available. To ensure less experienced athletes, who may be less in touch with their own needs, do not significantly over or under consume simple techniques such as monitoring urine frequency, volume and colour should be advised.

References

[1] D.J. Casa, P.M. Clarkson, and W.O. Roberts, "American College of Sports Medicine Roundtable on Hydration and Physical Activity: Consensus Statements." Current Sports Medicine Reports, vol. 4, pp.115-127, 2005.

[2] E.F. Coyle, "Fluid and fuel intake during exercise." Journal of Sports Sciences, vol. 22, pp.39-55, 2004.

[3] M.N. Sawka, "Physiological consequences of hypohydration: exercise performance and thermoregulation." Medicine and Science in Sports and Exercise, vol. 24, pp.657-670, 1992.

[4] H.R. Clark, M.E. Barker, and B,M. Corfe, "Nutritional Strategies of Mountain Marathon Competitors – An Observational Study." International Journal of Sport Nutrition and Exercise Metabolism, vol. 15, pp. 160-172, 2005.

[5] T.D. Noakes, Lore of Running. Champaign, IL: Human Kinetics, 2003.

[6] American College of Sports Medicine (ACSM), "Position Statement of the American College of Sports Medicine: prevention of heat injuries during distance running." Medicine and Science in Sports and Exercise, vol. 7, pp. vii-ix, 1975.

[7] T.D. Hew, J.N. Chorley, J.C. Cianca, and J.G. Divine, "The incidence, risk factors, and clinical manifestations of hyponatremia in marathon runners." Clinical Journal of Sports medicine, vol. 13, pp.41-47, 2003.

[8] International Olympic Committee (IOC). "IOC consensus statement on sports nutrition 2010." Journal of Sports Sciences, vol. 29:sup1, pp. S3-S4, 2011.

[9] B. Murray, "Hydration and physical performance." Journal of the American College of Nutrition, vol. 26, pp. S542-S548, 2007.

[10] G.K. McConnell, C.M. Burge, S.L. Skinner, and M. Hargreaves, "Influence of ingested fluid volumes on physiological responses during prolonged exercise." Acta Physiologica Scandinavica, vol. 160, pp.149-156, 1997.

[11] J.L. Fallowfield, C. Williams, J. Booth, B.H. Choo, and S. Growns, "Effect of water ingestion on endurance capacity during prolonged running." Journal of Sports Sciences, vol. 14, pp.497-502, 1996.

[12] W.F. Kao, C.L. Shyu, and X.W. Yang, "Athletic performance and serial weight changes during 12- and 24-hour ultra-marathons." Clinical Journal of Sports Medicine, vol.18, pp.155-158, 2008.

[13] H.R. Lieberman, "Hydration and Cognition: A critical review and recommendations for future research." Journal of the American College of Nutrition, vol.26, pp.555S-561S, 2007.

[14] P.N. Ainslie, I.T. Campbell, K.N. Frayn, S.M. Humphreys, D.P.M. MacLaren, T. Reilly, and K.R. Weserterp, "Energy balance, metabolism, hydration and performance during strenuous hill walking: the effect of age." Journal of Applied Physiology, vol.93, pp.714-723, 2002.

[15] K.J. Ellis, "Selected body composition methods can be used in field studies." Journal of Nutrition, vol.131, pp.1589S-1595S, 2001.

[16] M. Stroud, "The nutritional demands of very prolonged exercise in man." Proceedings of the Nutrition Society, vol.57, pp.55-61, 1998.

[17] L.E. Armstrong, "Hydration Assessment Techniques." Nutrition Reviews, vol.63, pp.S40-S54, 2005.

[18] S.M. Shirreffs, "Markers of hydration status." European Journal of Clinical Nutrition, vol.57, pp.S6-S9, 2003.

[19] American College of Sports Medicine, "Position stand: Exercise and fluid replacement." Medicine and Science in Sports and Exercise, DOI: 10.1249/mss.0b013e31802ca.597, 2007.

[20] L.E. Armstrong, J.A. Soto, F.T. Hacker, J.R. Casa, S.A. Kavouras, and C.M. Maresh, "Urinary indices during dehydration, exercise and rehydration." International Journal of Sports Nutrition, vol.8, pp.345-355, 1998.

[21] M. Collardeau, J. Brisswalter, F. Vercruyssen, M. Audiffren, and C. Gaubault, "Single and Choice Reaction Time during Prolonged Exercise in Trained Subjects: Influence of Carbohydrate Availability." European Journal of Applied Physiology, vol.86, pp.150-156, 2001.

[22] A.J. Hill, and J.E. Blundell, "Sensitivity of appetite control system in obese subjects to nutritional and serotoninergic challenges." International Journal of Obesity, vol.14, pp.219-233, 1990.

[23] P.N. Ainslie, I.T. Campbell, K.N. Frayn, S.M. Humphreys, D.P.M. MacLaren, T. Reilly, and K.R. Westerterp, "Energy balance, metabolism, hydration and performance during strenuous hill walking: the effect of age." Journal of Applied Physiology, vol.93, pp.714-723, 2002.

[24] G. Borg, "Perceived Exertion as an indicator of somatic stress." Scandinavian Journal of Rehabilitation Medicine, vol.2, pp.92-98, 1970.

[25] E. Blomstrand, P. Hassmen, B. Ekblom, and E.A. Newsholme, "Influence of ingesting a solution of branched-chain amino acids on perceived exertion during exercise." Acta Physiologica Scandinavica, vol.159, pp. 41-49, 1997.

[26] P.N. Ainslie, K. Abbas, I.T. Campbell, K.N. Frayn, M. Harvie, M.A. Keegan, D.P.M. MacLaren, I.A. MacDonald, K. Paramesh, and T. Reilly, "Metabolic and appetite responses to prolonged walking under three isoenergetic diets." Journal of Applied Physiology, vol.92, pp.2061-2070, 2002.

[27] A.C. Utter, J.I.E. Kang, R.J. Robertson, D.C. Nieman, E.C. Chaloupka, R.R. Suminski, and C.R. Piccinni, "Effect of carbohydrate ingestion on perceived exertion during a marathon." Medicine and Science in Sports and Exercise, vol.34, pp.1779-1784, 2002.

[28] M. Kruesman, S. Bucher, M. Bovard, B. Kayser, and p.A. Bovier, "Nutrient intake and performance during a mountain marathon: an observational study." European Journal of Applied Physiology, vol. 94, pp. 151-157, 2005.

[29] N. Tam, T. Hew-Butler, E. Papadopoulou, H. Nolte, and T.D. Noakes, "Fluid intake and changes in blood biochemistry, running speed and body mass during an 80km mountain trail race." Medicina Sportiva, vol.13, pp.108-115, 2009.

[30] N.E. Kimber, J.J. Ross, S.L. Mason, and D.B. Speedy, "Energy balance during an ironman triathlon in male and female triathletes." International Journal of Sport Nutrition and Exercise Metabolism, vol. 12, pp. 47-62, 2002.

[31] G.W. Mack, C.A. Weseman, G.W. Langhans, H. Scherzer, C.M. Gillan, and E.R. Nadel, "Body fluid balance in dehydrated healthy older men: thirst and renal osmoregulation." Journal of Applied Physiology, vol.76, pp.1615-1623, 1994.

[32] P.A. Phillips, B.J. Rolls, J.G. Ledingham, and J.J. Morton, "Body fluid changes, thirst and drinking in man during free access to water." Physiology and Behaviour, vol.33, pp.357-363, 1984.

[33] W.L. Kenney, and P. Chiu, P. "Influence of age on thirst and fluid intake." Medicine and Science in Sports and Exercise, vol.33, pp.1524-1532, 2001.

[34] K.E. Fallon, E. Broad, M.W. Thompson, and P.A. Reull, "Nutritional and fluid intake in a 100-km ultramarathon." International Journal of Sports Nutrition, vol. 8, pp. 24-35, 1998.

[35] R.J. Maughan, S.M. Shirreffs, and J.B. Leiper, "Errors in the estimation of hydration status from changes in body mass." Journal of Sports Sciences, vol.25, pp.797-804, 2007.

[36] R.F.G.J. King, C. Cooke, S. Carroll, and J. O'Hara, "Estimating changes in hydration status from changes in body mass: Considerations regarding metabolic water and glycogen storage." Journal of Sports Sciences, vol.26, pp. 1361-1363, 2008.

[37] F.E. Marino, J. Kannon, and D. Kay, "Neuromuscular responses to hydration in moderate to warm ambient conditions during self-paced high-intensity exercise." British Journal of Sports Medicine, vol.44, pp.961-967, 2010.

[38] T. Mundel, "To drink or not to drink? Explaining "contradictory findings" in fluid replacement and exercise performance: evidence from a more valid model for real-life competition." British Journal of Sports Medicine, vol.45, pp.1-2, 2011.

[39] E.D.B. Goulet, "Effect of exercise-induced dehydration on time-trial exercise performance: a meta-analysis." British Journal of Sports Medicine, vol.45, pp.1149-1156, 2011.

[40] M.MG. Wilson, and J.E. Morley, "Impaired cognitive function and mental performance in mild dehydration." European Journal of Clinical Nutrition, vol.57, pp.S24-S29, 2003.

[41] K.E. D'Anci, F. Constant, and I.H. Rosenberg, I.H. "Hydration and cognitive function in children." Nutrition Reviews, vol.64, pp.457-464, 2006.

[42] H.R. Lieberman, G.P. Bathalon, C.M. Falco, F.M. Kramer, C.A. Morgan, and P. Niro, "Severe decrements in cognitive functions and mood induced by sleep loss, heat, dehydration, and undernutrition during simulated combat." Biological Psychiatry, vol.57, pp.422-429, 2005.

[43] A. Adan, "Cognitive performance and dehydration." Journal of the American College of Nutrition, vol.31, pp.71-78, 2012.

[44] C. Cian, N. Koulmann, P. Barraud, C. Raphel, C. Jimenez, and B. Melin, "Influence of variation in body hydration on cognitive function: effect of hyperhydration, heat stress, and exercise-induced dehydration." Journal of Psychophysiology, vol.14, pp.29-36, 2000.

[45] D.S. Moran, S.J. Montain, and K.B. Pandolf, "Evaluation of different levels of hydration using a new physiological strain index." American Journal of Physiology: Regulatory, Integrative and Comparative Physiology, vol.275, pp.R854-R860, 1998.

[46] R.J. Maughan, "Impact of mild dehydration on wellness and on exercise performance." European Journal of Clinical Nutrition, vol.57, pp.S19-S23, 2003.

[47] M.P. Schwellnus, "Muscle Cramping in the Marathon: Aetiology and Risk Factors." Sports Medicine, vol.37, pp.364-367, 2007.

[48] A.P. Jung, P.A. Bishop, A. Al-Nawwas, and B. Dale, "Influence of hydration and electrolyte supplementation on incidence and time to onset of exercise-associated muscle cramps." Journal of Athletic Training, vol.40, pp.71-75, 2005.

[49] T.A. Robinson, J.A. Hawley, G.S. Palmer, G.R. Wilson, D.A. Gray, and T.D. Noakes, "Water ingestion does not improve 1-h cycling performance in moderate ambient temperatures." European Journal of Applied Physiology and Occupational Physiology, vol.71, pp.153-160, 1995.

[50] S.M. Shirreffs, and M.N. Sawka, "Fluid and electrolyte needs for training, competition and recovery." Journal of Sports Sciences, vol.29, pp.S39-S46, 2011.

Designing Iran sport for all model

Mohammad Javadipour[1], Monireh Ali[2], Rezvan Hakimzadeh[1]

[1]Psychology & Education, Tehran University, Tehran, Iranian
[2]Physical Education Organization (PEO), Tehran, Iranian

Email address:
javadipour846@yahoo.com (M. Javadipour), m_everlady@yahoo.com (M. Ali)

Abstract: The purpose of this research is to describe and diagnose Iran Sport For All status and to design a model. The population of the research includes: Sport For All Federation managers, its strategic Council members, its sub sport Associations and Sport For All provinces Units. TO benefit the experts and authorities' point of view effectively, a questionnaire within the framework of the federation strategic plan content was designed and sent to the target population including: different federations and associations managers, the provinces sports units and the federation strategic Council members. A five –level Likert scale (strongly agree /agree/ neutral/ disagree/ strongly disagree) was designed. After Investigating and analyzing the results; regarding a Pathological view and approach; Sport For All strong & weak points, treats and opportunities (SWOT) were recognized. Then considering the proportion of Sport For All processes role to the other sports and its relationship with procurement, management and processing control components and culture & religious values, Iran Sport For All development model was designed noticing sport management scientific structure, processing structure and its relationship with other sports and macro management circles for macro policy-making, planning and procurement & executive levels.

Keywords: Theoretical Framework, Model (Pattern) Designing, Iran Sport for All

1. Introduction

As science and technology develops management and planning play effective roles in social and executive organizations. The experts, who introduce development as the only principled and logical way to economical growth and blossoming, science and technology progress, achieving public welfare and improvement of living conditions, have frequently spoken on this subject and encouraged statesmen to run along the development programs framework. Development is a purposeful process which is started by human being and its goal is to improve all the people's living conditions in a society.

Considering development based on any definition, interpretation or view finally leads to a single concept to get to happiness, growth, justice, economic, social and cultural dynamism & freedom. So we should accept that development isn't a spontaneous phenomenon but a matter which we need to have a goal and a plan and hard attempt to achieve it. In this way, studying the developed countries reveals that achieving the sustainable development isn't possible without any attention to the young, rational, creative, dynamic and open –minded people. And those countries which had remarkable success, has based their development on their people's physical and mental education and training progress. The effect of thinking method on one's performance and the necessity of establishing a regular and coherent system for the individuals' thinking so that they could play the best role in making decisions, problem solving and leading organizations, themselves and others to get a successful result for their country is a vital and necessary matter. Real development and progress in countries have different indexes which one of the most important is sport. According to the well-known slogan: "A healthy mind locates in a healthy body", the argument on sport applications to human resources development in different economic, social and cultural fields, is more noticed.(1) Civilization and increasing progress in modern technology have resulted in "Sedentary behavior". This inactivity and Sedentary behavior causes some disorders which affect different physical, psychological and social aspects of life. Changing the status quo needs suitable and deserving tools like physical activity as a multidimensional tool with vast health, economic, social effects which helps healthy leisure time and creates liveliness and vitality. The undeniable educating and training role of physical activities specially among teenagers and young people ,its role in prevention of diseases , social corruptions and obliquities are just some of the functions of this valuable phenomenon.(2,3)Those people, who do regular sport exercises, have less risk of heart attack. At the same time their brain relaxes more, their heartbeats decrease while resting and they feel less stress and more self-confidence. They are more optimistic and feel less depressed as well. (2,4) Although there are different approaches toward sport as a phenomenon which some of them focus on competitive perspective and the others focus on public health and the vitality of the society and some of the other ones notice the economic perspective, but regardless of all these matters ,the importance of physical education and sport is increasing day by day. The relationship between sport and other cultural, social, political and economic phenomena reveals its importance and role in the countries national development programs and in a general point of view, sport development and progress in each country has a close relationship with the power and authority of that country.(5) Sport For All or Sport For all groups of people is a main part of sport which has close relationship with the health and the vitality of the society and a lot of sport main approaches are located in it. A lot of developed countries have chosen and accepted the health approach as their sport policy and run on the basis of this approach. These countries haven't mentioned the medal achievement (competing) in international fields or championships and professional approaches in their sport policies.

Among all kinds of sports especially in comparison with competitive (athletic) and professional sports, Sport For All has had a main and basic role which includes a great number of functions. (Mull 2005) Sport For All has been defined as all forms of extensive and comprehensive sport activities among all ages, genders, races, religions and nations with different physical and psychological abilities.(1)According to this definition , Sport For All isn't a duty, but an opportunity. It's not a collective sport but an individual and team one. In fact the people's motivation to participate in sport activities isn't getting to high ranks and achieving the Olympic motto (Faster, Higher and Stronger).Health, vitality and social relations are the main factors in taking part in these activities. Competition and wining & losing play the least role in their tendency toward sport.(5) Sport For All approaches are as follow: Getting vitality and joy feeling , enrichment of leisure time, getting health and physical fitness, improvement of job relations ,connection and social relations and life style, ,prevention and treatment of diseases , achieving the sport results and benefits, happiness and safety, energy balance and detoxifying ,controlling and losing the weight and getting to physical fitness, achieving social emotions and improving interaction and social relations.(1)

The researches on the effect of sport activities on physical and psychological health, longevity, vitality, improvement of social relations and enrichment of leisure time have caused an increase in people's participation in different sports specially in their participation in different forms of Sport For All in the world. This is why nowadays most of the world developed countries are competing with each other for their Sport For All organizations and arrangements and are delivering creative programs to improve this sport regularly. It's obvious that each country which cant cross this increased wave will never be able to fill this gap and so its differences with other countries to benefit from the advantages of sport and motor activities will be completely clear.(Dr. Ghare's Plan)Moreover, physical activity improves psychological health and decreases psychological problems.(6,7) Inspecting physical education organization published statistics; we can find that only 10 percent of people participate in sport & physical activities. This percent is too low in comparison with other countries like Australia where 52 percent do exercise. This Sedentary behavior and insufficient physical activity which comes from development and improvement of facilities, modern comforts and new lifestyles reveal the necessity of planning for physical activities which are needed in the society more.(8) According to UE published data, at least 30 percent of the world teenagers and young people don't have insufficient physical activity. This is a lot more in our country according to the available information. So the sport policy maker's most important duty or responsibility is paying attention to sport development among different people from walks of life. On the other hand sport is considered as a social human right. In 2003, UN has mentioned sport as a social right and expresses that the opportunity to take part in Sport and physical activity is a human right and the governors have to provide this opportunity for all of the people in the society. In some of the countries like Sweden and Finland, the number of sport participants is more than 80 percent of their population. Regarding the history of the world Sport For All and its new approaches and obvious philosophy in a lot of countries and also its focus on multiple approaches like health, vitality of the society, enrichment of leisure time, improvement of job relations, connection and social relations, prevention and treatment of diseases, happiness and energy balance and detoxifying ,achieving social emotions and getting to the sport results and benefits, it seems that using all the potentials of the society is necessary to improve and develop Sport For All. Moreover, increasing the awareness of the people in the society can play an important role to form it as a habit. The experience of the well-known countries in this field reveals that Sport For All development and improvement in these countries result from both the government and people's investment and their close cooperation. As the Constitution and Acts of Islamic Republic of Iran demonstrate that making the sport popular among people is the first duty of each sport organization, so it is believed that the result of this research will help the sport authorities to make their strategies out of these results and to be able to do effective measures to improve Sport For All programs. (2, 7, 22, 23, 24) Through studying the world experience and investigating our country status, this research has designed a model to improve sport and physical education.

This model includes 4 great components (sub-systems) as follow:

*The process of strategies and policies development

* Development of Sport and healthy Recreation

*Supporting Sport development and healthy Recreation and

*Coordination and Supervision

Sport and healthy Recreation are considered as the main process in "Sport and Physical Education Comprehensive System"(Plan). This process has been divided into 4 groups: Sport for All and Recreation, Educational Sport, Competitive (Athletic) and Professional Sport. Sport For All Movement in the world was started in 1960 in Europe by organizing Trim Associations (A Norwegian word means fit and fresh).International Sport For All Committee was established in 1964 and Sport For All Federation was formed in 1992 in our country.(17) In a study among 126 countries in the world, it was revealed that although 92 percent of these countries know physical education as a necessary and obligatory phenomenon for all different groups of the society ,but only in 71 percent of them physical education is in harmony with social needs and in 29 percent, its just a mean to get to other non-sport goals.

In 60 percent of developing countries, sport policies just remain on papers and as a motto. This study also shows that there is a big gap between what has been approved and the activities. (7) Razavi et al.(2009) studied Sport For All participants' social and Economical Status(SES) in Mazandaran province. The result of this study, among 384 Sport For All participants in Mazandaran showed that there is a meaningful relation between the number of Sport For All participants and their economical status. However, it seems that these participants mostly belong to mid-level or low-mid level groups. So it seems necessary to plan to omit the available obstacles for increasing the participation among low-level groups and attracting the high-mid level people's attention toward this field. Because this can result to improvement of all Sport For All participants' sports health levels. (3)

Ghafoori(2007) in his research studied different kinds of favorite Sport For All activities and Recreations in the society and offered a model for future plans. The result of his research revealed that the most obstacles in doing sport among the research samples in order of

Priorities are as follow: "The lack of motivation", "The extensive cost of doing sport ", "The lack of space and facilities" and "Time limitation". The result of studying priorities in sport divisions was also considerable. The research participants believed that in the next sport plans "Sport for All and Recreation" should be more focused. Then sport in the schools and universities; "Educational Sport" was located in a short distance and then it came to "Competitive (Athletic) Sport " and "Professional Sport" which were located next to each other in the third and fourth level but in a long distance from the first and second ones.(7) Ghare(2005) conducted the research of "Iran Sport For All status and its comparison with some of the world selected countries". The result of his research indicated that 5/92 percent of Iran population take part in sport activities under the supervision of Men & Women Sport for All Province Units which was the least percent among 23 countries in the world. Regarding the date of organizing Iran Sport for All official organization, Iran had the lowest rank among 20 countries in the world too. The percentage of participants in Iran Sport For All activities was more than the number of participants in Africa and less than this number in other continents.(2)

Afarinesh(2005) in his research compared different universities faculties, coaches, athletes and managers' points of view on the ways of improving Sport For All. According to the results of his research, the most important factors to improve Sport For All are as follow: Economic improvement of different people from walks of life, Using multimedia, Noticing the family status (number of children, marriage), Holding the sport competitions and awarding the prizes, Increasing public transportation services, Regarding sport as the first priority and at the top of the leisure time list and attracting the private and non-governmental investments. (10) Gholiniya(2004) in his research studied Iran total Sport For All status and challenges facing participation in the sport and planning for making the sport popular among the people. He chose 70 physical education organization managers and experts and 524 citizens living in 10 different provinces as his research sample. The results indicate the use of multiple approaches like Socio-Cultural and Group-Individual Salutary approaches (for implementation), multiple approaches of Active Interference, Participation & Supervising, Recreation-Naturalistic and Cultural & Local approaches (for finding priorities among sport disciplines), Spaces Combining Ability approaches (using sport places)

The approaches of Obligation for binding the rules (legal dimensions), the approaches of Modeling from bottom and making culture from top (performing), approach of Ultra mural Activity (cooperation of centers) and etc. in the frame of Offensive-Development and Diversity Strategy. (11) Atighechi(2004) also in a study on the way of spending leisure time found it about 3 to 5 hours per head. He who was studying 2301 university students (like Saneee) revealed the top students' extreme eagerness toward Sport For All rather than Competitive (Athletic) Sport as their popular pastime.(12) Saneee(1994) studied the university students' attitudes on sport regarding the way of spending their leisure time. He studied 700 Teacher Training university students and investigated their way of spending their leisure time. He found that their leisure time was about 3 to 4 hours and most of them were dissatisfied with their way of spending it. The students who answered his questionnaire emphasized paying attention toward Sport for All rather than Competitive (Athletic) Sport. Shafiee(1994) studied the socio-economical status of Sport For All participants .He studied 900 Sport For All participants and concluded that the most percent (% 31/1) of participants belonged to the middle or higher class of socio-economical category. Considering their living place, most of the participants (% 28/3) were living at the north of Tehran. (14) Ramezani Khalilabadi (1994) studied Sport for All participants' motivation in his research. He achieved the data through collecting the questionnaires answered by 975 participants in Sport for All Stations. The result included: Their first motivation was achieving vitality and joy feeling. Then there were sport advantages and positive effects and also Sport for All enjoyment and safety. Cheap expenses, no need to special sport equipments and facilities and filling their leisure time were as some of their motivations as well. The participants mentioned that multimedia had 42/2 percent role in their eagerness toward sport. Finally their inability to participate in Competitive (Athletic) Sport is mentioned as one of the peoples' motivation toward Sport for All.(15)

Studying Sport for All status in countries like Australia, Germany, Japan, Malaysia, Finland and Denmark reveals that regular plan to develop and improve Sport for All in these countries has a background of about 50 years. There are different factors to get to this success which the first can be mentioned as: Sport for All growth in the framework of these countries national plans and their governments' effective support of the plans. Furthermore, the clubs and sport public places development and establishing and organizing Sport for All forums can be mentioned too. (1)

The main factors in developing Sport for All in these countries are:

1-The governments' support of sport clubs development

2-Rgular development of Sport for All programs

3-Dvelopment of sport places

4-Dvelopment of Sport for All forums

5-Role of governmental institutes

6-Holding festivals and different social events

7-Marketing

8-Making culture to develop Sport for All

9-The national and state governments' financial support

10-Increase in target groups' activities including: The Youth, Old, Disabled, Schools, Women, Workers and Employees…

11-Having codified and clear strategy and policies to develop Sport for All

12- The role of private organizations

Strategic Planning is a tool for organizing the present on the basis of the projections of the desired future. That is, a strategic plan is a road map to lead an organization from where it is now to where it would like to be in five or ten years. It is a systematic planning process involving a number of steps that identify the current status of the organization including its mission, vision for the future, operating values, needs (strengths, weaknesses, opportunities and threats), goals, prioritized actions and strategies, action plans, and monitoring plans. Strategic planning has long been used as a tool for transforming and revitalizing corporations, government agencies and nonprofit organizations. Recently, however, skepticism about planning has been on the rise. Political and economic uncertainty is the norm and the space of technological and social change has accelerated. Each strategic planning includes three main components as: Plan development, Plan execution, and Plan review. Many of the functional areas within these components are similar in that all three require a team concept that is based on: ensuring the member's roles are defined, educating team members about the process, and using quality communication when interacting. Strategic planning is the cornerstone of every common-interest community. Without strategic planning, the community will never know where it is going—much less know if it ever got there. An important concept of strategic planning is an understanding that in order for the community to flourish, everyone needs to work to ensure the team's goals are met. (22, 23, 24)

Regarding the high frequency of different subjects on Sport For All and its theories and opinions all around the world which indicate its main components and their type of interaction and its relation to different sports, which theoretically is a guide for planning Sport for All development, mainly the growth and development of Sport For All among developed countries is caused by codified plans and the scientific method of performing them.

In our country in spite of different studies in this field, there aren't many scientific and exact studies on Sport for All methodology and designing models for its development. Planning System in our country has a different structure comparing with other countries. Dividing national Sport for All responsibilities and analyzing the government's missions into governing division, organizations and governmental & non- governmental centers basically needs a model which can make the relationship between Sport for All components and the extramural components which are focused on other sports and the supporting components of Sport for All System. In this research through identifying and studying Sport for All in Iran, we offer a model for its development. Two subjects are investigated in this survey: 1- Revealing Sport for All weak and strength points & its treats and opportunities.2- Designing a Sport for All development model.

2. The Research Methodology

As the nature of this survey is a kind of management and strategic planning survey, we have used different research methods to design a Sport for All development model. Achieving a study model and finalizing it to make a plan, Investigating the history and the available documents, Studying the previous researches and upper level documents, Comparative Studying and obtaining the authorities and experts' point of view need different approaches including management, descriptive or analyzing .This is an applied research and its necessary data, with paying attention to the available Sport For All indexes, have been collected through preparing and sending statistics forms to different provinces Sport Units, Sub-Sport Associations and Physical Education Centers. There are Statistics information and data on human resource status, the number and frequency of Sport Units all over Iran, Sport places which are under the supervision of the state and sport events like(competitions, mass walking events, national meetings,…)in this part of the research.

2.1. Population

The population of this research includes: Sport for All Federation managers, its strategic Council members, its sub-sport Associations and Sport for All provinces Units.

2.2. Sample and Sampling Method

In this research the number of Samples is the same as population.

2.3. Data Collecting Tool

TO benefit the experts and authorities' point of view effectively, a questionnaire within the framework of the federation strategic plan content was designed and sent to the target population including: different sport federations and associations managers, the provinces sports units and the federation strategic Council members. As a five –level Likert scale (strongly agree /agree/ neutral/ disagree/ strongly disagree) was designed to answer the questionnaire, it has been decided to accept an idea if it has been achieved %70 strongly agree or agree opinions. On the other hand, the idea with %50 disagree or strongly disagree opinions will be omitted.

2.4. Data Collecting Method

The necessary data, with paying attention to the available Sport for All indexes, have been collected through preparing and sending statistics forms to different provinces Sport Units, Sub-Sport Associations and Physical Education Centers.

3. Results

As it has been mentioned the population of this research includes: Sport for All Federation & Associations managers, the directors of the committees, the directors of different provinces Sport Units and the Federation strategic Council members. In this part we are going to show their formal education status and their experiences in Sport for All field.

Table 1. *The research population status regarding their Education.*

Education / Sex	DIP.		BA	MA	PhD
Female	3	0	4	1	0
Male	5	6	24	10	5

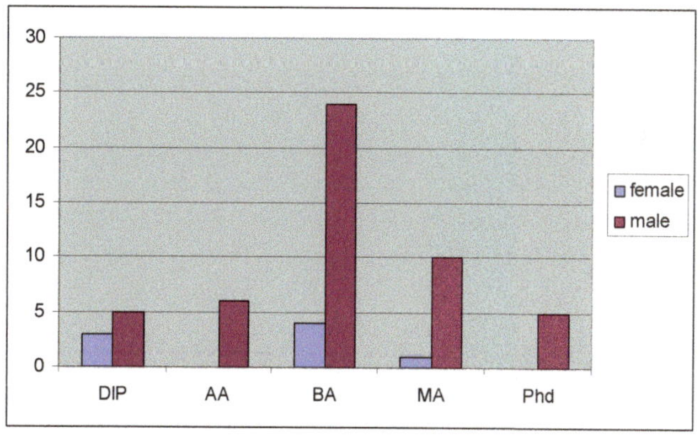

Chart 1. *The research population status regarding their Education.*

Table 2. *The research population status regarding their participation experiences in Sport For All activities.*

participation experiences in Sport For All activities / sex	Up to 5 years	Up to 10 years	Up to 20 years	20 year and more
female	3	4	1	0
male	9	17	10	8

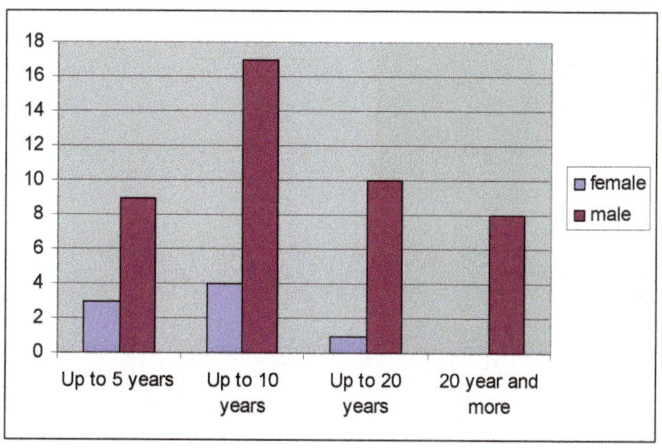

Chart 2. *The research population status regarding their participation experiences in Sport for All activities.*

According to a pathological approach, after studying and analyzing the results we found the following Sport For All weak and strength points & its treats and opportunities as follow:

3.1. Strength Points

- Individual and organizational motivation and eagerness toward Sport For All and Recreation development and improvement
- Having an independent legal entity and the possibility of using suitable financial and economical mechanisms
- Having the benefit of valuable, experienced human resources (managers, experts, teachers and coaches…)
- Having 32 active provinces Sport Units and 131 active

towns Sport Units

- Governing more than 22 different sport disciplines which are related to Sport For All and Recreation
- Connecting and being a member of TAFISA(The Association For Sport For All) & ASFAA(Asian Sport For All Association)
- Close relationship and special notice to National Broadcasting Media and other audio, written ones, ...
- Having the possibility of holding national events like Family Walking, Run Day & mass walking events on challenge days and so on, Official employees' competitions, Local & Traditional Festivals, etc.
- Active participation in international Sport For All events
- Having the benefit and cooperation of offices, organizations and governmental or non-governmental and private centers
- Signing memoranda with governmental & private organizations and centers

3.2. Weak Points

- Weakness of information and communication system in Sport For All Federation and adverse use of individual & organizational information and communication
- Traditional management in Sport For All Federation and its Sport Units
- Insufficient Sport For All governmental budget offering by Physical Education Organization(PEO)and NOC
- The lack of an economic outlook and disability for earning new income sources from the federation activities through marketing and business
- The shortage in Sport For All income and its great dependence to the government and Physical Education Organization public budget
- The lack of a systematic relationship with offices, organizations and governmental and private centers
- The lack of a national comprehensive plan for Sport For All
- The lack of both Sport For All TV channel and a unit management thinking and a central plan
- The lack of Sport For All managers, athletes and authorities' sufficient financial support
- The lack of a common definition of Sport For All and Recreation ,which is in harmony with the society needs, among the experts and managers in organizations and centers about sport views and applied concepts
- The lack of a Coherent organization and a structure to provide efficient human resource in the federation related organizations and units

3.3. Opportunities

- Focus on Physical Education in Islamic inspiration instructions
- Focus on free Physical Education development and improvement in Iran Constitution
- The Leathers' speeches in the start of the new year (1389: 2010) in Razavi Haram(Mashad)
- The senior authorities, clergymen and medical community's Special notices toward Physical Education development in Iran
- The community attitudes toward sport activities as an effective psychological, physical, cultural, educational and moral factor
- The young population of our country and the great number of sport talents
- Iran four climate variability and natural-sport attractions
- Iran geographical and climatic potentials for Tourism, Ecotourism and Fishing, ...
- Providing the possibility of using the offices, organizations and centers potentials and facilities through signing memoranda
- New and effective views of main organizations toward Sport For All development
- All walks of life people's great participation in weakly Family Walking events within provinces and towns
- Good support of companies and economical institutes to provide the needed financial resources of performing the federation activities

3.4. Treats

- The lack of necessary motivation in private divisions for developing facilities and improving national sport activities
- The intrusion of undesirable social and behavioral abnormalities in sport environment
- The lack of a coherent planning system to attract financial and economical nongovernmental resources
- Insufficient recognition of public physical education and Sport For All international potentials
- Inadequate quality and quantity of Asian, World and Olympic standings in Sport For All among the related authorities and experts
- Planning and performing parallel and non-normative activities in national organizations and centers

To design a Sport For All & Recreation development model in Iran, we have used different sources among them the two most important will be mentioned. It has been noticed that in addition to using the scientific sources to design the final model, with paying attention to social and cultural atmosphere of our society and the administrative and management structure of sport in Iran and the need for Iran Sport For All development model, a realistic and directional model will be used in Sport For All planning system. One of the most important classifications is Mull et al.'s model.(Mull, 2005) He has divided sport into four levels in his book "sport management and Leisure time."

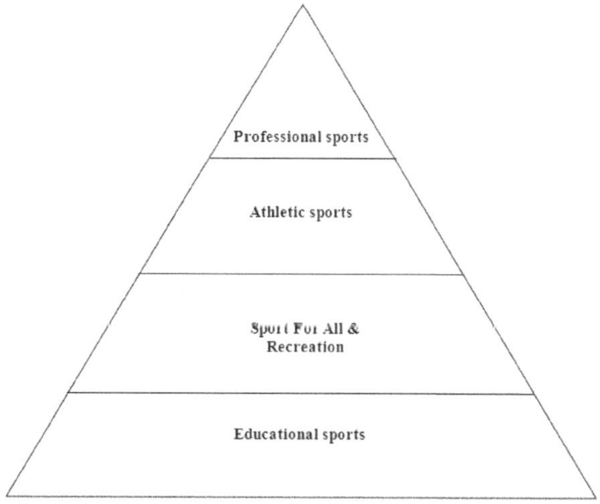

Chart 3. Mull et al. divided sport into four levels (Mull ,2005)

Mull et al. (Mull, 2005) then divided Sport For All & Recreation concepts into five levels (Chart 4)

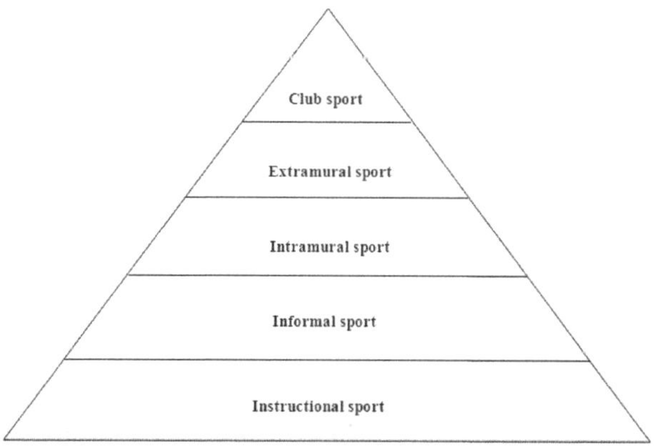

Chart 4. Mull et al. divided sport into five levels (Mull ,2005)

Then Iran Sport For All development model along with a sports management scientific structure and process structure and its relationship with other sports and high management circles for policy making and designing master (strategic) plans and supportive & executive levels- was designed with paying attention to the role of Sport For All processes in other sports and its relationship with components like: supporting, management, process control and culture and religious values.

3.5. Final Suggested Model for Sport For All & Recreation in Iran

This model, using the available background in Sport For All scientific sources and for the sake of making the performance of Sport For All_available concepts easier and with paying attention to the management structure attributes and specialties in planning system and Iran socio cultural atmosphere has been designed. To finalize the model the experts and the authorities' opinions have been used. The first level of this study includes Sport For All & Recreation development and the second level includes the following main processes in chart 5.

1) Sport for health and motion
2) Sport for treatment and reduction in the effects of chronic diseases
3) Educational sport with approach of training sports disciplines and paving the road to Athletic (Competitive) Sport.

In supporting processes of Sport For All development, some components like human resources, centers, Legal environment, sport places, scientific and research components, management and planning and ICT have been designed.

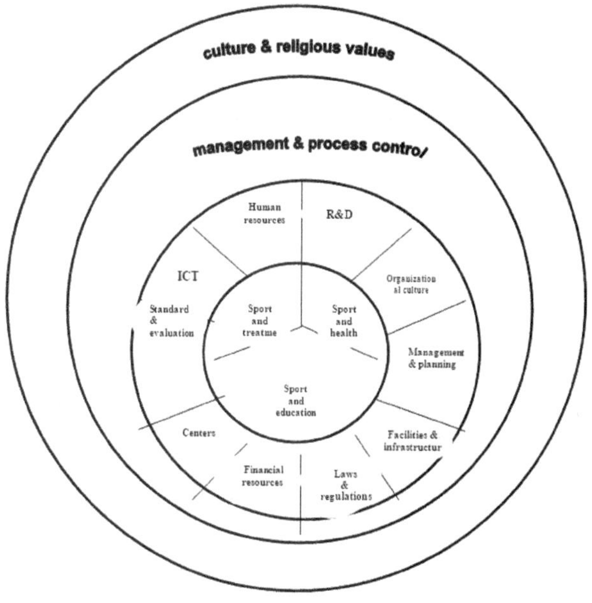

Chart 5. Final suggested model for Sport For All & Recreation development

4. Conclusion

The percentage of participants in Sport For All activities in different countries can show a clear image of the world Sport For All status. Studies show that most of the countries aren't satisfied with their Sport For All and mobility status. In this regard a special notice has been paid to social demands. People's priorities in doing sport activities are very important in these countries and measures are done by paying attention to this point. People's interest to Athletic (Competitive) Sport or Recreation ones can play an important role in performing Sport For All development programs and mobility in these countries. The government budget is one of the important governmental tools in developing this sport. In most of the countries Sport For All budget is more than the others which shows its importance in human societies. The studies reveal that in best situation the number of participants in Sport For All activities isn't more than %10 in our country.(A Local Strategic Plan For Iran Sport and Physical Education Comprehensive System 2002) Of course in some of the researches you can find it more and even about %60.(Tondnevis 2002)This is while the percentage of participants in sport activities in some of the countries like Finland and Sweden is more than %80 .(Bottenburg et al 2005, koski 2000, European commission 2004)So it is necessary to perform different micro and macro(master)plans to develop Sport For All in Iran. Paying attention to social demands and people's priorities & interests is very important too. (Girginov 2001, Echberg & Midol 1992, Australian sport commission 1999, Gholiniya(2004), Islamic Republic of Iran Broadcasting 1996) These priorities, social demands and interests determine which strategies, plans, sports and structures can be effective at the present time and future. Ghafoori(2007) In this research after studying Sport For All in Iran and some other countries(with similar socio cultural attributes and the same level of development)Strength &Weak points and Opportunities & Treats(SWOT)are analyzed and Sport For All Federation Strategic Plan was designed which hadn't been noticed separately in other Sport For All researches before. In "Iran Sport and Physical Education Comprehensive Plan" the processes of this sport has been studied completely and its different parts as SWOT analysis, vision, goals and strategies have been used in designing it. The studies in" Iran Sport and Physical Education Comprehensive Plan" are some of the most important and strategic studies among Sport For All ones. Saminiya (2009) studied the pathology and development of Sport For All in Iran based on SWOT model.(2009)A final model to develop Sport For and recreation is designed in this research as well. Ghafoori(2007) in his research titled as:" Different kinds of favorite Sport For All activities and Recreations in the society and offering a model for future plans" designed a model for future Sport For All Federation planning to increase the number of participants in Sport For All activities. Any way no Sport For All model in other researches is designed. In other researches on Sport For All, the status of this sport in people's leisure time and the participants' economic status are focused more. The first level of the designed model in this research emphasizes on Sport For All development and the second level focuses on Sport for health and motion, Sport for treatment and reduction in the effects of chronic diseases, Educational sport with approach of training of sports disciplines and paving the road to Athletic (Competitive) Sport. In a research by Kashef (1996) on Sport For All in West Azerbayjan, Keeping healthy was the participants' main aim and treatment was the less important one. In another research Kashef (2000) studied Iran Sport For All status and suggested some recommendations to develop it. In this research the most participants' motivations were public health, recreation, weight loss and treatment of diseases in turn. Having a review on the performed researches out of the country shows that the people's eagerness toward Sport For All is increasing. Countries like Australia, Germany, Canada, Sweden, Japan, Holland, Switzerland and France are more active in Sport For All. This reveals that personal and social health is more important in developed countries and they have paid attention to people's satisfaction & participation to have healthy life, Social solidarity and economic development among People of all walks of life in writing their strategic plan. If we are going to profit Sport For All advantages we should invest for it.

5. Suggestions and Solutions

- The Institutions affecting Sport For All specially The Ministry of Youth & Sport and Sport For All Federation should use strategic models to design their strategic plans.
- The main process of Sport For All development on the base of the suggested model and the scientific models has been designed in three parts as health, education and prevention of the diseases. It is necessary to have a written and scientific plan to connect and coordinate them to each other and to Educational and Athletic (Competitive) Sport.
- In spite of great similarities among these concepts, it should be noticed that because of their natural differences in Sport For All, their supporting components should be selected separately.
- The pathology of Sport For All in Iran shows that Sport For All system in Iran, in spite of its opportunities, should overcome its weaknesses.
- According to this pathology, Iran Sport For All strategic position is in growth and development level. To improve this strategy in Sport For All we need a Sport For All Development Model.
- It is necessary to determine some mechanisms which bind the performance of the rules and regulations, plan documentations in upper level documents, task orientation in Sport For All and make the sport popular in the society.
- Involving private and nongovernmental centers in policies while binding both profitable and non profitable approaches.
- Notice and focus on Customer Access Multistage Model with an emphasis on contingency and cultural infrastructures.
- Prediction of both Offensive - Development and Diversity Strategies considering SWOT.

References

[1] Mohammad .Javadipour, (2011).Sport For All Federation Strategic Plan, Research Design; Ministry of Youth & Sports, Sport For All Federation.

[2] Mohammad Ali. Ghare, (2004). Iran Sport For All status and its comparison with some of the world selected countries; PhD. Dissertation. Tehran Teacher Training University, Sport and Physical Education Collage.

[3] Mohammad Hosein. Eshkooh, Reza. Razavi, Taheri, (2010).Sport For All participants' social and Economical Status (SES) in Mazandaran province; Move Sport Management Journal, (2010/ summer), 5th Vol., pp 21-34.

[4] Fatemeh. Niknejad, (1996) Asking Tehran women's idea about Women Sport; Deputy of Women Sport and Physical Education in Physical Education Organization.

[5] Sport For All and Recreation Development detailed studies ;(2002).Iran Physical Education Organization, 1st version.

[6] Hasan. Asadi, Mohammad Reza. Ahmadi, (2000). Comparing the athletes and non- athletes students' psychological health in Sanandaj town high schools; Movement Issue, pp 36-46.

[7] Farzad. Ghafoori, (2007) .Different kinds of favorite Sport For All activities and Recreations in the society and offering a model for future plans; Research design.

[8] Mir Mohammad. Kashef, (2000). Studying Iran Sport For All status and suggesting some recommendations to develop it; Abstract. Essays of the 4th Physical Education and Sport Sciences National Meeting. pp 86-87.

[9] Maryam. Momtazbakhsh, (2006). Investigating the strategies of developing and improving Sport For All among women working in Military Sciences University; Military Knowledge Journal, 9th year.2nd no, pp53-62.

[10] Akbar. Afarinesh Khaki, Fereydoon. Tondnevis, Seyed Amir Ahmad. Mozafari, (2005). Comparing different universities faculties, coaches, athletes and managers' points of view on the ways of improving Sport For All ; Sport and Movement Sciences Issue, (2005/ summer); 3(5):22-1.

[11] Mohammad Javad. Gholiniya, (2004).Paving the road and Planning for making the sport popular among the people; Research design, Physical Education Organization.

[12] Atighechi,Akram,(1995). Investigating the ways of spending Zanjan city female university students' leisure time focusing on physical education role. MA Thesis. Tehran Central Branch Islamic Azad University.

[13] Saeed. Saneee, (1995). Investigating the ways of spending Tehran Teacher Training University students' leisure time focusing on physical education role; MA Thesis, Tehran Teacher Training University.

[14] Mohsen. Shafiee, (1994). Investigating the socio-economical status of Sport For All participants in Tehran city. MA Thesis. Tehran Teacher Training University.

[15] Gholam Reza. Ramezani Khalilabadi, (1994). Investigating the Sport For All participants' motivation in Tehran city; MA Thesis, Tehran Teacher Training University.

[16] Mona. Saminiya, (2011). The pathology and development of Sport For All in Iran based on SWOT model; MA Thesis, Mashhad Central Branch Islamic Azad University.

[17] Bottenburg, van M.; Rijnen, B. and van Sterkenburg, J. (2005). Sports participation in the European Union; Trends and differences. Arko Sports Media, Nieuwegein, Netherlands.

[18] European Commission (2004b) *The citizens of the European Union and sport.* Special Eurobarometer 62.0 213.TNS Opinion and Social c/o EOS Gallup Europe.

[19] Koski, P. & Heikkala, 1. (1998) Suomalaisten urheiluorganisaatioiden muutos. [National sports organisations in the process of professionalisation]. Jyvaskylan yliopisto, liikunnan sosiaalitieteiden laitos, tutkimuksia no.63. Jyvaskyla.

[20] United Nations (2003) "Sport for Development and Peace: Towards Achieving the Millennium Development Goals"; Report to Inter-Agency Task Force on Sport for Development and Peace; Available on: www.undp.bg.

[21] Council of Europe (2005). "Sport for all". Available on: www.coe.int

[22] Strategic planning. Report #3. Published by the foundation for community association research.

[23] Strategic planning handbook.(2001).Compiled by special libraries association.

[24] Richard A.Mittenthal. (2002). Ten keys to successful straregic planning for nonprofit and foundation leaders.

The effect of natural and artificial grass on sprinting performance in young soccer players

Vasileios Kanaras[1, 2], Thomas I. Metaxas[1, *], Athanasios Mandroukas[1], Ioannis Gissis[2], Andreas Zafeiridis[2], Christos S. Riganas[1], Evaggelos Manolopoulos[2], Vassilis Paschalis[3, 4], Ioannis S. Vrabas[2]

[1]Department of Physical Education and Sports Sciences, Aristotle University of Thessaloniki, Thessaloniki, Greece
[2]Department of Physical Education and Sports Sciences at Serres, Aristotle University of Thessaloniki, Greece
[3]Department of Physical Education and Sports Sciences, University of Thessaly, Greece
[4]Laboratory of Exercise, Health and Human Performance, Research Center, European University of Cyprus, Nicosia, Cyprus

Email address:
tommet@phed.auth.gr (T. I. Metaxas)

Abstract: The sprint performance on natural and artificial grass of 5th generation was assessed. Sixty eight young male soccer players, which were divided in two groups according to their age [children (n=36; 12.1±0.5y) and adolescents (n=32; 14.2±0.4y)], performed 30-m sprint tests with and without handling the ball on natural and artificial grass. The performance was recorded during 0-10m, 10-30m, and 0-30m running distances. It was found that children were significantly faster during 0-10m running distance on the artificial compared to natural grass when handling the ball while adolescents revealed no differences in sprint performance between the surfaces irrespectively of the ball condition. In running distances 10-30m and 0-30m, children were significant faster in the artificial compared to the natural grass either with or without ball, while the adolescents were significantly faster in the artificial grass only without handling the ball. Children run faster on artificial than natural grass while adolescent soccer players are faster in artificial grass when they do not have to handle the ball. It is clear that children should be more careful when play soccer on artificial grass because the ball is moving faster and greater skill is needed in order to avoid injuries.

Keywords: Adolescent, Artificial, Children, Natural Grass, Sprint Ability, Turf

1. Introduction

Sprinting constitutes a multidimensional and complex motor skill, being probably the most significant physical element of performance in modern soccer. Numerous studies have reported that in a 60 min soccer game, young players completed over 30 maximal sprints (i.e. speed higher than 18km/h), while the total distance covered during maximal sprints may reach 250m [1-3]. For this reason, coaches include at least two training sessions focusing on the improvement of maximal speed performance with and without handling the ball [4].

Traditionally, soccer games take place on natural grass; however, in many European countries, the use of artificial grass is continuously increased either for official soccer games or for training. Since 2005, UEFA and FIFA have approved the use of artificial grass of 3rd generation in their official tournaments [5, 6]. The last few years' research has focused on technical aspects and the physical conditioning of soccer players when training or competing on artificial grass. Anderson et al. [7] compared technical characteristics of soccer players on two different surfaces (i.e. natural grass vs. 3rd generation artificial grass) and was observed that players exhibited better technical skills on artificial compared to natural grass. Moreover, Di Michelle et al. [8] and Sassi et al. [9] reported that both heart rate and blood lactate were elevated when a game was performed on a 3rd generation artificial grass compared to natural grass.

The widely used artificial grass led Meyers and Barnhill [10] to examine the frequency, the causes, and the severity of injuries compared to natural grass. It was found that, there is a greater chance for of epidermal injuries and muscle strains on artificial grass compare to natural grass

[10] because of the greater fatigue potential of muscles [11], while the greater incidence of concussion and ligament tears on natural grass compared to the artificial grass may be related to the harder and drier surface [12]. Moreover, it was found that during a soccer game on artificial grass the mechanical load developed at the middle plantar portion and in the 5th toe was significantly higher compared to natural grass [13].

An increasing number of young soccer players compete and/or train on artificial grass. However, there is no data available regarding the effect of artificial grass on sprint performance while controlling the ball compared to natural grass in soccer players of developmental ages. Thus, the purpose of this study was to compare the sprint performance of children and adolescent soccer players on natural grass and artificial grass of 5th generation without or with handling the ball.

2. Methods

2.1. Participants

Sixty eight male children and adolescent soccer players participated in the present investigation (Table 1). All subjects participated regularly (i.e. 4-5 times/week) in soccer training or competitive matches. Participants were reported no injury of the lower limbs during the last year and they did not use any nutritional supplement. A written informed consent was provided by their parents after they were informed about all risks, discomforts, and benefits involved in the study. The procedures were in accordance with the 1975 Declaration of Helsinki, as revised in 2000, and approval was received from the institutional review board.

Table 1. *Demographic characteristics of the children and the adolescents group (mean ± SD).*

	Children n=36		Adolescents n=32	
Age (years)	12.0	± 0.5	14.0	± 0.5
Training age (years)	5.5	± 1.0	7.0	± 1.5
Body mass (kg)	39.4	± 6.1	57.1	± 9.9
High (cm)	146	± 7	165	± 7

2.2. Procedures

All measurements were conducted under field conditions on natural grass or artificial grass of 5th generation. Upon arrival the participants' body mass and height were measured on a digital height-weight scale (Seca, 703, Hamburg, Germany). Consequently, participants performed a standardized 25 min warm-up consisting of 5 min sub-maximal running, 5 min of stretching exercises, ball handling exercises for 5 min, three repetitions of 15m run-outs at approximately 90% of maximal speed, and 4 min of active recovery. Speed performance was assessed using a multidirectional 30m sprint test. During the test, the participants had to run 10m with maximal speed in a straight line (0-10m) followed by a 10m double change of direction right or left (10-20m), and finished with a 10-m maximal sprint in a straight line (20-30m). The sprint performance was assessed in running distances 0-10m, 10-30m, and 0-30m with the use of photocells (Newtest Powertimer, Finland) placed at the start, at 10m and at 30m marks. Each participant performed two efforts with and without handling the ball on the natural grass and the artificial grass while there was 5 min rest between the sprints. All efforts were randomized in respect to both conditions that is the ball handling and the surface of the field. During the trials, continuous verbal encouragement was provided to the players. All tests were performed on non-raining days and the wind speed not exceeding 1m/s. The ambient temperature and the relative humidity during the testing days ranged from 20° to 23°C and from 50 to 60%, respectively.

2.3. Statistical Analysis

A 3 way ANOVA [age (children and adolescents) × grass (natural and artificial) × ball (with and without handling)] with repeated measures on field surface and ball condition was used for analyzing the performance for each running distance (0-10m, 10-30m, and 0-30m). Significant main effects were followed by Tukey post hoc tests to locate the significantly different means. All data are presented as means±SD and were analyzed by Statistica version 7.0 (StatSoft Inc., Tulsa, USA). The level of significance was set at $\alpha=0.05$.

3. Results

A significant age × ball × grass interaction was detected on sprint performance in distances 0-10m ($F_{1,66}=2.47$; $p<0.001$; Figure 1A), 10-30m ($F_{1,66}=17.09$; $p<0.001$; Figure 1B) and 0-30m ($F_{1,66}=17.37$; $p<0.001$; Figure 1C).

Pair-wise comparisons between the field surface conditions at 0-10m running distance revealed that children when handling the ball are faster on artificial grass compared to natural grass ($p<0.01$; Fig 1A). In contrast, no differences in the performance at the same running distance were observed between artificial and natural grass of 0-10m in adolescents irrespective of ball condition.

Regarding the running distance of 10-30m (Figure 1B) and 0-30m (Figure 1C), the performance in children was significantly better ($p<0.01$) on the artificial compared to the natural grass with or without handling the ball (Figure 1B and 1C). In adolescents, sprint performance was significantly better ($p<0.01$) on the artificial compared to the natural grass only without handling the ball.

The performance was better ($p<0.05$) without handling the ball than handling the ball irrespectively of age and field surface while the adolescents were significantly faster ($p<0.05$) compared to children irrespectively of field surface with or without handling the ball (Figure 1).

4. Discussion

The main finding of this study is that sprinting performance is superior on artificial grass than natural grass in young soccer players. This superiority on artificial grass, however, is affected by age and handling or not a ball during the test. More specifically, children ran faster in 0-10m running distance on the artificial grass compared to the natural grass while handling the ball. In the same running distance the field surface did not affect the performance of adolescents. Regarding the sprint performance in 10-30m distance, children run faster on the artificial vs. the natural grass irrespective of handling or not the ball, whereas adolescents achieved better sprinting performance on the artificial vs. natural grass only without handling the ball. Overall, the adolescents run faster compared to the children irrespectively of field surface with or without handling the ball.

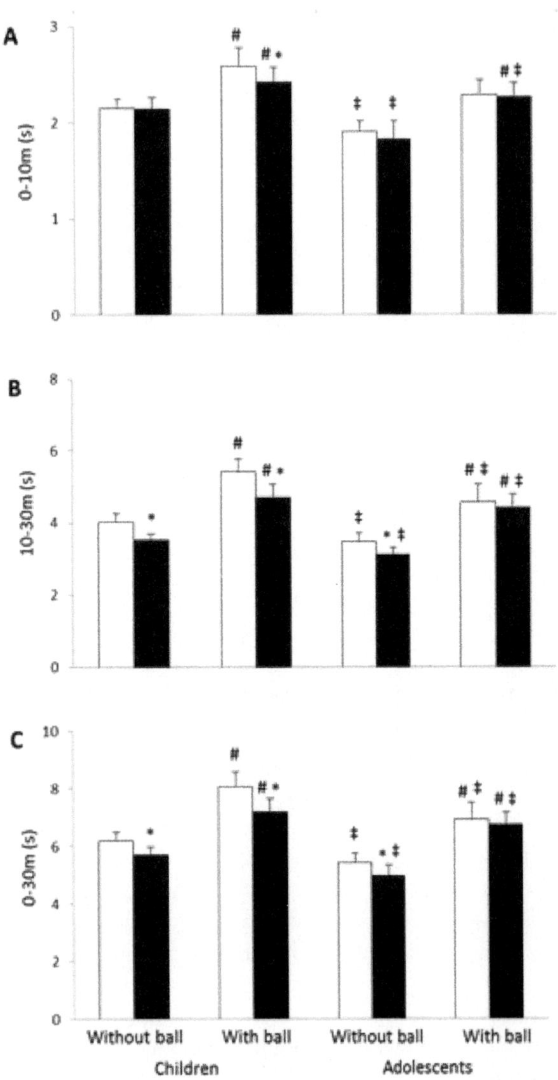

Figure 1. *Speed performance for children and adolescents in running distances 0-10m (A), 10-30m (B) and 0-30m (C), with and without handling a ball on a natural (open bars) and an artificial (closed bars) grass. * significant difference between the two field surfaces. # significant difference between with and without handling the ball. ‡ significant difference between children and adolescents*

The better sprinting performance found on artificial grass is in line with previous reports revealing that soccer players can perform faster sprints, accelerations and decelerations on artificial compared to natural grass [10, 14, 15]. It was suggested that the greater force exerted on artificial compared to natural grass results in the faster movement ability [16]. Indeed, a greater reduction in peak torque was reported on the hamstrings after a game on natural compared to artificial grass [16].

In an early investigation in this research field it was found that the ball bounce and the ball roll were greater in artificial compared to natural grass [17]. Moreover, it was more difficult for the players to start, turn, and stop on artificial grass while handling the ball [17]. Similarly, in a more recent investigation using questionnaires, a negative overall impression for the artificial grass, poorer ball control, and greater subjective physical effort was reported by the players. This was despite the fact that the total distance, the intensity and the number of sprints were similar between natural and artificial grass [7]. On the contrary, in the present investigation children and adolescents exhibited either better or no different sprinting performance on the artificial grass compared to the natural grass. It is possible that the different age of the participants between the present study and the previous investigations explain the diverse outcomes.

It is clear that the higher speed of the ball developed on the artificial grass makes increases the difficulty of controlling it [7], leading to changes in the play style [18]. Indeed, players on artificial grass are frequently complaining for poorer ball control and greater subjective physical effort compared to the natural grass [7]. As a result, it is common for soccer players to perform less aggressive defense as the fewer sliding tackles suggests [7]. On other hand, no differences were observed in injury rate between natural and artificial grass [19]. Nevertheless, between the two field surfaces there are differences in the sites of injuries as well as in the type of tissue sustaining an injury [13]. For instance, the medial forefoot region had a significantly higher relative load on natural grass when compared to artificial grass while the central forefoot as well as the lesser toes exhibited higher pressure while cutting on the artificial grass surface compared to the natural grass [13]. In addition, in regards to the type of tissue injury, it was found a higher frequency of muscle tissue injury on artificial grass compared to natural grass [10]. More studies are required in order to reveal the differences in performance characteristics between juveniles and adults during a soccer training/game on artificial grass.

In the present investigation the recruitment of more age groups could give additional information regarding the effects of different turf surfaces on sprinting performance.

5. Conclusions

It is concluded that the sprinting performance of young soccer players on artificial grass is superior to natural grass.

In fact, children ran faster on the artificial grass even when they had to handle the ball while adolescents ran faster on the artificial grass only without the ball. Therefore, caution should be paid when children play soccer on artificial grass because the ball is moving faster and greater skill is needed in order to avoid injuries. Considering that playing soccer on artificial grass affects playing style, more investigations in children and adolescences during a soccer game on different field surfaces are needed.

References

[1] C. Castagna, S. D'Ottavio, and G. Abt. Activity profile of young soccer players during actual match play. J Strength Cond Res. 2003, 17, 775-80.

[2] J. A. Harley, C. A. Barnes, M. Portas, R. Lovell, S. Barrett, D. Paul, and M. Weston. Motion analysis of match-play in elite U12 to U16 age-group soccer players. J Sports Sci. 2010, 28, 1391-7.

[3] C. Williams. Physiological demands of sprinting and multiple-sprint sports, R. J. Maughan. The Olympic Textbook of Science in Sport. Blackwell Publishing, 2009.

[4] A. Nummela, T. Keranen, and L. O. Mikkelsson. Factors related to top running speed and economy. Int J Sports Med. 2007, 28, 655-61.

[5] UEFA. FIFA quality concept: Handbook of test methods and requirements for artificial turf football surfaces, Nyon, Switzerland: UEFA, 2005.

[6] FIFA. FIFA quality concept for artificial turf quide, FIFA, Zurich, 2005.

[7] H. Andersson, B. Ekblom, and P. Krustrup. Elite football on artificial turf versus natural grass: movement patterns, technical standards, and player impressions. J Sports Sci. 2008, 26, 113-22.

[8] R. Di Michele, A. M. Di Renzo, S. Ammazzalorso, and F. Merni. Comparison of physiological responses to an incremental running test on treadmill, natural grass, and synthetic turf in young soccer players. J Strength Cond Res. 2009, 23, 939-45.

[9] A. Sassi, A. Stefanescu, P. Menaspa, A. Bosio, M. Riggio, and E. Rampinini. The cost of running on natural grass and artificial turf surfaces. J Strength Cond Res. 2011, 25, 606-11.

[10] M. M. Meyers, and B. Barnhill. Incidence, causes, and severity of high school football injuries on fieldturf versus natural grass. American Journal of Sports Medicine. 2004, 32, 1626-38.

[11] R. J. Lysens, W. de Weerdt, and A. Nieuwboer. Factors associated with injury proneness. Sports Med. 1991, 12, 281-9.

[12] J. Orchard. Is there a relationship between ground and climatic conditions and injuries in football? Sports Med. 2002, 32, 419-32.

[13] K. R. Ford, N. A. Manson, B. J. Evans, G. D. Myer, R. C. Gwin, R. S. Heidt, Jr., and T. E. Hewett. Comparison of in-shoe foot loading patterns on natural grass and synthetic turf. J Sci Med Sport. 2006, 9, 433-40.

[14] G. L. Gains, A. N. Swedenhjelm, J. L. Mayhew, H. M. Bird, and J. J. Houser. Comparison of speed and agility performance of college football players on field turf and natural grass. J Strength Cond Res. 2010, 24, 2613-7.

[15] C. L. Stanitski, J. H. McMaster, and R. J. Ferguson. Synthetic turf and grass: a comparative study. J Sports Med. 1974, 2, 22-6.

[16] M. Nedelec, A. McCall, C. Carling, F. Le Gall, S. Berthoin, and G. Dupont. Physical performance and subjective ratings after a soccer-specific exercise simulation: comparison of natural grass versus artificial turf. J Sports Sci. 2013, 31, 529-36.

[17] W. Winterbottom. Artificial grass surfaces for association football. Report and recommendations. . London: Sport Council. 1985,

[18] T. Lindholm, P. Olsson, and P. Balsom. Fysiska och tekniska krav vid fotbollspel med olika antal spelare. . Svensk Idrottsforskning, Swedish Sports Research Magazine. 1998, 4, 30 - 1.

[19] J. Ekstrand, T. Timpka, and M. Hagglund. Risk of injury in elite football played on artificial turf versus natural grass: a prospective two-cohort study. Br J Sports Med. 2006, 40, 975-80.

The effects of dietary nitrate (beetroot juice) supplementation on exercise performance

Andreas Zafeiridis

Exercise Physiology and Biochemistry Laboratory, Department of Physical Education and Sport Sciences at Serres, Aristotle University of Thessaloniki, Greece

Email address:
zafeirid@phed-sr.auth.gr

Abstract: Nitric oxide (NO) is a potent vasodilator that increases blood flow and induces various intracellular actions such as increased mitochondrial and contractile efficiency. NO bioavailability may be increased by direct consumption of dietary nitrate and its sequential reduction to nitrite, a regulator of NO-induced hypoxic signaling. Dietary nitrate consumption reduces blood pressure, protects from ischemia-reperfusion injury, and improves endothelial dysfunction. Recently, the popularity of dietary nitrate as an ergogenic aid has been increased dramatically. Most exercise studies have administered dietary nitrate in the form of beetroot juice containing 5-8 mmol of nitrate and a few studies have used sodium and potassium nitrate (8-10 mg/kg). The most prominent and consistent effects of dietary nitrate supplementation is a reduction in the oxygen cost of exercise and an increase in exhaustion time at submaximal workloads. This effect was observed after either a single bolus (2-3 h prior to exercise) or a long-term (2-15 days) supplementation. The ergogenic effects of beetroot supplementation appear to be dose-dependent and are most often observed after long-term ingestion (approximately 6 days), at high exercise intensities and in less fit individuals. The ergogenic value of beetroot supplementation in endurance athletes is not clear; many studies have documented no improvements and a few studies an enhanced performance (0.4% to 3%) in time- and distance-trials. Clearly, more research is needed to document (i) the optimal dosage of beetroot ingestion for enhancing exercise performance in athletes, (ii) the effects of dietary nitrate consumption on training adaptations, (iii) the efficacy of beetroot supplementation in increasing exercise tolerance in individuals with chronic disease, and (iv) the safety of long-term beetroot consumption.

Keywords: Dietary Nitrate, Nitric Oxide, Nitrite, Beetroot, Endurance, Exercise, VO2, Performance, Supplements

1. Introduction

Nitric oxide (NO) is a molecule that has been implicated in numerous vascular, contractile, and metabolic physiological processes (1-3). NO is biosynthesized by endogenous and exogenous processes. Endogenously, NO is produced by enzymatic and non-enzymatic pathways. The first pathway includes the oxidation of L-arginine to NO, a reaction catalyzed by the enzyme nitric oxide synthase (NOS); the second pathway involves a non-enzymatic (NOS-independent) reduction of inorganic nitrate to NO via the "nitrate-nitrite-NO" pathway. It should be noted that the L-arginine-NOS system contributes to recycling of nitrate and nitrite for the operation of the endogenous non-enzymatic "nitrate-nitrite-NO" pathway (4).

The NOS-independent processes occur also exogenously, by the direct consumption of dietary nitrate and its sequential reduction to nitrite and then to NO, enabling the "nitrate-nitrite-NO" pathway. In fact, it is believed that the biological effects of dietary nitrate are mediated by its conversion to NO. After ingestion, the nitrate is rapidly absorbed from the upper part of the small intestine into the plasma reaching the peak concentration in about 1 to 2h (5). About 25% of the ingested dietary nitrate is absorbed from the plasma by the salivary glands and undergoes metabolic conversion to nitrite in the oral cavity. Portion of the swallowed salivary nitrite is reduced to NO in the stomach and the remaining enters the systemic circulation and is converted to NO in the blood and body tissues (6, 7). This pathway is of great importance for production of NO under hypoxic conditions (mismatch of O_2 delivery and utilization).

Green leafy vegetables are the major dietary sources of nitrate. Particularly, plants grown in low exposure to sunlight, such as roots, have higher nitrate content compared to nitrate present in leaves and stems. Among leafy vegetables and roots with high nitrate concentration (>1000 mg/kg) is arugula (rocket), spinach, lettuce, radish, and beetroot that contain 140-260 mg of nitrate per 100 g (62 mg of nitrate equal 1 mmol) (8, 9). Numerous studies have pointed out the beneficial effects of dietary nitrate consumption on reducing blood pressure, on inhibiting platelet aggregation, on protecting from ischaemia-reperfusion injury, and on improving endothelial dysfunction (6, 7, 9).

Over the last five years, however, the popularity of dietary nitrate as an ergogenic aid has been increased dramatically. The rationale for the possible ergogenic effects of dietary nitrate is based on several facts *collectively*. First, NO and nitrite, the products of nitrate, are potent vasodilators that increase blood flow (1, 10, 11) and hence the O_2 delivery and oxygenation in working muscles (2, 12). Second, the ingestion of dietary nitrate increases the plasma nitrite bioavailability which acts as a reservoir for the "nitrate-nitrite-NO" pathway and as a regulator of hypoxic signaling for NO-induced vasodilatation (6, 10, 13). Third, the hypoxic and acidic conditions, as those observed during exercise, facilitate the reduction of nitrite to NO and potentiate the physiological effects of exogenously administered nitrite (11). Finally, the beneficial effects of nitrate/nitrite/NO on muscle blood flow and on mitochondrial and contractile efficiency (2, 14-17) may alter the muscle's hemodynamic and metabolic responses to exercise (18-20). In fact, there is evidence that pre-exercise plasma nitrite concentrations are independent predictors of exercise capacity and performance (12, 21-24).

In this review we include studies that have examined the effects of dietary nitrate on physiological responses and exercise performance in relation to exercise intensity (submaximal, maximal), training status (trained, untrained) and type of nitrate administration (acute, long-term). Furthermore, we discuss the possible mechanistic approaches for the improved exercise performance after dietary nitrate supplementation.

2. The Larsen's et al. Study (2007)

The pioneering study showing that dietary nitrate consumption may reduce energy cost during exercise was performed by Larsen et al. (2007)(25). Nine healthy, well-trained men performed cycling exercise at exercise intensities ranging from 45% to 100% of VO_2max after a 3-day sodium nitrate supplementation (0.1 mmol/kg/d). Dietary nitrate reduced VO_2 and increased gross efficiency at work rates corresponding from 45% to 80% of VO_2max compared with placebo. In contrast, dietary nitrate supplementation had no effect on VO_2 at maximal or near-maximal work rates (85% and 100% of VO_2max); neither effect was evident on heart rate, blood lactate, cycling cadence, ventilation, and respiratory exchange ratio (RER) at sub-maximal and maximal work rates. Interestingly, Larsen et al. showed that the increase in metabolic efficiency was elicited after dietary nitrate ingestion that is attainable through a consumption of leafy vegetables and roots.

The observation by Larsen et al. (2007) was followed by a bulk of studies investigating the effects of acute (single dose) and long-term (repeated doses) dietary nitrate supplementations on metabolic and circulatory responses and on exercise capacity and performance in healthy, non-athletic, population and in athletes. It should be noted that in the vast majority of studies dietary nitrate was administered in the form of beetroot juice.

3. Acute (Single dose) Nitrate Supplementation

For the purposes of this review, acute administration is considered the ingestion of dietary nitrate within 24h prior to exercise. Of the 19 studies that examined the effects of an acute (single-dose) of dietary nitrate supplementation, 8 were conducted in untrained to moderately trained individuals (Table 1), 10 in well-trained or elite athletes (Table 2) and only 1 in pathological population (Table 1). The dose of nitrate and the time of supplementation prior to exercise in these studies ranged from 5 to 19.5 mmol and from 75 to 180 min, respectively.

3.1. Supplementation in Untrained to Moderately Trained (Non-Athletic) Population

In the first study examining the ergogenic effects of a *single dose* of beetroot juice, Vohhatalo et al. (2010) administered in two occasions beetroot juice (5.2 mmol NO_3^-) and blackcurrant juice (negligible NO_3^-), 2.5h prior to exercise (26). Beetroot juice supplementation significantly reduced the O_2 cost at the completion of moderate exercise and improved metabolic efficiency (less increase in VO_2 relative to the increase in external work). In the same study, the participants performed a maximal ramp incremental test until exhaustion. The results showed that a single-dose of beetroot juice during maximal effort had no effects on physiological, metabolic, and performance parameters. In line, recent studies reported that VO_2 was significantly reduced at the completion of 5 min of cycling at 40%, 60%, and 80% of VO2max (27, 28); whereas, VO_2max did not change (29) after a single dose of nitrate supplementation compared to placebo. The above studies also examined the effects of acute nitrate supplementation on systemic and cerebrovascular hemodynamics (27, 28) and on cerebral and muscle de-oxygenation levels (29) during moderate-high intensity exercise. In Bond's et al. studies, a single bolus of nitrate (750 mg) administered 2 h before exercise significantly increased cerebral arterial blood flow velocity and reduced the cerebrovascular resistance (CVR), the rate-pressure product (RPP, an index of myocardial oxygen demand) and the systolic blood pressure compared to placebo, during cycling at 40%, 60%, and 80% of VO_2max. The reduced RPP and CVR have important clinical implications for heart failure and hypertensive patients, respectively, in order to exercise with less cardiac strain and reduced risk for stroke. The responses for cardiac output, heart rate, and diastolic blood pressure were not affected by nitrate ingestion. Thompson et al. (2014) reported reduced cerebral and muscle HHb concentration during exercise at 50% and 70% of VO_2max. This finding implies a reduced O_2 extraction response supporting the evidence of a reduced O_2 cost (25) and increased mitochondrial efficiency (15) after nitrate supplementation.

A few studies have examined in non-athletic population the effects of an acute nitrate supplementation on exercise capacity and performance (24, 29, 30). Murphy et al. (2012) documented that moderately trained individuals improved the performance in an all-out 5-km treadmill run by 3% after a single consumption of 200 g baked beetroot (≥500 mg of nitrate). More specifically, consumption of baked beetroot increased both the mean and the peak running velocities (by 3% and 5%, respectively); average rating of perceived exertion and heart rate were not different between the beetroot and the placebo conditions. In line, Thompson et al. (2014) showed that a single dose of beetroot juice supplementation (5.0 mmol NO_3^-) increased by 16% the time to exhaustion at 90% VO_{2max} compared with placebo. Wylie et al. (2013) evaluated the effects of acute nitrate supplementation on performance in team sport-specific exercise (24). Consumption of large doses of nitrate (28.6 mmol) over 30 h, in form of concentrated beetroot juice, increased the distance covered in the Yo-Yo intermittent recovery test by 4.2%.

Two studies completed by the same group of scientists examined the effect of acute nitrate supplementation on skeletal muscle metabolism. More specifically, Vohhatalo et al. (2011) evaluated whether potentiating the nitrate-nitrite-NO cycle with a single bolus of beet root juice would attenuate the deleterious effect of hypoxia on muscle metabolism and performance (20). They administered 0.75 L of beetroot juice (9.3 mmol of nitrate) or nitrate-depleted beetroot juice, in three equal doses, to 9 healthy moderately fit individuals 24 h, 12 h and 2.5 h prior exercise. Twenty-four hours following the first supplementation the participants performed knee-extension exercise until exhaustion, in three occasions: in hypoxia after beetroot ingestion (BR), in hypoxia after placebo (PL) ingestion, and in normoxia after placebo (PL). In support to authors' hypothesis, beetroot administration increased the time to exhaustion in hypoxia and abolished the deleterious effects of hypoxia on exercise performance. The ergogenic effects of nitrate were attributed to the reduced muscle metabolic perturbation, as observed by the smaller and slower reduction during exercise for phosphocreatine (PCr), inorganic phosphate (Pi) and pH, as well as to faster PCr recovery in BR-hypoxia and PL-normoxia versus PL-hypoxia. The authors suggested that the PCr-sparing effect of nitrate supplementation is possibly due to the improved matching of O_2 supply to demand. In their next study, the same group of scientists examined the effects of acute administration of nitrate-rich beetroot juice on muscle force production and muscle metabolism during repeated isometric maximum voluntary contractions (31). In two different occasions, the participants consumed 2.5 h prior exercise beetroot juice with (0.25 L with 10.2 mmol nitrate) and without nitrate (0.25 L with 0.17 mmol nitrate). The two exercise protocols consisted of (i) two bouts of continuous one-leg extension for 24 s, at 1 kg below the maximum, with 4 min recovery between bouts, and (ii) 50 isometric maximum voluntary contractions of 6.6 s intercepted by 2.2 s of rest. The force production (peak, mean, end, and fatigue index), as well as mean PCr changes (mean cost, mM; mean force/PCr depletion, N/mM) were not affected when a single dose of nitrate-rich beetroot juice was administered 2.5 h before exercise. The reason for the contrasting results regarding the PCr responses between the Vohhatalo et al. (2011) and Fulford et al. (2013) studies maybe attributed to the hypoxic conditions of exercise in beetroot supplemented group in the first study. It is possible that the hypoxic environment, in the Vohhatalo et al. (2011) study, favored the reduction of nitrite to NO. This in turn, could increase the NO-induced vasodilation, resulting to better matching of VO_2 supply to demand, and hence, increased oxidative function and PCr-sparing.

To the best of our knowledge, only one study to date, has investigated the effects of acute nitrate administration in a pathological population (32). The authors reasoned that the documented effects of nitrate supplementation on increasing muscle blood flow would improve muscle oxygenation in patients with peripheral arterial disease delaying the claudication pain and improving the exercise tolerance. Indeed, the participants increased their walking time (by 18%) before the onset of claudication pain and time to exhaustion (by 17%) during a maximal incremental test after the consumption of beetrout juice (750 mg of nitrate) compared with placebo treatment (orange juice). The enhanced exercise capacity, after nitrate ingestion, was accompanied by increased oxygenation (O_2Hb) and blood volume (tHb), and reduced O_2 extraction (HHb) during walking, suggesting an enhanced bulk muscle blood flow and an improved matching of O_2 delivery to utilization. In line with previous studies in healthy individuals, acute nitrate supplementation reduced diastolic blood pressure during a maximal incremental test.

3.2. Supplementation in Athletes

Several studies over the last four years have evaluated the ergogenic effects of acute nitrate supplementation in cyclists, skiers, runners, rowers, kayakers, and team-sport athletes. Surprisingly, 5 out of 10 studies were performed in cyclists. Lansley et al. (2011) was the first to examine the effects acute nitrate supplementation on exercise performance in athletes highlighting its potential use as an ergogenic aid

(33). Nine competitive cyclists (VO_2max: 56 ml/kg/min) significantly improved performance in a 4 km and a 16.1-km time-trials following ingestion of beetroot juice (6.2 mmol of nitrate) compared with placebo. Beetroot consumption increased also the mean power output and the power output to VO_2 ratio, supporting previous findings of increased contractile and mitochondrial efficiency following nitrate supplementation (15, 19). In contrast to results obtained in untrained individuals, no reduction in VO_2 was observed across both distances. Bescós et al. (2011) had competitive cyclists (VO_2max: 65 ml/kg/min) cycle for 4 bouts of 6 min at submaximal intensities (35%-65% of peak power) and then perform a maximal incremental test (34). Sodium nitrate ingestion, 3 h prior to trials, had no significant effect on submaximal O_2 cost, on time to exhaustion, on maximal power, and on blood lactate; VO_2max, however, was significantly reduced by 3.7%. It should be noted that despite the substantial increase in plasma nitrate (86%) in this study, nitrite, the regulator of NO-induced hypoxic signaling, was increased only by 16%. Cermak et al. (2012) also failed to document an ergogenic effect of a single bolus of nitrate administration (8.7 mmol of nitrate) in well-trained cyclists (VO_2max: 60 ml/kg/min) (35). Performance parameters (time, average power and cycling cadence), as well as body fuel selection and metabolites (glucose, free fatty acids, and lactate) were not different after ingestion of nitrate-rich and nitrate-depleted supplements.

Table 1. *Studies on the effects of acute (single–dose) dietary nitrate supplementation on physiological responses and indices of exercise tolerance and exercise performance in non-athletic population*

Study	Participants	Dose of Nitrate (NO_3^-)	Change in NO_2^- or NO	Time of ingestion	Study Design	Effects of BR ingestion
Vanhatalo (2010)	8 healthy, moderately fit men and women	BR juice (5.2 mmol NO_3^-)	↑36% NO_2^-	2.5h pre-exercise	Cycling: 2×5-min at 90% VT and a maximal test	At 90% VT: ↓VO_2 (~4%); ↓ VO_2/ work At Maximal: ↔VO_2max, peak and VT power, La_b, RERmax, VEmax, HRmax
Vanhatalo (2011)	9 healthy, moderately fit men and women	BR juice (9.3 mmol NO_3^-) in 3 equal doses	↑50% NO_2^-	24h, 12 h and 2.5h pre-exercise	Knee-extension in hypoxia and normoxia	In hypoxia: ↑ time to exhaustion, ↓ PCr breakdown, ↓ (faster) PCr recovery time
Fulford (2013)	8 healthy, moderately fit men	BR juice (10.2 mmol NO_3^-)	↑86% NO_2^- (from placebo)	2.5h pre-exercise	Knee-extension and Isometric	↔ peak force, mean force, ↔end-exercise force; ↔PCr responses
Murphy (2011)	11 healthy, moderately fit men and women	Baked BR (>500mg NO_3^--)	Not reported	75 min pre-exercise	5-km run trial	↑ mean and peak velocity; ↔ average RPE, HR; ↓ RPE at 1.8 km
Bond (2013)	12 healthy, active women	BR juice (750 mg NO_3^-)	↑300% NO	2h pre-exercise	Cycling at 40%, 60%, and 80% of VO_{2max}	↓ VO_2, RPP, SBP, CVRI; ↑ CBFV; ↔ CO, DBP, HR
Bond (2014)	12 healthy, active women	BR (750mg NO_3^-)	↑300% NO	2h pre exercise	Cycling at 40%, 60%, and 80% of VO_{2max}	↓ VO_2, RPP, SBP; ‹› HR, DBP,VE, RER
Thompson (2014)	16 healthy, moderately fit men	BR juice (5.0 mmol NO_3^-)	↑79% NO_2^-	2h pre-exercise	Cycling at 50% and 70% VO_{2max}; All-out trial at 90% VO_{2max}	↔ VO_{2max} At 50% and 70%: ↔ VO_2; ↔ RPE, HR; ↓ HHb All-out trial (90%): ↑ time to exhaustion
Wylie (2013)	14 recreational team-sport players	Multiple doses of BR juice (total of 28.6 mmol NO_3^-)	↑400% NO_2^-	Over 30h pre-exercise	Yo-Yo recovery 1 test	↑ Distance (by 4.2%) ↔ La_b
Kenjale (2011)	8 males and females with peripheral arterial disease	BR juice (~9 mmol NO_3^-)	↑186% NO_2^-	3h pre-exercise	Maximal incremental test	↑ Walking distance (by 17%); ↓ VO_2; ↓ HHb (reduced O_2 extraction)

↑ = increase; ↓ = decrease; ↔ = no change; NO_2^- = nitrite; NO = nitric oxide; BR = beetroot; VT = ventilatory threshold; VO_2 = oxygen consumption; La_b = blood lactate concentration; PCr = phosphocreatine; RPE = rate of perceived exertion; HR = heart rate; HHb = deoxygenated hemoglobin (index of O_2 extraction); RPP = rate-pressure product (index of myocardial work); SBP = systolic blood pressure; DBP = diastolic blood pressure; CVRI = cerebrovascular resistance index; CBFV = cerebral blood flow velocity; CO = cardiac output; VE = ventilation; RER = respiratory exchange ratio

Wilkerson et al. (2012) evaluated the efficacy of beetroot juice on improving performance in a longer event (23). Endurance cyclists (VO_2max: 63 ml/kg/min) executed a 50-mile time-trial following administration of nitrate-rich (6.2 mmol of nitrate) and nitrate-depleted beetroot juice. In line with the two previous studies, they did not observe a significant effect of beetroot juice on exercise performance and on average power, VO_2, HR, and lactate, but did document a 3% increase in mechanical efficiency (more power per VO_2). Interestingly, the increase in plasma nitrite and improvement in performance time were significantly correlated (r = -0.83). This observation encouraged the authors to separate the participants in "responders" and "non-responders", based on the % increase in plasma nitrite following nitrate supplementation. They observed that analyzing the results only for "responders" to beetroot supplementation (>30% increase in nitrite), there was a significant improvement in the time (-2%) of completion of the 50-mile trial after beetroot ingestion. In contrast, in a study by Bescos et al. (2012) repeated doses of sodium nitrate administered for 3 days, failed to discriminate between responders (>50% increase in nitrite) and non-responders (<30% increase in nitrite) on the effects of nitrate supplementation on exercise performance (36). It should be also pointed out that several studies have reported no changes in exercise performance after a single-dose of dietary nitrate, even though almost all of them have evidenced increases of more than 30% in plasma nitrite.

The possible reason for the equivocal results of the ergogenic value of a single dose of beetroot juice ingestion between Lansley et al. (2011) and the subsequent studies, may be the dependency of the beetroot-effect on the intensity or the duration of exercise (23, 35). In the Lansley et al. (2011) study, the participants performed the trial at a higher intensity for a shorter time. It has been previously suggested that the ergogenic effects of beetroot juice supplementation on exercise performance would be more apparent during high-intensity exercise, when greater hypoxia is developed and a greater % of type II muscle fibers is activated (18). The hypoxic and acidic environment at higher intensity exercise may potentiate the conversion of nitrite to NO and thus, the physiological effects of nitrate supplementation. Furthermore, the effects of beetroot on the augmentation of blood flow and vascular conductance was evident mostly in muscles comprised of primarily type IIb fibers. The increase in blood flow and vascular conductance after beetroot supplementation was highly correlated with the percentage of type IIb muscle fibers (18). Thus, the beneficial effects of beetroot on exercise performance maybe more apparent during high-intensity exercise, when a greater % of type IIb muscle fibers is activated and greater hypoxia is developed. A recent study in trained cyclists partially supports the ergogenic value of beetroot juice in hypoxic conditions. Muggeridge et al. (2014) investigated the effects of a single-dose of beetroot ingestion on cycling performance in simulated altitude (2,500 m) (37). This is of significant practical value, since many cycling competitions are performed at altitude. Consumption of beetroot juice (5 mmol of nitrate) reduced O_2 cost and enhanced the 16.1-km performance at normobaric hypoxia.

Studies performed in elite skiers (VO_2max: 70 ml/kg/min), kayakers, runners (VO_2max: 80 ml/kg/min), and team-sport (VO_2max: 57 ml/kg/min) athletes agree that a single-dose of beetroot juice (5 and 19.5 mmol of nitrate) has no effect on exercise performance (time-trials) (38-40) and on all-out sprints (39, 41). The effect, however, on energy cost was unclear, with studies reporting either no change (38, 40) or reduction (39). Hoon et al. (2014) examined the effects of two different doses of beetroot juice on simulated 2,000 m rowing performance. The authors reported that the moderate dose of nitrate (4.3 mmol) had no effect of 2,000 m rowing performance, whereas the high dose (8.4 mmol) improved performance (-1.8s) (42).

4. Long-Term Nitrate Supplementation

The ergogenic effects of nitrate supplementation have been partially attributed to the increased mitochondrial metabolic efficiency. This is in context with reports showing that continuous exposures of mammalian cells to NO for more than 6 days stimulate mitochondrial biogenesis (43, 44), which is unlikely to be observed with a single nitrate dose. Therefore, several studies examined the effects of long-term dietary nitrate (several doses over 2 to 15 days) supplementation on physiological responses and exercise performance in untrained to moderately trained individuals (Table 3) and in well-trained or elite athletes (Table 4).

4.1. Supplementation in Untrained to Moderately Trained (Non-Athletic) Population

Two years after Larsen's et al. (2007) study, Bailey et al. (2009) examined the effects of a 6-day beetroot supplementation (11.2 mmol/d of nitrate) on indices of muscle oxygenation and on VO_2 responses in healthy recreationally active men (45). Dietary beetroot reduced O_2 extraction (as evidenced by HHb response) and VO_2 during moderate intensity exercise (80% of ventilatory threshold), suggesting that the beneficial effects of repeated dietary nitrate consumption on reduced energy cost during exercise are attributed to mechanisms located within the muscle cell. The effects of beetroot supplements were different during severe exercise (70% between ventilatory threshold and VO_2max); that is, muscle oxygenation was unaffected after beetroot consumption, whereas, the exercise tolerance significantly increased (by 16%). In their follow up study, Bailey et al. (2010) attempted to study the mechanisms underlying the reduced energy cost after a short-term beetroot ingestion (5.1mmol/d of nitrate for 6 days). Muscle contractile efficiency was examined during knee-extension at low- and high-intensity work rates (19). There was a clear PCr-sparing effect and a reduced VO_2 response during low- and high-intensity exercise, after beetroot supplementation. Later studies, however, in elderly and young individuals failed to confirm the PCr-sparing effect of long-term (3-6 days) beetroot supplementation, during low (walking) and high (running) intensity exercise (46, 47). Furthermore, irrespective of the exercise intensity, the turnover rate for ATP_{total} was reduced after beetroot ingestion in Bailey et al. (2010) at expense of reduced ATP hydrolysis from the oxidative pathway and PCr breakdown. The reduced metabolic perturbation after beetroot ingestion tended to be related to the increased exercise tolerance. Interestingly, the reduction in PCr amplitude during the low-intensity exercise and in the PCr slow component during the high-intensity exercise, were analogous to changes in the respective VO_2 parameters. The authors suggested that that the beneficial effects of dietary nitrate on the reduced O_2 cost during exercise, are elicited through improved coupling of skeletal muscle ATP hydrolysis and force production rather than by increased mitochondrial ATP production per O_2 consumed.

Table 2. *Studies on the effects of acute (single–dose) dietary nitrate supplementation on physiological responses and indices of exercise tolerance and exercise performance in athletes*

Study	Participants	Dose of Nitrate (NO_3^-)	Change in NO_2^- or NO	Time of ingestion	Study Design	Effects of beetroot ingestion
Lansley (2011)	9 competitive male cyclists	BR (6.2 mmol NO_3^-)	$\uparrow$39% NO_2^-	2.5h pre-exercise	4km and 16.1km time-trials	$\leftrightarrow$ VO_2; $\uparrow$Power output (4.5%-6%); $\uparrow$ work/VO_2 (7-11%); $\uparrow$performance (~3.0%)
Bescós (2011)	11 competitive male cyclists	Sodium nitrate (10 mg/kg)	$\uparrow$16% NO_2^-	3h pre-exercise	4×6-min at 35%-65% of PPO and a maximal test	At 35%-65% PPO: $\leftrightarrow$ VO_2, VE, RER, La_b; Maximal: $\downarrow VO_{2max}$ (3.7%); $\downarrow VO_2$/ work; $\leftrightarrow$ time to exhaustion
Cermak (2012)	20 competitive male cyclists or triathletes	BR juice (8.7 mmol NO_3^-)	$\uparrow$124% NO_2^-	2.5h pre-exercise	~1 h time trial (75% PPO)	$\leftrightarrow$ Performance, average power, average cadence; $\leftrightarrow$HR, glucose, free fatty acids, La_b, insulin
Wilkerson (2012)	8 well-trained male cyclists	BR juice (6.2 mmol NO_3^-)	$\uparrow$25% NO_2^-	2.5h pre-exercise	50-mile time-trial	$\leftrightarrow$ Performance time; $\leftrightarrow$ average power, VO_2, HR, RPE, La_b; $\uparrow$ power/VO_2 (3.2%)
Muggeridge (2014)	9 trained male cyclists	BR juice (5 mmol NO_3^-)	$\uparrow$134% NO_2^-	3h pre-exercise	Altitude: 15 min at 60% W_{max} 16.1 km time-trial	$\downarrow$ VO_2; $\downarrow$ time ($\uparrow$performance) by 2.2%
Peacock (2012)	10 junior elite cross-country skiers	Potassium nitrate (614mg NO_3^-)	$\uparrow$127% NO_2^-	2.5h pre-exercise	55%VO_{2max} 75%VO_{2max} 5-km time-trial	$\leftrightarrow$ Performance time; $\leftrightarrow$ VO_2, HR, RER, La_b
Muggeridge (2013)	8 trained kayakers	BR juice (5 mmol NO_3^-)	$\uparrow$32% NO_2^-	3h pre-exercise	60%W_{max} all-out sprints 1-km time-trial	At 60%W_{max}: $\downarrow$ VO_2 Sprints: $\leftrightarrow$ Peak Power 1-km: $\leftrightarrow$ Performance time
Boorsma (2014)	8 elite 1,500-m runners	BR juice (19.5 mmol NO_3^-)	$\uparrow$17-fold in *nitrate*	AWAD	55-80%VO_{2max} 1,500 m time-trial	$\leftrightarrow$ Performance time $\leftrightarrow$ VO_2
Martin (2014)	16 team-sports males and females	BR juice (300 mg, ~5.0 mmol, NO_3^-)	AWAD	2h pre-exercise	all-out sprints on cycle ergometer	$\downarrow$ Number of sprints $\downarrow$ Total work; $\leftrightarrow$ Mean power
Hoon (2014)	10 highly trained rowers	BR juice (4.2 and 8.4 mmol NO_3^-)	AWAD	2h pre-exercise	Simulated 2,000-m rowing	At 4.2 mmol: $\leftrightarrow$ Performance At 8.4 mmol: $\uparrow$ Performance

$\uparrow$ = increase; $\downarrow$ = decrease; $\leftrightarrow$ = no change; NO_2^- = nitrite; NO = nitric oxide; BR = beetroot; PPO = peak power output; VO_2 = oxygen consumption; La_b = blood lactate concentration; HR = heart rate; VE = ventilation; RER = respiratory exchange ratio; AWAD = information from abstracts without adequate data

In line, 7 days of beetroot juice supplementation increased the contractile properties of human skeletal muscle. Nitrate supplementation improved the evoked peak force at low frequencies and the explosive force at maximal twitch; there were no beetroot-effects on voluntary maximum or explosive force production (48). Subsequent studies showed that the ergogenic effects of long-term dietary nitrate supplementation are also evident during high-intensity exercise. More specifically, dietary nitrate ingestion (2 to 5 days) reduced O_2 cost during maximal exercise (49), and increased exercise tolerance across a range of severe-intensity exercise bouts performed above the ventilatory threshold (50). The critical power, however, which corresponds to the highest power output that can be supported mainly by aerobic pathways, was unaffected by long-term beetroot administration (50).

What was not clear from preceding studies (prior to 2011), is whether the beneficial effects of beetroot juice consumption on reducing the energy cost was attributed to dietary nitrate *per se,* and not to other bioactive compounds, such as bitaine and polyphenols, present in beetroot juice. Lansley et al. (2011) investigated this issue by using a nitrate-depleted beetroot juice as placebo (46). They confirmed previous findings of reduced O_2 cost during moderate- and high-intensity running, and of increased exercise tolerance (time to exhaustion) in nitrate-rich vs. nitrate-depleted beetroot juice. The novel important observations in that study were that 6 days of beetroot administration (i) reduced the energy cost during very-low intensity exercise (walking), and (ii) did not change the mitochondrial oxidative capacity, suggesting that the improvement in aerobic exercise tolerance is not attributed to NO-induced mitochondrial biogenesis. Masschelein et al. (2012) examined the effects of a 6-day of beetroot supplementation on energy cost and oxygenation of muscle and brain in simulated severe hypoxia (51). Beetroot consumption for 6 days significantly ameliorated the deleterious effects of hypoxia increasing both muscle oxygenation during submaximal exercise (45% of VO2max), and time to exhaustion during maximal incremental testing; there were no effects of dietary nitrate on cerebral oxygenation. Resting energy expenditure and energy cost during submaximal exercise were significantly reduced (51).

VO_2 kinetics may alter the contribution of fuel utilization to energy production and affect the development of fatigue. More specifically, faster VO_2 kinetics during transition from rest to the first 2 min into exercise, may reduce the contribution of PCr and anaerobic glycolysis to energy production, whereas, a reduced VO_2 slow component delays the attainment of VO_2max during severe-intensity exercise increasing exercise tolerance (52, 53). Studies that evaluated the effect of long-term beetroot consumption on the primary amplitude of VO_2 kinetics revealed equivocal findings. Some studies reported that long-term administration of beetroot juice significantly reduced the primary amplitude of VO_2 during low-moderate exercise intensity (19, 45, 46), whereas other studies reported no effects (47, 54). Similarly, for high intensity exercise, there are reports showing increased primary amplitude of VO_2 after beetroot supplementation (45) and reports showing no changes (19, 46, 50, 54). The results for the phase II time constant are consistent for low-moderate intensity exercise, reporting no effects of beetroot juice (19, 45, 46, 54), and are contrasting for high-intensity, showing no effects (19, 46, 50), faster kinetics (54) or slower kinetics (45). Finally, the effect of beetroot juice on the VO_2 slow component also appears to divide the researchers into those observing (19, 45) and those not observing a beetroot-effect (46, 50, 54). Despite the divergent results on the effects of dietary intake on VO_2 slow component, all four studies reported an increased exercise time to fatigue. Collectively, long-term beetroot juice supplementation improved at least one parameter of VO_2 kinetics. That is, beetroot speeded VO_2 uptake in the first 1-2 min into exercise and/or reduced the magnitude of the VO_2 slow component or the mean response time (47, 54). The faster kinetics of VO_2 coincided with faster kinetics for HHb (faster O_2 extraction) (54). It should be also noted, that the effects of beetroot juice supplementation on VO_2 kinetics appear to be exercise-intensity dependent, with greater and more consistent effects observed during high intensity exercise.

4.2. Supplementation in Athletes

At the time of this review preparation, only seven studies examined the effects of long-term dietary nitrate supplementation on physiological responses and exercise performance in athletes. Three studies demonstrated an improved performance and four studies reported no effect of repeated beetroot supplementation of dietary nitrate (3-8d). The first two studies, performed in well trained athletes, showed that a 6-day beetroot ingestion (5.5 to 8 mmol of nitrate) improved the10-km cycling (55) and the 6 × 500 rowing (56) performance by 1.2% and 0.4% (by 1.7% in 4-6 reps), respectively. Finally, a recent study in master swimmers showed that beetroot juice (5.5 mmol of nitrate) consumed for 6 days, significantly increased the workload (by 6%) and reduced the energy cost (by 11%) at exercise intensity corresponding to the anaerobic threshold (57). Three points, however, should be considered before drawing conclusions from the above studies on the ergogenic value of long-term dietary nitrate supplementation in elite athletes. First, the within subject day-to-day variability in time trial performance was 1.0% that is very close to the reported effect of beetroot (55). Second, the worthwhile difference, index of practical significance, is very small for elite athletes (about 0.3% for rowers) (58). Third, the participants in Pinna's et al. study were master athletes with VO_2max values (43 ml/kg/min) comparable to those seen in young fit males; hence, it is not clear whether the documented effects in their study could be applied to athletes with higher aerobic fitness.

In contrast to the above results, more recent studies performed in endurance athletes and cyclists (VO_2max: 60-80 ml/kg/min) failed to observe an effect of repeated dietary nitrate supplementation in the form of either beetroot juice or sodium nitrate on exercise performance (36, 40, 59, 60). More specifically, Bescos et al. (2012) after a 3-day administration of sodium nitrate (10mg/kg/d) to endurance athletes reported no effect of dietary nitrate on mean distance covered and mean power exerted during the 40-min distance trial (36). Furthermore, no differences in respiratory parameters and blood lactate concentrations were observed between the nitrate and the placebo groups. In agreement, three subsequent studies also showed that beetroot administration for 4-8 days to elite 1500-m runners and cyclists had no effect on time-trial performance (40, 59, 60), on mean and peak power (59, 60), on submaximal VO_2 (40), on blood lactate (60), and on VO_2 kinetics and repeated sprinting ability (59). Furthermore, there was no effect of beetroot supplementation on adaptations to hypoxic training (60). In conclusion, the observations for the effects of repeated dietary nitrate supplementation on exercise performance in athletes remain largely divided.

***Table 3.** Studies on the effects of long-term (several doses over 2-15 days) dietary nitrate supplementation on physiological responses and indices of exercise tolerance and exercise performance in non-athletic population*

Study	Participants	Dose of Nitrate (NO_3^-)	Change in NO_2^- or NO	Study Design	Effects of beetroot ingestion
Larsen (2007)	9 well-trained men	Sodium nitrate (0.1 mmol/kg /d for 2 d)	↑82% NO_2^-	Cycling maximal incremental test	At 45%-80% VO_2max: ↓ VO_2 cost and gross efficiency; ↔ HR, VE, RER At VO_2max: ↔ VO_2max, HR, VE, RPE, work
Bailey (2009)	8 healthy, recreationally active men	BR juice (5.5 mmol NO_3^-/d for 6d)	↑96% NO_2^- (6 d rise)	Cycling at moderate (<VT) and severe (>VT) work rates	At Moderate: ↓ HHb amplitude (reduced O_2 extraction); ↔ O_2Hb, tHb; ↓ VO_2 cost At Severe: ↔ HHb, O_2Hb, tHb; ↓VO_2 kinetics; ↓ VO_2 slow component; ↑ exercise tolerance
Bailey (2010)	7 healthy, recreationally active men	BR juice (5.1 mmol NO_3^-/d for 6d)	↑137% NO_2^- (4-6d rise)	Knee-extension at low (15% of MVC) and high (30% of MVC) intensity	At Low: ↓ VO_2 cost and ↑ work efficiency; ↓ PCr and Pi amplitudes and ↔pH; ↓ATP_{total}, ATP_{ox}, ATP_{PCr} and ↔ATP_{Gly} At High: ↓ VO_2 cost and ↑ work efficiency and exercise tolerance; ↓ PCr and VO_2 slow components and ↔pH; ↓ATP_{total}, ATP_{ox}, ATP_{PCr} and ↔ATP_{Gly}
Larsen (2010)	9 healthy men and women	Sodium nitrate (0.1 mmol NO_3^-/kg/d, 2d)	↑133% NO_2^-	Combined arm and leg maximal exercise	↓ VO_{2max} and O_2 pulse; ↔ VEmax, HRmax, RER, La_b, and time to exhaustion
Vanhatalo (2010)	8 moderately fit men and women	BR juice (5.2 mmol NO_3^-/day for 15 d)	↑46% NO_2^- at 15th d	Cycling: 2×5-min at 90% VT and a maximal test	At 90% VT: ↓VO_2 (~4-5%); ↓ VO_2/ work At Maximal: ↔ VO_{2max} and La_b; ↑ VT and peak power
Lansley (2011)	9 healthy active men	BR juice (6.2 mmol NO_3^-/d for 6d)	↑104% NO_2^-	Walking and running at moderate (<VT) and severe (>VT) exercise intensities	↓VO_2 at walking (-12%), at moderate-intensity (-7%) and at high-intensity running (-7%); ↑VO_2 primary amplitude at moderate intensity; ↑ time to exhaustion; ↔ mitochondrial oxidative capacity and ↔ PCr and pH changes
Masschelein (2012)	15 healthy active men	BR juice (0.07 mmol/kg/d NO_3^- for 6d)	↑40% NO_2^-	Cycling in hypoxia and normoxia at 45% VO_{2max} for 20 min and maximal test	In hypoxia: ↓ VO_2 at rest (-9%) and at 45% VO_{2max} (-4%); ↑ muscle oxygenation (+4-5%); ↑ exhaustion time at maximal test (+5%); ↔ brain oxygenation
Kelly (2013)	9 habitually active men	BR juice (8.2 mmol NO_3^-/d for 5d)	↑197% NO_2^-	Cycling above the ventilatory threshold	↑ exhaustion time; ↔ La_b; ↔ resting metabolic rate; ↔ critical power; ↔VO_2 kinetics
Kelly (2013)	12 older men and women	BR juice (9.6 mmol NO_3^-/d for 3d)	↑418% NO_2^-	6-min walking test	↑ VO_2 kinetics (faster); ↔ walking distance; ↔ VO_2 cost, ↔ PCr response,
Breese (2013)	9 healthy men and women	BR juice (8 mmol NO_3^-/d for 6d)	↑435% NO_2^-	Cycling at moderate (<VT) and severe (>VT) exercise intensities	Moderate: ↔ O_2 extraction (HHb) and tHb; ↔VO_2 kinetics Severe: ↑ HHb kinetics;↓ HHb levels (reduced O_2 extraction); ↔ tHb; ↑VO_2 kinetics and ↔ VO_2 slow component; ↑ exercise tolerance
Fulford (2013)	8 moderately fit men	BR juice (10.2 mmol NO_3^- for 15d)	↑76% NO_2^- (vs. placebo)	Knee-extension and Isometric	↔ peak, mean, end-exercise force production; ↓PCr cost/mean force at end-exercise;
Haider (2014)	19 healthy men	BR juice (9.7 mmol NO_3^-/d for 7d)	AWAD	Voluntary and involuntary isometric contractions	↑ excitation-contraction coupling; ↑ evoked peak and explosive force; ↔ voluntary maximum and explosive force

↑ = increase; ↓ = decrease; ↔ = no change; NO_2^- = nitrite; NO = nitric oxide; BR = beetroot; VT = ventilatory threshold; VO_2 = oxygen consumption; La_b = blood lactate; PCr = phosphocreatine; Pi = inorganic phosphate; HHb = deoxygenated hemoglobin (index of O_2 extraction); O_2Hb = oxygenated hemoglobin; tHb = total hemoglobin (index of blood volume); VE = ventilation; RER = respiratory exchange ratio; AWAD = abstract without adequate data

***Table 4.** Studies on the effects of long-term (several doses over 2-15 days) dietary nitrate supplementation on physiological responses and indices of exercise tolerance and exercise performance in athletes*

Study	Participants	Dose of Nitrate (NO_3^-)	Change in NO_2^- or NO	Study Design	Effects of beetroot ingestion
Cermak 2012)	13 competitive male cyclists or triathletes	BR juice (8.0 mmol NO_3^- /day for 6 d)	↑ 20-fold in *nitrate*	2 × 30-min at 45% and 65% of PPO 10-km time-trial	At 45%-65% PPO: ↓ VO_2 cost; ↔ fuel selection, La_b and insulin: 10-km trial: ↑ Performance (1.2%) and average power output (2%);

Study	Participants	Dose of Nitrate (NO_3^-)	Change in NO_2^- or NO	Study Design	Effects of beetroot ingestion
Bond (2012)	14 well-trained male rowers	BR juice (5.5 mmol NO_3^- /day for 6 d)	Not reported	6 × 500-m with 90 s rest	↑ Performances in 4-6 repetitions (1.7%) and 1-6 (0.4%); ↔ HR, La_b, pH
Bescos (2012)	13 male cyclists and triathletes	Sodium nitrate (10 mg/kg) for 3 days	↑79% NO_2^-	40-min cycling distance-trial	↔ distance covered and mean power output; ↔ VO_2, VE, RER, and La_b
Christensen (2013)	10 elite cyclists	BR juice (500 ml, ~8 mmol NO_3^- for 6 d)	↑298% of *nitrate* +NO_2^-	3 × 6-min Endurance trial (120 min) Repeated sprints (6×20 s)	↔ performance time and mean power output; ↔ repeated sprinting ability; ↔ VO_2, gross efficiency, HR, RER, and RPE; ↔ VO_2 kinetics
Puype (2014)	22 well fit men (VO2max: 60 ml/kg/min)	BR juice (0.07 mmol/kg NO_3^-/d for 4 d)	↑ 7.5-fold in *nitrate*	30-min cycling time-trial Incremental test	↔ time to exhaustion and VO_2max; ↔ peak and mean power output; ↔ submaximal and peak La_b; ↔ adaptations to hypoxic training
Pinna (2014)	14 master swimmers	BR juice (5.5 mmol NO_3^-/day for 6 d)	Not reported	Incremental test	↑ workload at AT; ↓ energy cost at AT
Boorsma (2014)	8 elite 1,500-m runners	BR juice (19.5 mmol NO_3^- for 8d)	↑ 24-fold in *nitrate*	Runs at 55-80%VO_{2max} 1,500 m time-trial	↔ Performance time ↔ VO_2

↑ = increase; ↓ = decrease; ↔ = no change; NO_2^- = nitrite; NO = nitric oxide; BR = beetroot; AT = anaerobic threshold; VO_2 = oxygen consumption; La_b = blood lactate concentration; RPE = rate of perceived exertion; HR = heart rate; VE = ventilation; RER = respiratory exchange ratio

There are several reasons for the less apparent ergogenic effects of nitrate supplementation in highly endurance trained individuals compared to their untrained or moderately trained counterparts. Athletes demonstrate increased NO-induced endothelial function and vascular control, higher muscle blood flow and are metabolically more efficient (consume less O_2 at a given workload) compared to untrained individuals. Since the ergogenic effects of dietary nitrate supplementation are primarily elicited by enhancing the metabolic efficiency, there is possibly less room for further improvements in exercise O_2 cost and performance in athletes. Furthermore, the effects of dietary nitrate supplementation on muscle contractile efficiency and blood flow were selectively documented in muscles with predominant type II fibers (> than 60%) (18). Thus, endurance trained athletes might not demonstrate the muscle fiber composition to obtain the effects of beetroot juice supplementation. Also, the mitochondrial content/activity and the aerobic potentials of type II muscle fibers are increased in endurance athletes (61). Furthermore, the increased capillarity in endurance athletes may reduce the extent and the likelihood of developing hypoxia at a given exercise intensity. Finally, endurance athletes have higher levels of basal nitrite (62, 63); hence they might require higher doses of nitrate to evidence an ergogenic effect (23, 35).

5. Potential Mechanisms for the Ergogenic Effects of Dietary Nitrate

One of the most prominent and consistently reported ergogenic effects of acute or long-term dietary nitrate supplementation is the reduced energy cost of exercise (increased exercise efficiency). The exact mechanisms for the ergogenic effect of nitrate administration have not been described in full. To the best of our knowledge, 7 studies (3 in humans and 4 in rodents) attempted to shed light into the mechanisms of nitrate-induced improvement in exercise efficiency. These mechanisms include: (i) increased muscle contractile efficiency, (ii) increased mitochondrial efficiency, and (iii) improved vascular control and blood flow.

Bailey et al. (2010) were the first to report an increased muscle contractile efficiency during exercise, after beetroot supplementation in healthy young males (19). They found that 6 days of nitrate supplementation (5.1 mmol/d of nitrate) resulted to analogous VO_2- and PCr-sparing effects and to reduced ATP turnover rate during low and high intensity exercise. The decreased total ATP turnover rate was attributed to reduced ATP hydrolysis derived from oxidative phosphorylation and PCr breakdown; the ATP turnover rate from the glycolytic pathway remained unchanged. It has been suggested that the possible mechanisms for the reduction in ATP cost after nitrate supplementation may be due to the effect of nitrate on contractile filaments (actomyosin-ATPase) or on Ca^{2+} handling (Ca^{2+}-ATPase) (3, 16, 19). To examine the above hypothesis, Hernandez et al. administered to rats inorganic nitrate (beetroot juice) for 7 days in a dose that is easily obtained by humans with high-nitrate diets and is similar to that eliciting an ergogenic effect (17). The authors observed a faster rate and greater magnitude of force production after nitrate, compared with placebo, only in fast-twitch (extensor digitorum longus) and not in slow-twitch (soleus) muscles. The enhanced muscular function was attributed to the improved Ca^{2+} handling, as documented by the increased myoplasmic free Ca^{2+} levels and overexpression of calsequestrin1 and dihydropyridine receptors proteins. Interestingly, the expression of these proteins did not change in the soleus muscle after the administration of beetroot, which was in line with the lack of changes in contractile force in the soleus muscle. The authors suggested that by lowering the threshold for fast-twitch muscle activation to achieve similar force production, the dietary nitrate supplementation may increase the muscle contractile efficiency and reduce the effort and the number of motor units required for a given task without affecting the rate of force development. These results were recently confirmed in humans. In a double-blind randomized study, nitrate-rich beetroot juice enhanced the contractile properties of human skeletal muscle by improving the excitation-contraction coupling at low stimulation frequency (48).

There is evidence from a recent study that mitochondria constitute the main targets for the effects of nitrate on reduced O_2 consumption and increased exercise tolerance (15). The authors evaluated the mitochondrial efficiency after 3 days of dietary nitrate supplementation (0.1 mmol/kg/d of sodium nitrate) in healthy young males. They observed that the number of ATP molecules produced per O_2 consumed (P/O ratio) in skeletal muscle mitochondria increased by 19% after dietary nitrate ingestion compared with placebo. Importantly, the improved mitochondrial efficiency was correlated to the reduction in whole-body O_2 cost during exercise. The increased mitochondrial efficiency (P/O ratio) after nitrate supplementation was possibly attributed to the reduction in proton leak across the inner mitochondrial membrane, as suggested by the downregulation of adenine nucleotide transporter and UCP-3 proteins. In particular, the adenine nucleotide transporter catalyzes the exchange of ATP and ADP across the mitochondrial inner membrane and the cytoplasm; two-thirds of the basal proton conductance of mitochondria is catalyzed by this carrier (64). It is unlikely that improved metabolic efficiency after nitrate ingestion was due to changes in mitochondrial density or power, since no changes were observed in mitochondrial copy number, in expression of genes involved in mitochondrial biogenesis, and in the activity of citrate synthase and cytochrome c oxidase (16).

Recent studies propose that the beneficial effects of dietary nitrate supplementation on the metabolic control and exercise performance may be elicited through a non-intracellular mechanism. Ferguson at al. (2013) documented that dietary nitrate supplementation (1 mmol/kg/d) for 5 days enhanced vascular control and elevated skeletal muscle O_2 delivery during exercise in rats (18). The authors proposed this finding as the potential mechanism for the improved metabolic control after dietary nitrate supplementation. Interestingly, the augmenting effects of beetroot ingestion on blood flow and vascular conductance were most evident in muscles comprised of primarily type IIb fibers. The authors reasoned that the nitrate-induced increase in blood flow during exercise, would improve muscle O_2 perfusion and hence, increase the O_2 delivery/utilization matching, and would enhance the pressure gradient for blood-muscle O_2 flux. This would increase the contribution of oxidative pathways for energy production, would reduce the contribution of glycolytic pathway and the accumulation of lactate in muscles, and would delay fatigue (18). The above idea of NO availability (the end product of nitrate) rising the microvascular O_2 driving pressure during exercise, was previously documented by Ferreira et al. (65). Thus, in their subsequent two studies Ferguson et al. administered beetroot juice to rats and examined the muscle hemodynamic responses during exercise. The authors reported that dietary nitrate supplementation improved skeletal muscle blood flow and O_2 delivery/utilization matching during exercise, and increased the microvascular O_2 pressure in a dose dependent manner (66, 67). More specifically, a low dose (0.3 mmol/kg/d; ~3.2mmol/d for humans) of beetroot juice, corresponding to a *typical* nitrate-rich diet consumed by humans, had no effects on muscle blood flow, vascular conductance, and microvascular (driving) O_2 pressure during exercise; whereas a high dose (1 mmol/kg/d; ~7.4 mmol/d for humans) significantly increased all parameters (67). The findings of Ferguson et al. are in line with an earlier report that the increased NO bioavalability after training is accompanied by a delayed fall in microvascular O_2 pressure during exercise (68). The improved microvascular O_2 pressure response during exercise, after nitrate supplementation may also well explain the reduced PCr degradation during high-intensity exercise (19, 20), and the improved exercise tolerance.

6. Conclusion

The vast majority of studies that examined the ergogenic value of dietary nitrate supplementation used beetroot juice and only a few administered sodium nitrate. The most prominent and consistent effects of dietary nitrate supplementation is a reduction in the oxygen cost of exercise, an increase in exercise tolerance at submaximal workloads, and an attenuation of the deleterious effects of hypoxic environment during exercise. The mechanistic bases for these effects are not clear yet, but appear to be of intracellular (increased contractile and mitochondrial efficiency) and hemodynamic (increased blood flow) origin. The ergogenic effects of beetroot ingestion were observed after a single bolus (2-3 h prior to exercise) and following long-term (several doses for 2-15 d) supplementation, and may be depended on the type of supplementation, the exercise intensity, and the fitness level. That is, the ergogenic beetroot-effects are more readily apparent after repeated ingestion (over approximately 6 days), during higher exercise intensities and in less fit individuals (69). Particularly for athletes, the ergogenic value of beetroot supplementation on exercise performance is not clear, with most studies documenting no significant improvements in time- and distance-trials. Given the paucity of data on the dose-response relationship between the effects of beetroot juice and exercise tolerance (70), studies should be conducted in various populations to establish the effectual dose for enhancing exercise performance. It is possible, for example, that athletes may require higher dosage to evidence an ergogenic effect. It should be noted, however, that most exercise studies exceeded the acceptable daily nitrate intake; yet, no adverse effects have been reported. Importantly, the ergogenic effects of beetroot supplementation should be examined in individuals with cardiovascular, respiratory, and metabolic diseases, since the potential of beetroot ingestion to reduce energy cost and increase exercise tolerance is of practical importance for these individuals.

References

[1] Stamler JS, Meissner G. Physiology of nitric oxide in skeletal muscle. Physiol Rev. 2001 Jan;81(1):209-37. PubMed PMID: 11152758. Epub 2001/01/12. eng.

[2] Joyner MJ, Tschakovsky ME. Nitric oxide and physiologic vasodilation in human limbs: where do we go from here? Can J Appl Physiol. 2003 Jun;28(3):475-90. PubMed PMID: 12955873. Epub 2003/09/06. eng.

[3] Ferreira LF, Behnke BJ. A toast to health and performance! Beetroot juice lowers blood pressure and the O2 cost of exercise. J Appl Physiol (1985). 2011 Mar;110(3):585-6. PubMed PMID: 21183624. Epub 2010/12/25. eng.

[4] Lundberg JO, Weitzberg E. The biological role of nitrate and nitrite: the times they are a-changin'. Nitric Oxide. 2010 Feb 15;22(2):61-3. PubMed PMID: 19919855. Epub 2009/11/19. eng.

[5] Miller GD, Marsh AP, Dove RW, Beavers D, Presley T, Helms C, et al. Plasma nitrate and nitrite are increased by a high-nitrate supplement but not by high-nitrate foods in older adults. Nutr Res. 2012 Mar;32(3):160-8. PubMed PMID: 22464802. Pubmed Central PMCID: PMC3319660. Epub 2012/04/03. eng.

[6] Lundberg JO, Carlstrom M, Larsen FJ, Weitzberg E. Roles of dietary inorganic nitrate in cardiovascular health and disease. Cardiovasc Res. 2011 Feb 15;89(3):525-32. PubMed PMID: 20937740. Epub 2010/10/13. eng.

[7] Gilchrist M, Winyard PG, Benjamin N. Dietary nitrate--good or bad? Nitric Oxide. 2010 Feb 15;22(2):104-9. PubMed PMID: 19874908. Epub 2009/10/31. eng.

[8] Alexander J, Benford D, Cockburn A, Cravedi J, Dogliotti E, Di Domenico A, et al. Nitrate in vegetables. The EFSA Journal. 2008 (689):1-79.

[9] Lidder S, Webb AJ. Vascular effects of dietary nitrate (as found in green leafy vegetables and beetroot) via the nitrate-nitrite-nitric oxide pathway. British Journal of Clinical Pharmacology. 2012;75(3):677-96.

[10] van Faassen EE, Bahrami S, Feelisch M, Hogg N, Kelm M, Kim-Shapiro DB, et al. Nitrite as regulator of hypoxic signaling in mammalian physiology. Med Res Rev. 2009 Sep;29(5):683-741. PubMed PMID: 19219851. Pubmed Central PMCID: PMC2725214. Epub 2009/02/17. eng.

[11] Totzeck M, Hendgen-Cotta UB, Luedike P, Berenbrink M, Klare JP, Steinhoff HJ, et al. Nitrite regulates hypoxic vasodilation via myoglobin-dependent nitric oxide generation. Circulation. 2012 Jul 17;126(3):325-34. PubMed PMID: 22685116. Pubmed Central PMCID: PMC3410747. Epub 2012/06/12. eng.

[12] Dreissigacker U, Wendt M, Wittke T, Tsikas D, Maassen N. Positive correlation between plasma nitrite and performance during high-intensive exercise but not oxidative stress in healthy men. Nitric Oxide. 2010 Sep 15;23(2):128-35. PubMed PMID: 20451646. Epub 2010/05/11. eng.

[13] Gladwin MT, Kim-Shapiro DB. The functional nitrite reductase activity of the heme-globins. Blood. 2008 Oct 1;112(7):2636-47. PubMed PMID: 18596228. Pubmed Central PMCID: PMC2556603. Epub 2008/07/04. eng.

[14] Casey DP, Beck DT, Braith RW. Systemic plasma levels of nitrite/nitrate (NOx) reflect brachial flow-mediated dilation responses in young men and women. Clin Exp Pharmacol Physiol. 2007 Dec;34(12):1291-3. PubMed PMID: 17973870. Epub 2007/11/02. eng.

[15] Larsen FJ, Schiffer TA, Borniquel S, Sahlin K, Ekblom B, Lundberg JO, et al. Dietary inorganic nitrate improves mitochondrial efficiency in humans. Cell Metab. 2011 Feb 2;13(2):149-59. PubMed PMID: 21284982. Epub 2011/02/03. eng.

[16] Larsen FJ, Schiffer TA, Weitzberg E, Lundberg JO. Regulation of mitochondrial function and energetics by reactive nitrogen oxides. Free Radic Biol Med. 2012 Nov 15;53(10):1919-28. PubMed PMID: 22989554. Epub 2012/09/20. eng.

[17] Hernandez A, Schiffer TA, Ivarsson N, Cheng AJ, Bruton JD, Lundberg JO, et al. Dietary nitrate increases tetanic [Ca2+]i and contractile force in mouse fast-twitch muscle. J Physiol. 2012 Aug 1;590(Pt 15):3575-83. PubMed PMID: 22687611. Pubmed Central PMCID: PMC3547271. Epub 2012/06/13. eng.

[18] Ferguson SK, Hirai DM, Copp SW, Holdsworth CT, Allen JD, Jones AM, et al. Impact of dietary nitrate supplementation via beetroot juice on exercising muscle vascular control in rats. J Physiol. 2013 Jan 15;591(Pt 2):547-57. PubMed PMID: 23070702. Pubmed Central PMCID: PMC3577528. Epub 2012/10/17. eng.

[19] Bailey SJ, Fulford J, Vanhatalo A, Winyard PG, Blackwell JR, DiMenna FJ, et al. Dietary nitrate supplementation enhances muscle contractile efficiency during knee-extensor exercise in humans. J Appl Physiol (1985). 2010 Jul;109(1):135-48. PubMed PMID: 20466802. Epub 2010/05/15. eng.

[20] Vanhatalo A, Fulford J, Bailey SJ, Blackwell JR, Winyard PG, Jones AM. Dietary nitrate reduces muscle metabolic perturbation and improves exercise tolerance in hypoxia. J Physiol. 2011 Nov 15;589(Pt 22):5517-28. PubMed PMID: 21911616. Pubmed Central PMCID: PMC3240888. Epub 2011/09/14. eng.

[21] Rassaf T, Lauer T, Heiss C, Balzer J, Mangold S, Leyendecker T, et al. Nitric oxide synthase-derived plasma nitrite predicts exercise capacity. Br J Sports Med. 2007 Oct;41(10):669-73; discussion 73. PubMed PMID: 17496072. Pubmed Central PMCID: PMC2465183. Epub 2007/05/15. eng.

[22] Totzeck M, Hendgen-Cotta UB, Rammos C, Frommke LM, Knackstedt C, Predel HG, et al. Higher endogenous nitrite levels are associated with superior exercise capacity in highly trained athletes. Nitric Oxide. 2012 Aug 15;27(2):75-81. PubMed PMID: 22609879. Epub 2012/05/23. eng.

[23] Wilkerson DP, Hayward GM, Bailey SJ, Vanhatalo A, Blackwell JR, Jones AM. Influence of acute dietary nitrate supplementation on 50 mile time trial performance in well-trained cyclists. Eur J Appl Physiol. 2012 Dec;112(12):4127-34. PubMed PMID: 22526247. Epub 2012/04/25. eng.

[24] Wylie LJ, Mohr M, Krustrup P, Jackman SR, Ermiotadis G, Kelly J, et al. Dietary nitrate supplementation improves team sport-specific intense intermittent exercise performance. Eur J Appl Physiol. 2013 Jul;113(7):1673-84. PubMed PMID: 23370859. Epub 2013/02/02. eng.

[25] Larsen FJ, Weitzberg E, Lundberg JO, Ekblom B. Effects of dietary nitrate on oxygen cost during exercise. Acta Physiol (Oxf). 2007 Sep;191(1):59-66. PubMed PMID: 17635415. Epub 2007/07/20. eng.

[26] Vanhatalo A, Bailey SJ, Blackwell JR, DiMenna FJ, Pavey TG, Wilkerson DP, et al. Acute and chronic effects of dietary nitrate supplementation on blood pressure and the physiological responses to moderate-intensity and incremental exercise. Am J Physiol Regul Integr Comp Physiol. 2010 Oct;299(4):R1121-31. PubMed PMID: 20702806. Epub 2010/08/13. eng.

[27] Bond V, Jr., Curry BH, Adams RG, Asadi MS, Millis RM, Haddad GE. Effects of dietary nitrates on systemic and cerebrovascular hemodynamics. Cardiol Res Pract. 2013;2013:435629. PubMed PMID: 24455404. Pubmed Central PMCID: PMC3886243. Epub 2014/01/24. eng.

[28] Bond V, Jr., Curry BH, Adams RG, Millis RM, Haddad GE. Cardiorespiratory function associated with dietary nitrate supplementation. Appl Physiol Nutr Metab. 2014 Feb;39(2):168-72. PubMed PMID: 24476472. Pubmed Central PMCID: PMC3909870. Epub 2014/01/31. eng.

[29] Thompson KG, Turner L, Prichard J, Dodd F, Kennedy DO, Haskell C, et al. Influence of dietary nitrate supplementation on physiological and cognitive responses to incremental cycle exercise. Respir Physiol Neurobiol. 2014 Mar 1;193:11-20. PubMed PMID: 24389270. Epub 2014/01/07. eng.

[30] Murphy M, Eliot K, Heuertz RM, Weiss E. Whole beetroot consumption acutely improves running performance. J Acad Nutr Diet. 2012 Apr;112(4):548-52. PubMed PMID: 22709704. Epub 2012/06/20. eng.

[31] Fulford J, Winyard PG, Vanhatalo A, Bailey SJ, Blackwell JR, Jones AM. Influence of dietary nitrate supplementation on human skeletal muscle metabolism and force production during maximum voluntary contractions. Pflugers Arch. 2013 Apr;465(4):517-28. PubMed PMID: 23354414. Epub 2013/01/29. eng.

[32] Kenjale AA, Ham KL, Stabler T, Robbins JL, Johnson JL, Vanbruggen M, et al. Dietary nitrate supplementation enhances exercise performance in peripheral arterial disease. J Appl Physiol (1985). 2011 Jun;110(6):1582-91. PubMed PMID: 21454745. Pubmed Central PMCID: PMC3119136. Epub 2011/04/02. eng.

[33] Lansley KE, Winyard PG, Bailey SJ, Vanhatalo A, Wilkerson DP, Blackwell JR, et al. Acute dietary nitrate supplementation improves cycling time trial performance. Med Sci Sports Exerc. 2011 Jun;43(6):1125-31. PubMed PMID: 21471821. Epub 2011/04/08. eng.

[34] Bescos R, Rodriguez FA, Iglesias X, Ferrer MD, Iborra E, Pons A. Acute administration of inorganic nitrate reduces VO(2peak) in endurance athletes. Med Sci Sports Exerc. 2011 Oct;43(10):1979-86. PubMed PMID: 21407132. Epub 2011/03/17. eng.

[35] Cermak NM, Res P, Stinkens R, Lundberg JO, Gibala MJ, van Loon LJ. No improvement in endurance performance after a single dose of beetroot juice. Int J Sport Nutr Exerc Metab. 2012 Dec;22(6):470-8. PubMed PMID: 23212319. Epub 2012/12/06. eng.

[36] Bescos R, Ferrer-Roca V, Galilea PA, Roig A, Drobnic F, Sureda A, et al. Sodium nitrate supplementation does not enhance performance of endurance athletes. Med Sci Sports Exerc. 2012 Dec;44(12):2400-9. PubMed PMID: 22811030. Epub 2012/07/20. eng.

[37] Muggeridge DJ, Howe CC, Spendiff O, Pedlar C, James PE, Easton C. A single dose of beetroot juice enhances cycling performance in simulated altitude. Med Sci Sports Exerc. 2014 Jan;46(1):143-50. PubMed PMID: 23846159. Epub 2013/07/13. eng.

[38] Peacock O, Tjonna AE, James P, Wisloff U, Welde B, Bohlke N, et al. Dietary nitrate does not enhance running performance in elite cross-country skiers. Med Sci Sports Exerc. 2012 Nov;44(11):2213-9. PubMed PMID: 22874535. Epub 2012/08/10. eng.

[39] Muggeridge DJ, Howe CC, Spendiff O, Pedlar C, James PE, Easton C. The effects of a single dose of concentrated beetroot juice on performance in trained flatwater kayakers. Int J Sport Nutr Exerc Metab. 2013 Oct;23(5):498-506. PubMed PMID: 23580456. Epub 2013/04/13. eng.

[40] Boorsma RK, Whitfield J, Spriet LL. Beetroot Juice Supplementation Does Not Improve Performance in Elite 1500-m Runners. Med Sci Sports Exerc. 2014 Apr 28. PubMed PMID: 24781895. Epub 2014/05/02. Eng.

[41] Martin K, Smee D, Thompson KG, Rattray B. Dietary Nitrate Does Not Improve Repeated Sprint Performance. Int J Sports Physiol Perform. 2014 Jan 15. PubMed PMID: 24436354. Epub 2014/01/18. Eng.

[42] Hoon MW, Jones AM, Johnson NA, Blackwell JR, Broad EM, Lundy B, et al. The Effect of Variable Doses of Inorganic Nitrate-Rich Beetroot Juice on Simulated 2,000-m Rowing Performance in Trained Athletes. Int J Sports Physiol Perform. 2014 Jul;9(4):615-20. PubMed PMID: 24085341. Epub 2013/10/03. eng.

[43] Clementi E, Nisoli E. Nitric oxide and mitochondrial biogenesis: a key to long-term regulation of cellular metabolism. Comp Biochem Physiol A Mol Integr Physiol. 2005 Oct;142(2):102-10. PubMed PMID: 16091305. Epub 2005/08/11. eng.

[44] Nisoli E, Falcone S, Tonello C, Cozzi V, Palomba L, Fiorani M, et al. Mitochondrial biogenesis by NO yields functionally active mitochondria in mammals. Proc Natl Acad Sci U S A. 2004 Nov 23;101(47):16507-12. PubMed PMID: 15545607. Pubmed Central PMCID: PMC534517. Epub 2004/11/17. eng.

[45] Bailey SJ, Winyard P, Vanhatalo A, Blackwell JR, Dimenna FJ, Wilkerson DP, et al. Dietary nitrate supplementation reduces the O2 cost of low-intensity exercise and enhances tolerance to high-intensity exercise in humans. J Appl Physiol (1985). 2009 Oct;107(4):1144-55. PubMed PMID: 19661447. Epub 2009/08/08. eng.

[46] Lansley KE, Winyard PG, Fulford J, Vanhatalo A, Bailey SJ, Blackwell JR, et al. Dietary nitrate supplementation reduces the O2 cost of walking and running: a placebo-controlled study. J Appl Physiol (1985). 2011 Mar;110(3):591-600. PubMed PMID: 21071588. Epub 2010/11/13. eng.

[47] Kelly J, Fulford J, Vanhatalo A, Blackwell JR, French O, Bailey SJ, et al. Effects of short-term dietary nitrate supplementation on blood pressure, O2 uptake kinetics, and muscle and cognitive function in older adults. Am J Physiol Regul Integr Comp Physiol. 2013 Jan 15;304(2):R73-83. PubMed PMID: 23174856. Epub 2012/11/24. eng.

[48] Haider G, Folland JP. Nitrate Supplementation Enhances the Contractile Properties of Human Skeletal Muscle. Med Sci Sports Exerc. 2014 Mar 27. PubMed PMID: 24681572. Epub 2014/04/01. Eng.

[49] Larsen FJ, Weitzberg E, Lundberg JO, Ekblom B. Dietary nitrate reduces maximal oxygen consumption while maintaining work performance in maximal exercise. Free Radic Biol Med. 2010 Jan 15;48(2):342-7. PubMed PMID: 19913611. Epub 2009/11/17. eng.

[50] Kelly J, Vanhatalo A, Wilkerson DP, Wylie LJ, Jones AM. Effects of nitrate on the power-duration relationship for severe-intensity exercise. Med Sci Sports Exerc. 2013 Sep;45(9):1798-806. PubMed PMID: 23475164. Epub 2013/03/12. eng.

[51] Masschelein E, Van Thienen R, Wang X, Van Schepdael A, Thomis M, Hespel P. Dietary nitrate improves muscle but not cerebral oxygenation status during exercise in hypoxia. J Appl Physiol (1985). 2012 Sep 1;113(5):736-45. PubMed PMID: 22773768. Epub 2012/07/10. eng.

[52] Jones AM, Burnley M. Oxygen uptake kinetics: an underappreciated determinant of exercise performance. Int J Sports Physiol Perform. 2009 Dec;4(4):524-32. PubMed PMID: 20029103. Epub 2009/12/24. eng.

[53] Jones AM, Grassi B, Christensen PM, Krustrup P, Bangsbo J, Poole DC. Slow component of VO2 kinetics: mechanistic bases and practical applications. Med Sci Sports Exerc. 2011 Nov;43(11):2046-62. PubMed PMID: 21552162. Epub 2011/05/10. eng.

[54] Breese BC, McNarry MA, Marwood S, Blackwell JR, Bailey SJ, Jones AM. Beetroot juice supplementation speeds O2 uptake kinetics and improves exercise tolerance during severe-intensity exercise initiated from an elevated metabolic rate. Am J Physiol Regul Integr Comp Physiol. 2013 Dec 15;305(12):R1441-50. PubMed PMID: 24089377. Epub 2013/10/04. eng.

[55] Cermak NM, Gibala MJ, van Loon LJ. Nitrate supplementation's improvement of 10-km time-trial performance in trained cyclists. Int J Sport Nutr Exerc Metab. 2012 Feb;22(1):64-71. PubMed PMID: 22248502. Epub 2012/01/18. eng.

[56] Bond H, Morton L, Braakhuis AJ. Dietary nitrate supplementation improves rowing performance in well-trained rowers. Int J Sport Nutr Exerc Metab. 2012 Aug;22(4):251-6. PubMed PMID: 22710356. Epub 2012/06/20. eng.

[57] Pinna M, Roberto S, Milia R, Marongiu E, Olla S, Loi A, et al. Effect of beetroot juice supplementation on aerobic response during swimming. Nutrients. 2014;6(2):605-15. PubMed PMID: 24481133. Pubmed Central PMCID: PMC3942720. Epub 2014/02/01. eng.

[58] Smith TB, Hopkins WG. Variability and predictability of finals times of elite rowers. Med Sci Sports Exerc. 2011 Nov;43(11):2155-60. PubMed PMID: 21502896. Epub 2011/04/20. eng.

[59] Christensen PM, Nyberg M, Bangsbo J. Influence of nitrate supplementation on VO(2) kinetics and endurance of elite cyclists. Scand J Med Sci Sports. 2013 Feb;23(1):e21-31. PubMed PMID: 23020760. Epub 2012/10/02. eng.

[60] Puype J, Ramaekers M, Van Thienen R, Deldicque L, Hespel P. No effect of dietary nitrate supplementation on endurance training in hypoxia. Scand J Med Sci Sports. 2014 Mar 20. PubMed PMID: 24646076. Epub 2014/03/22. Eng.

[61] Hopker J, Passfield L, Coleman D, Jobson S, Edwards L, Carter H. The effects of training on gross efficiency in cycling: a review. Int J Sports Med. 2009 Dec;30(12):845-50. PubMed PMID: 19941249. Epub 2009/11/27. eng.

[62] Jungersten L, Ambring A, Wall B, Wennmalm A. Both physical fitness and acute exercise regulate nitric oxide formation in healthy humans. J Appl Physiol (1985). 1997 Mar;82(3):760-4. PubMed PMID: 9074960. Epub 1997/03/01. eng.

[63] Schena F, Cuzzolin L, Rossi L, Pasetto M, Benoni G. Plasma nitrite/nitrate and erythropoietin levels in cross-country skiers during altitude training. J Sports Med Phys Fitness. 2002 Jun;42(2):129-34. PubMed PMID: 12032406. Epub 2002/05/29. eng.

[64] Brand MD, Pakay JL, Ocloo A, Kokoszka J, Wallace DC, Brookes PS, et al. The basal proton conductance of mitochondria depends on adenine nucleotide translocase content. Biochem J. 2005 Dec 1;392(Pt 2):353-62. PubMed PMID: 16076285. Pubmed Central PMCID: PMC1316271. Epub 2005/08/04. eng.

[65] Ferreira LF, Padilla DJ, Williams J, Hageman KS, Musch TI, Poole DC. Effects of altered nitric oxide availability on rat muscle microvascular oxygenation during contractions. Acta Physiol (Oxf). 2006 Mar;186(3):223-32. PubMed PMID: 16497201. Epub 2006/02/25. eng.

[66] Ferguson SK, Hirai DM, Copp SW, Holdsworth CT, Allen JD, Jones AM, et al. Effects of nitrate supplementation via beetroot juice on contracting rat skeletal muscle microvascular oxygen pressure dynamics. Respir Physiol Neurobiol. 2013 Jul 1;187(3):250-5. PubMed PMID: 23584049. Pubmed Central PMCID: PMC3753182. Epub 2013/04/16. eng.

[67] Ferguson SK, Hirai DM, Copp SW, Holdsworth CT, Allen JD, Jones AM, et al. Dose dependent effects of nitrate supplementation on cardiovascular control and microvascular oxygenation dynamics in healthy rats. Nitric Oxide. 2014 May 30;39:51-8. PubMed PMID: 24769046. Epub 2014/04/29. eng.

[68] Hirai DM, Copp SW, Ferguson SK, Holdsworth CT, McCullough DJ, Behnke BJ, et al. Exercise training and muscle microvascular oxygenation: functional role of nitric oxide. J Appl Physiol (1985). 2012 Aug 15;113(4):557-65. PubMed PMID: 22678970. Pubmed Central PMCID: PMC3424059. Epub 2012/06/09. eng.

[69] Hoon MW, Johnson NA, Chapman PG, Burke LM. The effect of nitrate supplementation on exercise performance in healthy individuals: a systematic review and meta-analysis. Int J Sport Nutr Exerc Metab. 2013 Oct;23(5):522-32. PubMed PMID: 24172997. Epub 2013/11/01. eng.

[70] Wylie LJ, Kelly J, Bailey SJ, Blackwell JR, Skiba PF, Winyard PG, et al. Beetroot juice and exercise: pharmacodynamic and dose-response relationships. J Appl Physiol (1985). 2013 Aug 1;115(3):325-36. PubMed PMID: 23640589. Epub 2013/05/04. eng.

Offensive process analysis in handball: Identification of game actions that differentiate winning from losing teams

Willian R. Ferrari*, João Valente dos Santos, Vasco Parreiral Simões Vaz

Faculty of Sports Science and Physical Education, University of Coimbra, Portugal

Email address:
willroque@hotmail.com (W. R. Ferrari), jvsantos@fcdef.uc.pt (J. V. dos Santos), vascovaz@fcdef.uc.pr (V. P. S. Vaz)

Abstract: This present study aims to show the main offensive differences between handball teams that lead to a win or a loss. The samples were collected through quantitative analyses of the Champions League 2011-2012 handball games. This study relied on non-descriptive and non-parametric statistics. The Mann-Whitney U test was used as the statistical method. The variables that show the significant differences in favour of the winners were the goals obtained in positioned attacks, 9-meter goals and 7-meter penalties, which, in the semi-finals and final decided who the winner would be. This study shows that the teams who reached the finals and came out victorious have a wide and well-defined range of offensive actions enabling them to involve all aspects of the game, in any situation. This tendency was particularly visible in positioned attacks, which was the main difference throughout the competition.

Keywords: Handball, Observational Methodology, Manual Notation, Winning and Losing Teams Profile, Sports Performance

1. Introduction

Today's Handball is being decided in small details, due to the big investments made in teams, turning the game analysis, as in most sports, into a game decisive factor. The direct observation is the most used method in game analysis, helping to better understand and explore the different relations within the game (1). In order to enhance the game comprehension, it's necessary to focus on the analysis that enables us to better understand the relationship between different factors, making the relation between the game dynamics and the success patterns of the winning teams understandable (2; 3). From this point of view, it is important that coaches consider, among other physical attributes, the player's ability to interact with the environment and the individual and group decision-making within the game (4).

The observation and analysis of play is essential to the evaluation of the fundamental characteristics of teams and players, resulting in the coach's intervention (5). The game analysis is defined by measuring individual performance, physical loads, tactical solutions, the study of interactions within and between staff, discovering talents, supporting the decision making of coaches and theoretical interest in the game's structure (6;7).

Various authors in various ways have carried out handball analysis. The predominance of tactical elements in the outcome of the winning team's attacks during the first Croatian Handball League was clearly characterized by rapid attacks against disorganized defences (8). Bilge compares data from the European Championships with other tournaments, considering the success of European teams in World Men's Handball. It was determined that in terms of efficiency, fast break goals, which is the key element of modern Handball, compared to the effectiveness of nine meters shots, remained relatively constant over the three years of competition.

Makes a game analysis where the winning and losing teams are distinguished by collecting variables from the autonomous male cadet (U16) team's championship, concluding that the main variables that differentiate the teams were goals, 6m goals, 6m pitches, counterattack goals and counterattack shooting (9). Also in this aspect, besides differentiating the winners from the losers, an assessment of male and female is made, indicating that the teams should concentrate more on the collective aspect of the game because the best teams are most effective when shooting near the goal, noting that the women's teams that had a higher shot efficacy reached victory. In men, the main difference is the number of balls lost due to a more balanced physical and evolutionary game (10).

Following the same type of study, Saez has collected data from the teams participating in the 2008 King's Cup in Spain by observing 7 games of 8 different teams, using, as the key differentiating factors between winning and losing teams, goals, failed 6m shots and counterattack goals. However, a study conducted in the ASOBAL Handball league in the 2008-2009 season with 240 games of 16 different teams has shown that there are significant differences between winners and losers in the following statistics: goals and shooting in actions counterattack (11).

This study aims to develop a characterization of the offensive process, evaluate the attack patterns, correlate the effectiveness of winning team's attacks and analyse the attack variables that differentiate the winning from the losing teams. At the end, verify if the performance of the winning teams follows a pattern that is likely to be a future standard.

After consultations articles made in this area, this study aims to take a different view from other studies due to the level of the teams in the competition to be very similar, there is no great disparity between teams and players.

2. Methods

2.1. Sample

The data for this study collected through observation of the official EHF Champions League games available online, containing the complete sets of all 2011/2012 season games. We observed 20 games throughout the finals from the "Last 16" teams that reached the "Final 4", 8 games in the "Last 16", 8 games in the "quarterfinals" and 4 more games in the "Final 4". With the main focus on the four teams (THW Kiel, Atletico de Madrid, and AG Kobenhavn Fusche Berlin) that reached the final stages of the competition

For the present study was constructed a grate collection. Data collected simultaneously with the losing team and the winning team of the respective game. Then the data placed in *Microsoft Excel 2013* program, for a better analysis of results. All games seen within one month aiming to minimize the discrepancy analysis.

2.2. Variables

The variables chosen according to studies, in which we identified as being most important to define the winners from losers.

- Number of possess: Number of the ball in offensive actions of each team. It considered that a team has possession of the ball when you have an uninterrupted and complete control of the ball (12).
- Time of posse: Number of the ball in offensive actions of each team.
- Total Attempts: Total number of attempts made by the team throughout the game.
- Attempts Positioned: Number of attempts made by the teams placed in the position of attack.
- Attempts Counter Attack: Number of trim held on the counterattack as described (13), which set against direct attack as a direct attack by 2 or 3 players, emerging from a long pass from the guard goalkeeper or an outfield player in their defensive zone to a player who isolates himself in front of the opponents.
- Attempts Sustained Attack: Number of shots played in supporting attack (13) is defined as an attack carried out by the rearmost players progress in the field passes through quick progression on in order to make an attack on a numerical superiority while the defense is not fully organized.
- Attempts 9m.: Total number of shots made the dashed line of 9 meters or behind it.
- Attempts 7m.: Total number of shots made in a game penalty.
- Attempts 6m.: Total number of shots made from the line of 6 meters.
- Total Goals: Total goals achieved by the teams.
- Positioned goals: Number of goals made by the teams when they positioned in attack.
- Goals Counterattack: Number of goals made by the teams using the counterattack.
- Attack Sustainable Goals: Number of goals made by the teams using the sustained attack
- Goals 9m.: Number of goals made by teams in shots 9 feet.
- Goals 7m.: Number of goals made by teams in penalty 7 meters.
- Goals 6m.: Number of goals made by the teams to trim 6 feet.
- % Attempts: Percentage of success of the teams on the total number of shots
- % Positioned: Percentage of correct teams positioned in attack.
- % Counter Attack: Percentage of success of the teams on the counterattack.
- % Sustainable: Percentage of success of teams in sustained attack.
- % Attempts 9m.: Percentage of success of the teams in the shot 9m.
- % Attempts 7m.: Percentage of correct teams in penalties of 7 meters.
- % Attempts 6m.: Percentage of success of the teams shots of 6m.

Initially a sample characterization with descriptive statistics including parameters of central tendency (mean) and dispersion (standard deviation and range) made. Then we used non-parametric inferential statistics through the Mann-Whitney U test (13). Newton and Rudestam (1999) define criteria for the choice of non-parametric statistical techniques. Statistical analysis performed using *IBM SPSS statistics 20.*

3. Results and Discussion

Something that contradicts the literature is that counterattack shots do not show statistically significant differences (p = 0.44) showing a mean difference of 0.88 shots. In terms of counterattack goals, we have a mean difference of 0.88 in favour of the losing teams (Table 1).

Table 1. *Results of the Mann-Whitney U test, concerning Possession and shots of the winning and losing teams.*

Variables	Losers (n=17) Mean	DP	*Mean Rank*	Winners (n=17) Mean	DP	*Mean Rank*	*z*	*p*
Number of Possess	56.59	2.83	17.15	56.71	2.84	17.85	-.21	.83
Time of Posse	32.42	2.96	19.50	30.91	3.40	15.50	-1.17	.24
Total Attempts	46.47	3.52	14.44	49.06	3.56	20.56	-1.80	.07
Attempts Positioned	34.53	4.69	17.24	34.59	3.26	17.76	-.16	.88
Attempts Counterattack	5.88	2.76	16.21	6.76	2.82	18.79	-.76	.44
Attempts Sustained	3.71	1.83	14.50	4.82	2.24	20.50	-1.79	.07
Attempts 9m.	21.94	3.13	16.06	23.35	4.27	18.94	-.85	.40
Attempts 7m.	3.18	1.55	15.26	4.06	1.89	19.74	-1.34	.18
Attempts 6m.	21.82	3.73	17.29	21.65	5.48	17.71	-.12	.90

(*) p<0.05 (**) p<0.01)

The total number of goal attempts that hit the target tended to be statistically significant (p = 0:07) (Table 1).

Statistical significances may be noted in the aspect of goals in positioned attacks (p = 0.03) and a difference between means of 8.22% about the percentage of successful shots in positioned attacks. The number of 9m goals scored by the winning teams (p = 0.00) and goals scored from 7m penalties (p = 0.04) were the main aspects that differentiated winning from losing teams (Table 2).

Table 2. *Results of the Mann-Whitney U test, referring to the Offensive Effectiveness in both winning and losing teams.*

Variables	Losers (n=17) Média	DP	*Mean Rank*	Winners (n=17) Média	DP	*Mean Rank*	*z*	*p*
Goals Total	24.35	3.46	11.03	30.06	4.17	23.97	-9.80	.00**
Goals Positioned	15.76	4.16	13.79	18.59	3.97	21.21	-2.18	.03*
Goals Counterattack	4.24	2.66	15.94	5.12	2.76	19.06	-.92	.36
Goals Sustained	2.24	1.56	15.26	3.00	1.70	19.74	-1.34	.18
Goals 9m.	8.88	2.59	12.21	12.12	2.59	22.79	-3.12	.00**
Goals 7m.	2.06	1.03	14.12	3.35	1.93	20.88	-2.03	.04*
Goals 6m.	13.59	2.98	16.15	14.59	4.56	18.85	-.80	.42
% Attempts	52.76	7.88	12.53	61.02	6.42	22.47	-2.91	.00**
% Positioned	45.69	10.33	13.50	53.91	9.61	21.50	-2.34	.02*
% Counterattack	65.31	26.62	15.91	72.00	22.98	19.09	-.93	.35
% Sustained	60.08	29.21	16.91	63.14	23.21	18.09	-.35	.73
% Attempts 9m.	40.99	11.97	13.18	52.34	9.25	21.82	-2.53	.01**
% Attempts 7m.	70.20	30.87	16.26	79.51	19.22	18.74	-.75	.45
% Attempts 6m.	62.96	9.82	15.76	67.70	13.49	19.24	-1.02	.31

(*) p<0.05 (**) p<0.01)

The total number of shots on target have shown a tendency to be statistically significant (p = 0.07), having an average difference between the teams of 2.59 shots (losing teams) per game (Table 1). Thus the percentage of Goal attempts as a statistically significant difference (p = 0.00) showed a mean difference between the teams of 8.26% for the winners (52.76% losers, 61.02% winners), (Table 2). The comparative study shows that winners have an average difference of 8.17% (41.01% losers, 51.18% winners) showing the quality of the observed games, where the percentage of successful shots (goals) in that particular study to be higher in the losing teams then in the winning ones by comparing both studies (14). These were the main aspects where winning and losing teams can be differentiated.

In another comparative study, losing teams have a 7.21 9m goals average, whilst the winning teams have a 8.41 average, resulting in a mean difference of 1.2 goals between them, this study showed numbers of 8.88 goals for losing teams and 12.12 for the winners with an average between them of 3.24 goals per game featuring the goal difference of the losing teams higher than the winners by comparing both studies. (10) shows 2.82 goals on 7m shots for the losers and 3.34 goals with a 0.52 mean between them, as this present study shows 2.06 for the losers and 3.35 for the winners with a 1.29 mean difference, being the number of goals scored by the losers the major difference between the studies which, in this study, presents an average number of 0.76 between the two comparative studies.

Something that contradicts the literature is that counterattack shots do not show statistically significant differences (p = 0.44) showing a mean difference of 0.88 shots Table 1. In terms of counterattack goals, we have a mean difference of 0.88 in favour of the losing teams and a percentage of hits of 65.31% for the losers and 72.00% for the winners. The same study mentioned above shows an average of 2.84 goals for the losers and 4.45 goals in counterattack situations whilst this present study shows 4.24 for the losers and 5.12 for the winners.

When we compare this present study with youth teams it shown that the winning teams have a higher 6m and counterattack goals rating, as the main differentiators between winning and losing teams (9). 9m goals which, in this present study, show significative values (p = 0.00), are not relevant in Saez's study (p = 0.41). The same applies to the study of Antunes where he makes a comparison between winning and losing teams in the children's category. Featuring a very low 9m scored goals index (5.78 ± 5:23 to 6:39 ± 6:09 and losers to winners) thereby not a statistically significant difference (p = 0.61).

4. Conclusion

Games won in positioned attack, unlike all the studies, where the literature points to the counter-attack as the main variable of differentiation between winners and losers. 7m penalties, 9m shots, and their efficacy are more and more the main differentiators between winning and losing teams. Due to this, and as an incentive for the youth teams and their coaches, there is no need to have only one offensive solution whether that solution is the counterattack or the positioned attack. This study shows that the all-round teams are the ones who come out victorious. With a positioned attack with a vast number of solutions and variations and well executed by quality players.

Encouraging the training teams and coaches of the same terms that not only have a choice of offensive play, as the counter attack or attack positioned. This study shows that victories made to the most complete teams in all these aspects. With an attack positioned with a greater number of options and variations and running well with high-level players. Having the counterattack as a variable attack and not your main offensive foundation. Complementing this sustained attack, which in turn ends up being a difference in winning teams.

This study hopes to change the coaches' who spend too much training time with the counterattack philosophies, not to forsake the counterattack, but to add a greater part for the all-round attack and enable shooting opportunities for every player in the team despite their position, because modern handball seeks the most complete players.

Acknowledgements

My family, friends and teachers who have helped me in this study, with support and help when needed.

References

[1] Silva, A., Sánchez, F., Garganta, J., & Anguera, M.T. (2005). Patrones de juego en el fútbol de alto rendimiento. Análisis secuencial del proceso ofensivo en el campeonato del mundo Corea-Japón 2002. Cultura, Ciencia y Deporte, 1 (2), 65-72.

[2] Volossovitch A. (2005). Analysis of the performance in handball: perspectives and tendencies. Technical Handball Magazine; Vol. 3 : 16-20.

[3] Warren W. (2006). The Dynamics of Perception and Action. Psychological Review; Vol. 113 : 358-89.

[4] Araújo, D. Davids, K. & Hristovski, R. (2006). The ecological dynamics of decision making in sport. Psychol Sport Exercices, 7: 653-676.

[5] Gomes R 2002. Análise de dados em pesquisa qualitativa. Pesquisa social: teoria, método e criatividade. Editora Vozes, p 67-80 Petrópolis.

[6] Garganta, J. (1998). Analisar o jogo nos jogos desportivos. Revista Horizonte XIV (83), 7-14.

[7] Garganta, J. (1996). Análise do jogo de futebol. Acta das II jornadas do CEJD. FCDEF-UP, Porto.

[8] Rogulj, N., Srhoj, V., & Srhoj, L. (2004). The contribution of collective attack tactics indifferentiating handball score efficiency. Coll. Antropol. 28 (2): 739-746.

[9] García J., Ibáñez S., Feu S., Cañadas M., Parejo I. (2008). Study of the differences y play between winning and losing teams in formative stages of team handball. CCD. 5 Vol. 3 (9) 195-200.

[10] Antúnez, A., García, J, Sáez, F.J., Valle, A., García, A. (2013) Differences in performance indicator between winning and losing team in formative stages according to sex and final score differences. Revista de Ciencias del Deporte, 9 (1), 5-16.

[11] Gutiérrez A., López P. (2010). Discriminant analysis between winners and losers in the asobal league 2008-2009. http://activities.eurohandball.com/web-periodicals [pesquisa efectuada em 20/10/12].

[12] Malarranha, J., Sampaio, J. (2007). Ritmo dos jogos das finais das competições europeias de basquetebol (1988-2006) e as estatísticas que discriminam os jogos mais rápidos dos jogos mais lentos. *Revista Portuguesa de Ciências do Desporto*; vol.7, 2: 202-208.

[13] Fernandez E. & Falkowski, M. (1988). Los sistemas de juego offensivos. *Coleccion Handball,* número 8 Editorial Esteban Sanz Martinez.

[14] Newton, R. R., & Rudestam, K. E. (1999). Your statistical consultant. Answers to your data analysis questions. Thousand Oaks: SAGE.

[15] Sáez, F.J., Roldán, A., Feu, S. (2009). Diferencias en las estadisticas de juego entre los equipos ganadores y perdedores de la copa del rey 2008 de balonmano masculino. Revista de Ciencias del Deporte, 5 (3), 107-114.

Lateral epicondylitis: A novel non-invasive treatment approach

Christopher Bui

Department of Physical Medicine and Rehabilitation, West Los Angeles Veterans Administration/UCLA, Los Angeles, CA, USA

Email address:
chrisbui.ucla@gmail.com

Abstract: Objective: To evaluate the effectiveness of the TheraPoint Focal Pressure Support (TP-FPS) as a non-invasive treatment for pain associated with lateral Epicondylitis (LE). Design: Prospective cohort study. Participants: $n = 25$ study subjects (20 males and 5 females) ranging in age from 18-65 with pain in one upper limb either dominant (23) or non-dominant (2) associated with lateral epicondylitis for a minimum of six months. Interventions: Study participants were tasked to wear the TP-FPS for 3 hours per day for two weeks except when bathing or during main sleep hours. Outcome measures: Visual analog scale (VAS) pain score pre- and post-treatment period. Results: The combined (male and female) cohort average pre-treatment VAS pain score was 7.44 +/- 0.57. Post-treatment VAS pain score was 1.07 +/- 0.42, with a total reduction of 6.37 points and reached significance with p=0.0005. Male cohort demonstrated an average pre-treatment VAS pain score of 7.45 +/- 0.56. Post-treatment VAS pain score was 1.40 +/- 0.45, with a total reduction of 6.05 points and reached significance with p=0.006. Female cohort displayed an average pre-treatment VAS pain score of 7.40 +/- 1.92. Post-treatment VAS pain score was 1.70 +/- 1.14, with a total reduction of 5.70 and reached significance with p=0.001. No statistically significant difference was observed in the VAS pain score reduction between the male and female groups. Conclusion: The TP-FPS may indeed be a non-invasive therapeutic option for reducing pain associated with lateral epicondylitis.

Keywords: Lateral Epicondylitis, Elbow Pain, Non-Invasive, Pain Management, Pain Reduction

1. Introduction

Lateral epicondylitis (LE), otherwise known as tennis elbow, is a common clinical complaint with an incidence of 4-7/1000 patients per year [4,8,11]. It is characterized by pain over the lateral humeral epicondyle, and commonly radiates into the dorsal forearm. This condition tends to be self-limiting, often resolving in 6-12 months irrespective of treatment; however, complaints may sometimes last up to two years or longer.

Although an exact cause on how lateral epicondylitis develops has yet to be determined, it is generally agreed that the overuse of wrist and hand functions contributes to the complaint of pain. Tissue-based pathology seen in cases of lateral epicondylitis includes degenerative changes at the proximal common extensor origin. In addition, myofascial trigger points in the muscles attached to the lateral epicondyle may also be a source of pain [6].

As described by Nirschl et al., workplace activities contribute to 35-64% of all cases [12]. Sports related injury is also a frequent culprit. This places a significant economic burden resulting in a high rate of missed workdays and productivity.

Multiple approaches for the treatment of lateral epicondylitis have been described in the medical literature. Analgesic medications such as oral or topical non-steroidal anti-inflammatory to opioid drugs have been used to treat the pain associated with lateral epicondylitis. In addition, a number of physiotherapeutic approaches including manipulation, therapeutic ultrasound, iontophoresis, phonophoresis, and low-level laser treatment have been described. More invasive interventional methods like corticosteroid, prolotherapy, and regenerative biologic injections have also been described. However, such interventions have not been shown to have consistent long-term clinical benefit [10, 11].

The aim of this paper is to determine the efficacy of a simple mechanical intervention utilizing the TheraPoint Focal Pressure Support (TP-FPS) in the treatment of pain associated with lateral epicondylitis.

2. Physiology and Mechanism of Action

The TheraPoint Focal Pressure Support (TP-FPS) provides focal pressure to the area of application. As mentioned prior, there are at least two major theories as to the cause of lateral epicondylitis. This brings to light the unique nature of the TP-FPS. The system is theorized to affect both pathophysiological etiologies of lateral epicondylitis:

1. Active focal pressure for myofascial trigger point [6] and
2. Proximal isometric stabilization of the common extensor tendon, specifically the extensor carpi radialis brevis (ECRB) tendon, to curtail further overuse injury [2,3,7,11].

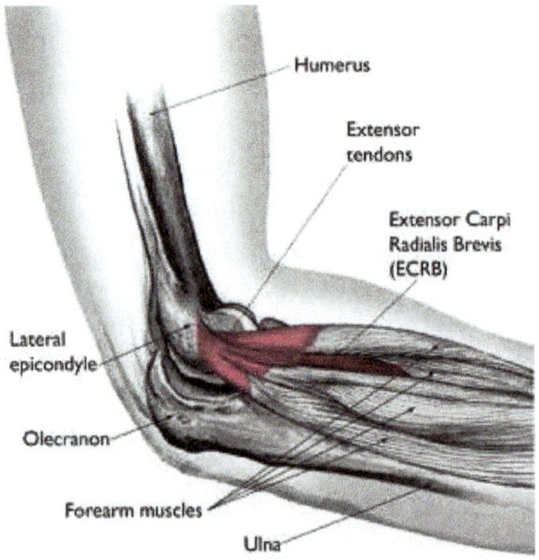

Figure 1. *Origin of Extensor Tendons. The Body Almanac. © American Academy of Orthopedic Surgeons, 2003*

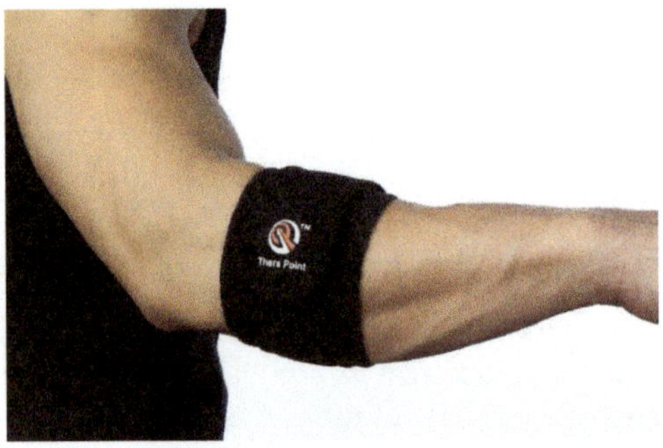

Figure 2. *Application of TP-FPS*

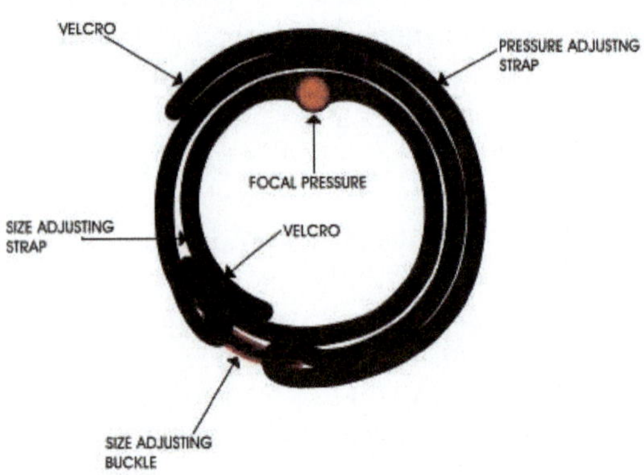

Figure 3. *TP-FPS Cutaway Schematic*

3. Methods

This was a prospective cohort study that took place over the course of six months.

Participants were recruited throughout the community. The following inclusion criteria was used: males and females between the ages of 18 and 65, pain in one dominant or non-dominant upper limb associated with lateral epicondylitis for a minimum of six months, and have no significant impairment in the use of the affected upper limb.

Exclusion criteria included: potential participants actively receiving physiotherapy for their lateral epicondyle pain, recent (≤6mo) interventional injection, history of surgery to the elbow region, significant functional impairment in the affected upper limb, and/or significant analgesic medication use.

Once participants were deemed eligible they were given a TP-FPS to be used for a two-week treatment period. Participants were trained on donning and doffing the support. They were to wear the support for three hours per day, and not during bathing and main sleep hours.

35 participants were screened and accepted into the study. 30 participants were included in the final analysis with 5 being lost to follow-up.

Table 1. *Subject Demographics*

	Male	Female
N	20	5
Median Age	44.5	48
Avg Duration of Pain Complaint (months)	11.4+/- 6	9.49+/- 5.1
Work:Sports Etiology	0.67	1.5

3.1. Measurements

Primary Outcome: Pre- and post-treatment visual analog scale (VAS) pain measurements were obtained and analyzed.

3.2. Statistical Analysis

SPSS Statistics ver. 20.0.1 was used for data analysis. Data was reported as means and standard deviations, medians and ranges. Two-sided, two-sample t-tests were used to compare pre- and post-treatment pain VAS scores with a significance level of 0.05. Cohort was analyzed as a whole. ANOVA was utilized in the Male-to-female group comparison.

4. Results

30 participants completed the two-week treatment period with the TP-FPS. In the combined (male and female) cohort the average pre-treatment VAS pain score was 7.44 +/- 0.57. Post-treatment VAS pain score was 1.07 +/- 0.42, with a total reduction of 6.37 points and reached significance with p=0.0005.

Male cohort demonstrated an average pre-treatment VAS pain score of 7.45 +/- 0.56. Post-treatment VAS pain score was 1.40 +/- 0.45, with a total reduction of 6.05 points and reached significance with p=0.006.

Female cohort displayed an average pre-treatment VAS pain score of 7.40 +/- 1.92. Post-treatment VAS pain score was 1.70 +/- 1.14, with a total reduction of 5.70 and reached significance with p=0.001.

Post-hoc analysis between the male and female group did not show significance between the magnitudes of reduction in their VAS pain scores.

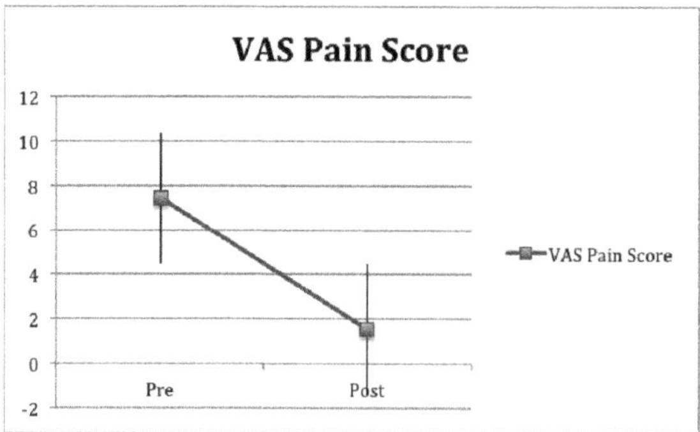

Graph 1. *Changes in VAS Pain Scores Pre- Post- Treatment*

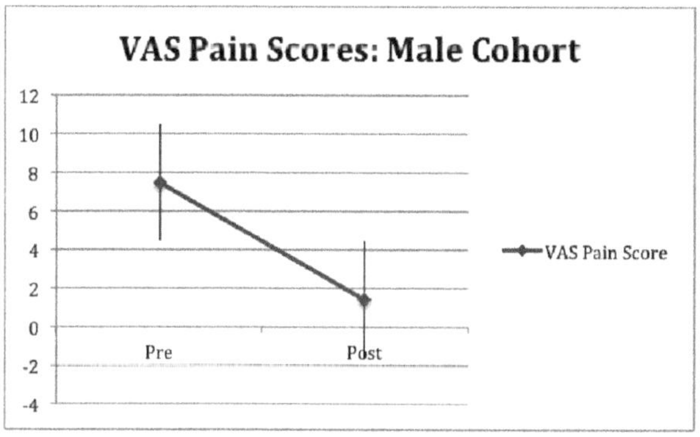

Graph 2. *Changes in VAS Pain Scores Pre- Post- Treatment in the Male Cohort*

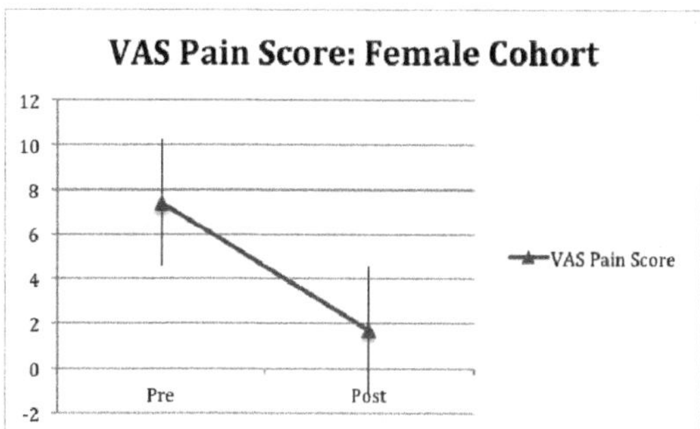

Graph 3. *Changes in VAS Pain Scores Pre- Post- Treatment in the Female Cohort*

5. Discussion

Lateral epicondylitis is a common clinical complaint, affecting 1-3% of the general population each year. A variety of treatments ranging from non-invasive physiotherapy techniques to analgesic medication and invasive therapies have been described in the medical literature. Most of these treatments exhibit significant pain reduction in the short term; however, lasting benefits are less clear.

The TheraPoint Focal Pressure Support aims to be a non-invasive treatment approach to reduce pain associated with lateral epicondylitis. The theorized mechanism of action includes both proximal stabilization of the wrist extensor tendons attaching at the lateral epicondyle, more specifically the ECRB tendon, as well as active focal pressure over the myofascial trigger point. It has been well studied that steadying the ECRB tendon lends to improvement in pain by limiting the amount of shear over the lateral epicondyle [18].

With regards to acupressure, there are a limited number of studies conducted on the effects of it on musculoskeletal pain, with most focusing on low back pain. According to Hsieh, et al. acupressure treatment six times over a one month period was significantly more effective in reducing chronic low back pain compared to a comparison group that was treated with physical therapy (n=146) [19]. In a subsequent study, the Hsieh group found that acupressure significantly reduced chronic low back pain when compared to a placebo acupressure group (n=129) [20]. Although the exact mechanism of acupressure has not been established, the dominant rationale is that it stimulates the release of neurochemicals associated with analgesia (i.e. endogenous opioid including ß-endorphins, enkephalins, dynorphins, and/or serotonin) [21]. Given that the elbow is also a component of the musculoskeletal system like the lumbar spine, it would be reasonable to extrapolate the analgesic effects of acupressure on the elbow.

This study demonstrated that use of the TheraPoint Focal Pressure Support was effective in reducing the VAS pain score of study participants. Post-treatment VAS pain scores decreased 86%, p=0.0005. No significant difference is pain score was observed between the male and female groups. Therefore, the TP-FPS may indeed be a viable non-invasive therapeutic option for reducing pain associated with lateral epicondylitis.

Limitations of this study include a small sample size and limited power. In addition, the absence of follow-up after the treatment period makes it difficult to determine long-term pain improvement. Participants were to only use the TP-FPS for the treatment of their pain. As a result, it is unknown if the TP-FPS has a synergistic effect with other non-invasive and invasive treatments. Lastly, our primary outcome was reduction in VAS pain score, which may provide us with a limited profile of the pain experienced by our study participants. Further studies are needed to evaluate and characterize the effectiveness of non-invasive therapeutic treatments, specifically the TP-FPS with regards to pain reduction in lateral epicondylitis.

6. Conclusion

Lateral epicondylitis, also known as tennis elbow, is a commonly seen musculoskeletal complaint. There are multiple approaches in the treatment of lateral epicondylitis. These include but are not limited to analgesic medication, physiotherapeutic modalities, and invasive interventions.

This study demonstrated that the TheraPoint Focal Pressure Support may indeed be an effective non-invasive therapeutic option for reducing pain associated with lateral epicondylitis. Further studies are needed to evaluate and characterize the utility of non-invasive therapeutic treatments, specifically the TP-FPS in the treatment of lateral epicondylitis.

References

[1] Ajimsha, M. S., Chithra, S., & Thulasyammal, R. P. (2012). Effectiveness of myofascial release in the management of lateral epicondylitis in computer professionals. *Arch Phys Med Rehabil, 93*(4), 604-609. doi: 10.1016/j.apmr.2011.10.012

[2] Ashe, M. C., McCauley, T., & Khan, K. M. (2004). Tendinopathies in the upper extremity: a paradigm shift. *J Hand Ther, 17*(3), 329-334. doi: 10.1197/j.jht.2004.04.002

[3] Blanchette, M. A., & Normand, M. C. (2011). Augmented soft tissue mobilization vs natural history in the treatment of lateral epicondylitis: a pilot study. *J Manipulative Physiol Ther, 34*(2), 123-130. doi: 10.1016/j.jmpt.2010.12.001

[4] Chard, M. D., & Hazleman, B. L. (1989). Tennis elbow--a reappraisal. *Br J Rheumatol, 28*(3), 186-190.

[5] Chaudhury, S., de La Lama, M., Adler, R. S., Gulotta, L. V., Skonieczki, B., Chang, A., . . . Fealy, S. (2013). Platelet-rich plasma for the treatment of lateral epicondylitis: sonographic assessment of tendon morphology and vascularity (pilot study). *Skeletal Radiol, 42*(1), 91-97. doi: 10.1007/s00256-012-1518-y

[6] Chop, W. M., Jr. (1989). Tennis elbow. *Postgrad Med, 86*(5), 301-304, 307-308.

[7] Gabel, G. T. (1999). Acute and chronic tendinopathies at the elbow. *Curr Opin Rheumatol, 11*(2), 138-143.

[8] Hamilton, P. G. (1986). The prevalence of humeral epicondylitis: a survey in general practice. *J R Coll Gen Pract, 36*(291), 464-465.

[9] Jensen, M. P., Turner, J. A., Romano, J. M., & Fisher, L. D. (1999). Comparative reliability and validity of chronic pain intensity measures. *Pain, 83*(2), 157-162.

[10] Khan, K. M., Cook, J. L., Bonar, F., Harcourt, P., & Astrom, M. (1999). Histopathology of common tendinopathies. Update and implications for clinical management. *Sports Med, 27*(6), 393-408.

[11] Kivi, P. (1983). The etiology and conservative treatment of humeral epicondylitis. *Scand J Rehabil Med, 15*(1), 37-41.

[12] Nirschl, R. P. (1992). Elbow tendinosis/tennis elbow. *Clin Sports Med, 11*(4), 851-870.

[13] Nourbakhsh, M. R., & Fearon, F. J. (2008). The effect of oscillating-energy manual therapy on lateral epicondylitis: a randomized, placebo-control, double-blinded study. *J Hand Ther, 21*(1), 4-13; quiz 14. doi: 10.1197/j.jht.2007.09.005

[14] Overend, T. J., Wuori-Fearn, J. L., Kramer, J. F., & MacDermid, J. C. (1999). Reliability of a patient-rated forearm evaluation questionnaire for patients with lateral epicondylitis. *J Hand Ther, 12*(1), 31-37.

[15] Rompe, J. D., Overend, T. J., & MacDermid, J. C. (2007). Validation of the Patient-rated Tennis Elbow Evaluation Questionnaire. *J Hand Ther, 20*(1), 3-10; quiz 11. doi: 10.1197/j.jht.2006.10.003

[16] Shiri, R., Viikari-Juntura, E., Varonen, H., & Heliovaara, M. (2006). Prevalence and determinants of lateral and medial epicondylitis: a population study. *Am J Epidemiol, 164*(11), 1065-1074. doi: 10.1093/aje/kwj325

[17] Simons, D. G., Hong, C. Z., & Simons, L. S. (2002). Endplate potentials are common to midfiber myofacial trigger points. *Am J Phys Med Rehabil, 81*(3), 212-222.

[18] Walz, D. M., Newman, J. S., Konin, G. P., & Ross, G. (2010). Epicondylitis: pathogenesis, imaging, and treatment. *Radiographics, 30*(1), 167-184. doi: 10.1148/rg.301095078

[19] Hsieh, L.L., et al., Treatment of low back pain by acupressure and physical therapy: randomised controlled trial. *BMJ, 2006.* 332(7543): p. 696-700.

[20] Hsieh, L.L., et al., A randomized controlled clinical trial for low back pain treated by acupressure and physical therapy. *Prev Med, 2004.* 39(1): p. 168-76.

[21] Luo, D., X. Wang, and J. He, A comparison between acute pressure block of the sciatic nerve and acupressure: methodology, analgesia, and mechanism involved. *J Pain Res, 2013.* 6: p. 589-93.

Effects of oral coenzyme Q_{10} on preventing the accumulation of lactic acid developing during the exercise performances of endurance skiing athletes

Nevzat Demirci[1], Ebru Beytut[2]

[1]Mersin School of Physical Education and Sports, Mersin University, Mersin, Turkey
[2]Department of Physiology, Faculty of Medicine, University of Erzincan, Erzincan, Turkey

Email address:
nevzatdemirci44@hotmail.com (N. Demirci)

Abstract: Aim: This study aims to examine the effects of oral coenzyme Q_{10} (CoQ_{10}) on preventing the accumulation of lactic acid developing during the exercise performances of endurance skiing athletes. Materials and Methods: The study population was composed of 15 volunteering male athletes. The blood samples thus collected were utilized for the measurement of athletes' $CoQ_{10,}$ lactate, lactate dehydrogenase (LDH), creatine phosphokinase (CPK), heart rate and blood pressure. Results: Significant decreases were identified in the systolic and diastolic blood pressures, pulses and plasma lactate levels of the athletes in the trial group when their pre- and post-exercise results were compared ($p<0,01$; $p<0,001$) while an increase of $p<0,01$ was observed in their plasma CoQ_{10} levels. However, plasma LDH and CPK levels of the trial group athletes using 100 and 200 mg CoQ_{10} were observed to increase less when compared to the results of the control group athletes in seven days ($p<0,001$; $p<0,01$). Conclusion: regular and gradual exercise is considered to enhance physical performance depending on the usage of CoQ_{10} while it decreases the accumulation of La and thus delays fatigue.

Keywords: Endurance skiing, CoQ_{10}, Lactic Acid, Exercise Performance

1. Introduction

The basic goal of regular exercise is to prevent the organic deficiencies caused by a sedentary lifestyle, to increase the physiological capacity and tolerances, both of which are the basis of a dynamic and balanced life as much as possible, and to maintain this healthy structure as long as possible [1]. The point at which cardiac output addresses mostly is skeletal muscle. However, energy used by the skeletal muscles as fuel changes depending on the intensity and duration of the exercise as well as the performance level and nutritional status of the individual. Organism cannot supply enough oxygen when short-time exercise with high intensity is in question, so Adenosine Triphosphate (ATP) is synthesized through anaerobic means. On the other hand, fat is used as fuel in long-term exercises and thus the need for energy is met at a level of 60-70% [2]. While these exercises mentioned above do not cause an excessive burden on skeleton muscle system, too much or unusual exercises cause muscle fatigue the next day after the exercise.

Fatigue is accepted to be a natural result of exercise and mental effort; however, muscle fatigue is defined as the deficiency in producing or maintaining certain strength by means of muscular contraction [3]. When intense exercise (maximal or supra-maximal) is in question, exceeding the limits of aerobic metabolism increases the speed of glucose and lactic acid (La) is formed inevitably. When the intensity of the exercise is higher than the capacity of the body to supply oxygen, La system is used as fuel, the accumulation of La in the blood causes a decrease in the pH level and fatigue comes out as a result of enzymatic activity [2]. In this case, it is necessary to have a rest in order to ensure that lactate is eliminated from the body and damage at cellular level arises at the muscles because of exercise. This is observed as an increase in serum CPK and LDH levels, which is the indicator of specific muscle damage in humans [4].

During the exercise, coenzyme Q_{10} (CoQ_{10}) is a basic catalyst necessary for the energy production at cellular level. CoQ10, which is produced and synthesized naturally by human body and which is a benzoquinone compound, is found in skeleton and cardiac muscular tissues that have a high level of physical activity as well as organs such as liver, kidney and brain [5]. Physical exercise increases the metabolic activity and oxygen consumption, and accordingly the production of reactive oxygen types, and thus it causes muscular fatigue and correspondingly oxidative damage. However, it is claimed that CoQ_{10} enhances the energy production in the mitochondria and so increases the performance and decreases the fatigue [6]. The primary duty of CoQ_{10} is its function as a part of mitochondrial respiratory chain and an important compound of cellular energy production [7]. This study aims to examine the effects of oral administration of CoQ_{10} at different dosages on LDH, CPK and lactate levels which are accepted to be as fatigue parameters of post-training, heart pulse and blood pressures to determine the effectiveness of CoQ_{10} during exercise performances.

2. Materials and Methods

This study is reproduced from thesis study carried out during September 2007 and June 2011 at Kafkas University, Health Sciences Institute, Department of Physiology. Thesis Protocol was accepted by Kafkas University Faculty of Medicine Ethics Committee with approval dated 09.06.2009 and numbered B.30.2.KAÜ.0.20.71.00. Conducted in line with the relevant directive specified in Helsinki Declaration, the study obtained approval from the Local Ethics Committee and ensured voluntary participation by providing study subjects with information on the objective of the study before the measurements.

The athletes were divided into3 groups in the study. Group 1 (n=5): Control Group, Group 2 (n=5): the group taking 100 mg CoQ_{10}, Group 3 (n=5): the group taking 200 mg CoQ_{10}. The age, weight and height averages of the respondents are stated in Table 1.

Table 1. *Comparison of age, weight and height of the respondent athletes. The data were expressed as mean ± standard deviation.*

	Control Group	1. Group (100 mg)	2. Group (200 mg)
Age:	21.60 ± 0.51	21.80 ± 0.73	21.60 ± 0.51
Weight:	64.20 ± 3.14	66.80 ± 2.97	63.80 ± 2.31
Height:	1.76 ± 0.02	1.76 ± 0.01	1.75 ± 0.01

2.1. The Implemented Training Program

The study subjects were divided into three groups, namely the control group and two subject groups taking 100 mg and 200 mg CoQ10. For a period of 1 week, each one of the 3 groups was made subject to a training load of 70-80% and repetitions making up 2 hours in total once every day. The exercise program started at $10.^{00}$ and was systematically adjusted specifically for each group to obtain the most suitable effects in physiological terms. Before the athletes started the training program, their heart beat rates and blood pressures were measured, blood samples were collected. Preparations of 100 and 200 mg of CoQ10 were given to the athletes to be taken after dinner. The exercises were repeated in the same manner as the first day for a period of a week.

2.2. Blood Sampling

The blood samples of the athletes were collected once before exercise, and immediately after the training for a period of 1 week. HPLC [8], lactic acid levels of CoQ_{10} levels were determined through lactate eassay kit II. Blood analysis of LDH and CPK blood samples were carried out at Kafkas University Faculty of Medicine Central Laboratory.

2.3. Determination of Plasma CoQ_{10} Levels

For the determination of CoQ10 levels, a 50 µl solution of 1,4-benzoquione was added to plasma of 200 µl (2 mg/ml) and the end product was vortexed for 10 seconds. 1 ml n-propanol was added to the product after 10 minutes. Following the vortexing of the tube for 10 seconds, 2 minutes of centrifugation was applied at 10.000 rpm to precipitate protein. The content was then injected into supernatant HPLC of two hundred micro-litres. It was transferred into a supernatant capped test tube that is capable of maintaining activity for 3 days at ambient temperature (22°C). The flow rate was 1 ml/minute following the composition of the mobile phase with ethanol-methanol (65-35%). The UV measurement was performed at 275 nm [8].

2.4. Measuring Blood Pressure

Systolic and diastolic blood pressures (tension) of the study subjects were measured from a. brachialisin of the arm by means of using mercurial sifigmo manometer device in terms of mmHg immediately before and after the training [9].

2.5. Measuring Heart Rate

Heart rates (pulse/min.) of the study subjects during rest time were determined before the training and after the athletes were ensured to have a rest, by means of putting carotid and radial arteries on forefinger and middle finger for 1 minute [9].

2.6. Statistical Analysis

The mean ($\overline{X}$) and standard deviation (sd) of the data obtained in the study were measured by means of using MINITAB statistics packet program (Minitab Inc. Pennsylvania, Version16.0 ABD). General Linear Model of the same program was used to determine the analysis in the study. Paired t-test was used to find out if there is a change between pre-substance and post-substance data. SAS 9.2 Proc GLM procedure was used to determine if there was any change among the Lactate and CoQ_{10} levels of all 3 groups in those 7 days and the measurements were compared in line with LSD procedures [10]. The changes of all 3 groups in 7 days and their regression curves were calculated using Excel 2007. P values lower than 0.05 were regarded as significant.

3. Results

Ages, weights and heights of the athletes who participated in the study and who were all male were compared among the groups which are control and CoQ10. The results are summarized in Table 1. At the end of the comparison, the groups did not demonstrate a significant difference in terms of their ages, weights and heights (p>0,05).

When systolic and diastolic blood pressures as well as heart rates of the trial groups during the training period of one week were compared separately with the control group, the related levels of trial groups which were high at the beginning were observed to decrease significantly in the following days and stay at a level lower than controls (p< 0,001) (Figures 1,2,3).

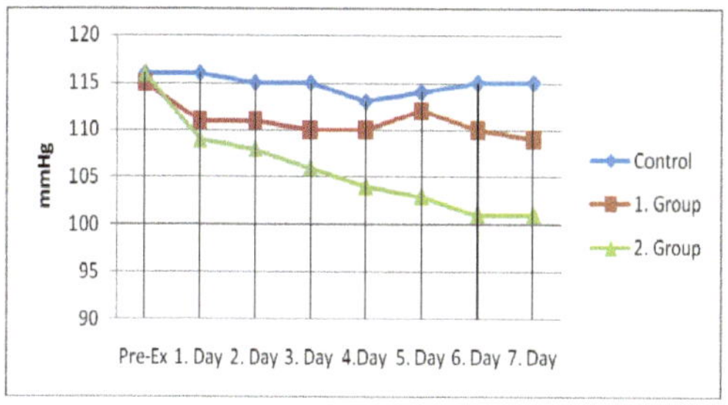

***: p<0.001, Pre-Exercise (Pre- Ex.)

***Figure 1.** Changes in Systolic Blood Pressure Values of CoQ_{10} Trial Groups During One-Week-Training Period*

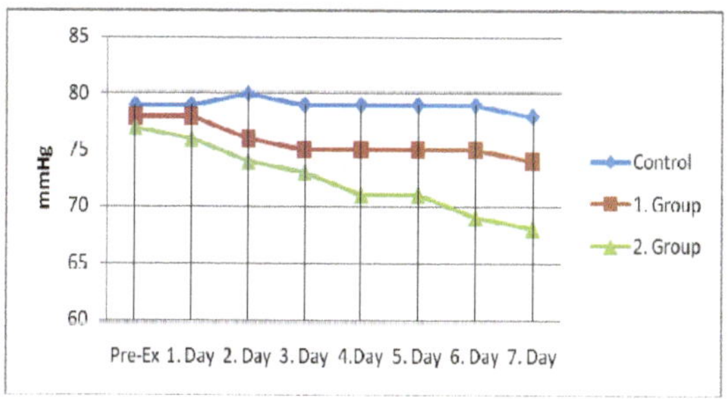

***: p<0.001, Pre-Exercise (Pre- Ex.)

***Figure 2.** Changes in Diastolic Blood Pressure Values of CoQ10 Trial Groups during One-Week-Training Period*

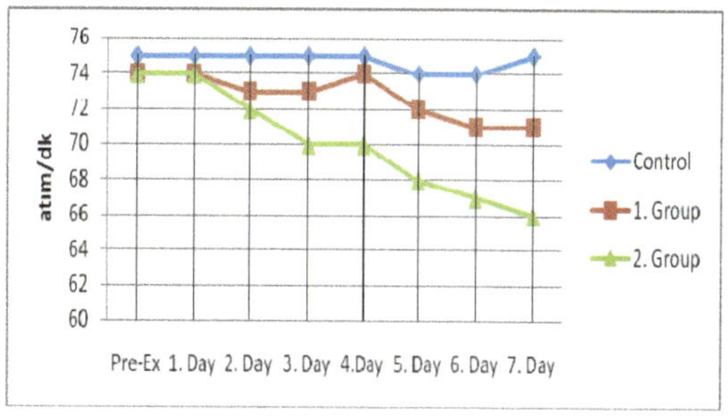

***: p<0.001, Pre-Exercise (Pre- Ex.)

***Figure 3.** Changes Heart Rates of CoQ10 Trial Groups During One-Week-Training Period*

There is no significant difference between pre-training systolic and diastolic blood pressures, and heart rates of skiing athletes in the trial groups (p>0,05); however, there are significant differences between post-training systolic and diastolic blood pressures (p<0,01), and heart rates (p<0,001) of the same groups. Table 2 summarizes the results of these measurements and their comparisons according to the groups.

The post-training levels of plasma LDH and CPK in all the groups were determined to increase continuously when compared to pre-training levels all throughout 7 days. However, the increase in the trial groups taking 100 and 200 mg CoQ_{10} was observed to be less than the increase in the control group. This increase was significant statistically and found in both of the trial groups at the level of p< 0,001 (Table 2).

Post-training increase in the control group was compared separately to the pre-training lactate levels of 100 and 200 mg CoQ_{10} trial groups, and significant decreases (p<0,01) were observed. However, the decrease in lactate levels of the trial group taking 200 mg CoQ_{10} was observed to be more relevant than the decrease in the lactate levels of the trial group taking 100 mg CoQ_{10}. When the pre- and post-training plasma CoQ_{10} levels of all the groups were compared, no change was observed in the control group whereas an increase of p<0,01 was observed in the trial groups (Table 2).

***Table 2.** Mean and Standard Deviation Values (±SD) of All Groups' Pre-Training and Post-Training Systole, Diastole, Pulse, LDH, CPK, Lactate and CoQ_{10} Levels*

Groups	Control Group		100 mg CoQ_{10} Group		200 mg CoQ_{10} Group	
	Pre-T	Post - T	Pre-T	Post - T	Pre-T	Post - T
Systole (mmHg)	116,2±1,92	115,0±1,00	111,6±1,14	109,2±0,83**	109,0±1,00	101,0±1,00**
Diastole (mmHg)	79,80±1,64	78,80±0,83	78,80±0,83	74,0±0,70**	76,60±1,14	68,40±1,14**
Pulse (atım/dak)	75,80±1,09	74,60±0,54	74,60±0,54	71,60±1,14***	74,20±0,83	65,80±0,83***
LDH (IU/L)	151,0±12,9	442,6±32,4***	146,2±13,7	271,4±11,2***	118,0±12,9	240,4±9,24***
CPK (IU/L)	135,0±15,6	648,4±19,5***	131,4±8,01	583,6±9,86***	129,0±2,01	499,6±13,2***
Lactate (nmol)	2,15±0,12	4,40±0,66**	2,59±0,26	1,21±033**	2,37±0,37	0,55±0,16**
CoQ_{10} (µmol/L	1,57±0,56	1,50±0,27	1,57±0,22	2,24±0,73**	2,12±0,32	3,80±0,54**

*** p<0.001, ** p<0.01, * p<0.05, Pre-Training (Pre.T.), Post-Training (Post.T.) coenzyme Q_{10} (CoQ_{10}), Lactate Dehydrogenase (LDH), Creatine phosphokinase (CPK)

Plasma lactate levels of the groups considering the time period were compared on the basis of days (for 1 whole week of training); plasma lactate levels of the control group on the specified days were observed to increase positively whereas a negative decrease was observed in other groups. This decrease was not found to be significant between the control group and trial group taking 100 mg CoQ_{10} on the first day while it was found to be significant in the trial group taking 200 mg CoQ_{10} at a level of $p<0.05$. During the time period starting from the second day to the seventh day, the decreases and increases in the plasma lactate levels were observed to be significant ($p<0.001$), (Table 3).

Table 3. *Changes in the Plasma Lactate Levels (nmol) on the Basis of Days During the Training Program of Seven Days When Control Group and Trial Groups Taking 100 and 200 mg CoQ_{10} Were Compared*

Groups	1. Day	2. Day	3. Day	4.Day	5.Day	6.Day	7.Day
	$\bar{X} \pm Sd$	$\bar{X} \pm Sd$	$\bar{X} \pm Sd$	$\bar{X} \pm Sd$	$\bar{X} \pm Sd$	$\bar{X} \pm Sd$	$\bar{X} \pm Sd$
Control	2.1 ± 0.11^a	2.65 ± 0.29^a	2.6 ± 0.34^a	2.94 ± 0.34^a	3.38 ± 0.61^a	3.72 ± 0.62^a	4.41 ± 0.67^a
1.Group	2.19 ± 0.49^a	1.65 ± 0.12^b	1.66 ± 0.36^b	1.39 ± 0.22^b	1.31 ± 0.23^b	1.3 ± 0.3^b	1.18 ± 0.19^b
2.Group	1.31 ± 0.22^b	1.22 ± 0.14^c	1.09 ± 0.25^c	0.91 ± 0.12^c	0.77 ± 0.31^c	0.67 ± 0.12^c	0.53 ± 0.1^c

* The difference between the groups expressed with different letters is significant statistically ($p<0.05$).

When plasma CoQ_{10} levels of the trial groups were compared to the first day of the control group, no change was observed in the plasma CoQ_{10} levels of the trial group taking 100 mg CoQ_{10} until the third day; however, significant increases were observed starting from the 4th day. On the other hand, plasma CoQ_{10} levels of the trial group taking 200 mg CoQ_{10} were observed to increase significantly in a positive way starting from the 1st day (Table 4).

Table 4. *Changes in the Plasma CoQ10 Levels (μmol/L) on the Basis of Days During the Training Program of Seven Days When Control Group and Trial Groups Taking 100 and 200 mg CoQ10 Were Compared*

Groups	1. Day	2. Day	3. Day	4.Day	5.Day	6.Day	7.Day
	$\bar{X} \pm Sd$	$\bar{X} \pm Sd$	$\bar{X} \pm Sd$	$\bar{X} \pm Sd$	$\bar{X} \pm Sd$	$\bar{X} \pm Sd$	$\bar{X} \pm Sd$
Control	1.43 ± 0.18^a	1.69 ± 0.52^a	1.65 ± 0.38^a	1.59 ± 0.25^a	1.86 ± 0.58^a	1.62 ± 0.43^a	1.5 ± 0.28^a
1.Group	1.83 ± 0.34^a	1.75 ± 0.54^a	2.03 ± 0.33^a	2.11 ± 0.44^b	2.02 ± 0.4^b	2.22 ± 0.36^b	2.4 ± 0.45^b
2.Group	2.75 ± 0.46^b	3 ± 0.72^b	3.4 ± 0.32^b	3.31 ± 0.5^c	3.7 ± 0.28^c	3.97 ± 0.53^c	4.2 ± 0.21^c

* The difference between the groups expressed with different letters is significant statistically ($p<0.05$).

4. Discussion

The limits of aerobic metabolism are exceeded during intense exercises and this increases the speed of glycolysis, which inevitably causes lactate formation. Because of this reason, energy consumption and metabolic activity increase to a great extent during physical exercise, in other words, intense muscular activity [11]. Accordingly, individual's need for energy increases depending on the exercise and it gets more and more difficult to continue trainings as muscular glycogen storage decreases; hence, a state of fatigue comes out quickly. However, it is also a well-known fact that CoQ10 is an important catalyst that increases the energy production at cellular level during exercise. CoQ_{10} can be effective in such a way because it increases the energy production in the mitochondria, decreases the plasma lactate level and thus lowers the feeling of fatigue [12]. In a study which was carried before [13], it was stated that taking CoQ10 for 2 to 5 months caused a decrease of 16 mmHg in the systolic blood pressure while it caused a decrease of 10 mmHg in the diastolic blood pressure. It was observed that taking different dosages of CoQ_{10} every day for 12 weeks caused a decrease in the systolic and diastolic blood pressures to a great extent [14]. And in this study, we observed significant decreases at the level of $p<0,01$'in post-training systolic and diastolic blood pressures of skiing athletes taking 100 and 200 mg CoQ_{10}. However, when systolic and diastolic blood pressures of the trial groups were compared separately to the ones in the control group during one-week training program, it was observed that these levels which were high in the trial groups at the beginning demonstrated a significant decrease of $p<0,001$'in the following days, staying at a level lower than the controls. Although all the cells in human body contain CoQ_{10}, its level is higher in heart and liver, where energy is produced intensely. Because of this reason, the high level of energy necessary for systole and diastole of heart during exercise ensures that the organism adapts to this intense physiological activity by means of joining krebs cycle and being supplied by CoQ_{10} which plays an important role in producing energy [15].

One of the most important factors that affect athletes' performances is heart beat rate. In the studies carried out by Wilmore et al. [16] and Digiesi et al. [17], taking CoQ_{10} was observed to decrease heart beat rates to a great extent. And in this study, we observed significant decreases in post-training heart beat rates for 1 week of skiing athletes which were administered 100 and 200 mg CoQ_{10}. The decrease of ATP in hypoxia, which affects heart beating in a negative way, damages heart functions and ATP is not synthesized again in mitochondria. CoQ10 given from outside starts ATP synthesis and normalizes heart functions by means of arriving at inner membranes of mitochondria and organizing enzymatic events playing a role in electron carrying chain in the mitochondria [18]. With regard to these results, it is possible to say that CoQ_{10} which has a crucial role in energy production can improve diastolic functions, that there can be significant improvements in blood pressure and pulse functions of people who are hypertensive patients and who have mitral valve prolapses, left ventricular hypertrophy, hypertrophic cardiomyopathy and dysfunctional diastolic depending upon taking CoQ_{10}.

Muscular fatigue usually comes out after exercise and muscular enzymes such as CPK and LDH are released because of the fatigue in muscular fibers during exercise. The increase in the level of serum CPK continues as muscular fatigue after exercise. Weakening energy storages and accumulation of metabolic waste products, which are listed among the reasons of fatigue, cause neural conduction and contractility to weaken [19]. In a study carried out with 17 volunteering healthy men and women in order to examine the effect of bicycle ergonometric on physical fatigue, orally administered 100 mg and 300 mg CoQ10 every day for 2 weeks were observed to cause a significant decrease in post-training serum CPK and LDH levels [5]. In this study, we observed that plasma CPK and LDH levels of all the trial groups increased gradually starting from the 2nd day of the one-week training, but the increase in the trial groups taking CoQ_{10} was less than the increase in the control group. In line with these results, it has been concluded that continuous and gradually-increasing training not only generates a physiological dilatation and hypertrophy in the athlete's heart but also helps circulation to be more harmonious, and regular training can ensure that CPK and LDH levels which get higher right after the training decrease to normal levels after a while.

During intense exercise, lactate that accumulates in the muscle and blood causes fatigue. In this case, it becomes necessary to have a rest to ensure that lactate is eliminated from the body [11]. In a study carried out with 25 elite skiing athletes [19], it was determined that adding CoQ_{10} decreases the level of muscle lactic acid, but it increases the level of plasma CoQ_{10} after the exercise. In this study, we determined that post-training plasma lactate levels of trial groups taking 100 and 200 mg CoQ_{10} demonstrated significant decreases. Porter et al. [20] carried out a study in which they made untrained men do bicycle ergonometric as well as giving them 150 mg CoQ_{10} every day for 2 months, and at the end of this period, they observed that lactate levels demonstrated significant decreases. Similar results were also observed by Fujimoto et al. [21]. In this study, we determined that post-training plasma lactate levels of trial groups taking 100 and 200 mg CoQ_{10} demonstrated significant decreases ($p<0,01$). However, a negative relation was observed between the increases in CoQ_{10} and decreases in plasma lactate values. On the other hand, a positive relation was observed between plasma lactate levels and days in the control group whereas this relation was observed to be negative in trial groups. We can say that the increase in plasma La levels of the control group depends on the balance between catabolism and production ratio. Because during exercise, glucose is turned into lactic acid through anaerobic respiration when the level of oxygen decreases or all oxygen is consumed, and this generates a state of fatigue. However, it is possible to say that CoQ_{10} taken at that moment carries electron to mitochondria, increases energy production in mitochondria, decreases the accumulation of lactate in the muscles, and thus increases physical performance. It was observed that CoQ_{10} that was administered to 25 elite skiing athletes before training decreases the level of lactic acid in the muscles, increases the physical performance, and does not change the amount of VO_2max, but increases plasma CoQ_{10} level [19].

Similarly, in a study carried out by Weston et al. [22] in order to examine the effects of CoQ_{10} on aerobic capacity, endurance and plasma CoQ_{10}, 18 volunteering athletes were administered to take 1 mg/kg CoQ_{10} every day for 28 days; and at the end of 28 days, plasma CoQ_{10} levels of these athletes demonstrated significant increases while their VO_2max levels did not demonstrate any change. Likewise, in a study carried out by Bonetti et al. [23], middle-aged respondents, all of whom ride a bicycle at least 1000 km a month, were administered to take CoQ_{10} for 8 weeks and at the end of this period, plasma CoQ_{10} levels demonstrated significant increases. Similar results were also obtained by Cooke et al. [24]. In this study, we observed significant increases in the post-training plasma CoQ_{10} levels of trial groups. Athletes that are dealing with endurance sports have low concentrations of CoQ_{10} in their blood; and this proves that taking CoQ_{10} is necessary for increasing physical performance in such sports. However, although plasma CoQ_{10} levels of trial groups demonstrated significant increases from the 1st to the 7th day, these increases were observed to be more distinct in 200 mg CoQ_{10} groups, which is quite interesting. So, it is possible to say that energy consumption and metabolic activity increases to a great extent during physical exercise, namely, intense muscular activity, and that muscular fatigue comes out after maximal exercise activities. Because the fact that CoQ_{10} concentration of athletes is low during exercise plays a crucial role as a main factor in the process of energy production that receives electron and gives proton in mitochondria wall.

5. Conclusions

It has been concluded that CoQ_{10} caused significant decreases in post-training systolic and diastolic blood pressures and heart beat rates of trial groups whereas it caused a relatively limited decreases in LDH and CPK levels when compared to the control group; these decreases and increases were mostly clear in skiing athletes taking 200 mg CoQ_{10}; lactate levels demonstrated a significant decrease in trial groups to the contrary of plasma CoQ_{10} levels; however, regular and gradual exercise increased physical performance depending on taking CoQ_{10} while it decreased La accumulation and delayed fatigue.

References

[1] E.L. Fox, R.W. Bowers and M.C. Foos. Physical Education and Physiological Basics of Sports. Translated By: Cerit, M. Ed: Yaman, H. Ankara, Bağırgan Yayınevi. 1999.

[2] G. Ersoy. Nutrition for Exercise and Sports Performance, Ankara, Ata offset. 2006.

[3] M. Günay. Exercise Physiology, Ankara, Bağırgan Yayım evi. 1998.

[4] J.A. Schwane, R.T. Buckley, D.P. Dipaolo, M. Atkınson and J.R. Shepherd. Plasma creatine kinase responses of 18- to 30-yr-old african-american men to eccentric exercise. Med. Sci. Sports Exerc 2000; 23 (2): 370-378.

[5] M. Kei, M. Tanaka, S. Nozaki, H. Mizuma, S. Ataka, T. Tahara, T. Sugino, T. Shirai, Y. Kajimoto, H. Kuratsune, O. Kajimoto and Y. Watanabe. Antifatigue effects of coenzyme Q10 during physical fatigue. Nutrition 2008; 24: 293–299.

[6] E.H. Wıtt, A.Z. Rezhıck, C.A. Vıguıe, P. Starke- Reed and L. Packer. Exercise, oxidative damage and effects of antioxidant manipulation. J. Nutr. 1992; 122: 766- 773.

[7] L. Frederick, PhD. Crane. Biochemical functions of coenzyme q10. Journal of the American College Of Nutrition 2001; Vol. 20, No. 6, 591–598.

[8] F. Mosca, D. Fattorini, S. Bompadre and GP. Littarru. Assay of coenzyme q10 in plasmaby a single dilution step. Anal. Biochem 2002; 305: 49-54.

[9] K. Tamer. Measuring and Evaluating Physical Physiological Performance in Sports Ankara, Bağırgan Yayın Evi. 2000.

[10] SAS Puphlishing, SAS/STAT 9.2 User's Guide The GLM Procedure (Book Excerpt), 2008.

[11] V.L. Billat. Use of blood lactate measure ments for prediction of exercise performance and forcontrol of training. Sports Med 1996; 22: 157-75.

[12] A.S. Gürkan, O. Bozdağ and O. Dündar. Coenzyme Q10, Ankara Journal Of Faculty Of Pharmacy 2005; 34 (2) 129 –154.

[13] F. Rosenfeldt, D. Hilton, S. Pepe and H. Krum. Systematic review of effect of coenzyme Q10 in physical exercise, hypertension and heart failure. Biofactors 2003; 18, 91- 100.

[14] J.M. Hodgson, G.F. Watts, D.A. Playford, V. Burke and K.D. Croft.Coenzyme Q10 improves blood pressure and glycaemic control: a control ledtrial in subjects with type 2 diabetes. European Journal of clinical Nutrition 2002; 56,1137-1142.

[15] A.W. Linnane, G. Kopsidas, C. Zhang, N. Yarovaya, S. Kovalenko, P. Papakostopoulos, H. Eastwood, S. Graves and M. Richardson. Cellular redoxactivity of coenzyme Q10: effect of CoQ10 supplementation on human skeletal muscle. Free Radic Res. 2002; 36:445–453.

[16] J.H. Wilmore, P.R. Stanforth, J. Gagnon, A.S. Leon, D.C. Rao, J.S. Skinner and C. Bouchard. Enduranc eexercise training has a minimal on resting heart rate the herltage study. Medicine And Science İn Sport And Exercise 1996; 28 (7): 829-35.

[17] V. Digiesi, F. Cantini, A. Oradei and G. Bisi. Coenzyme Q10 in essential hypertension. Mol. Aspects. Med 1994; 15, 257-263.

[18] K. Salbaş, R. Karaoguz and A. Sonel. The Effect of coenzyme q10 on hypoxia and reoxijenation insulated rabbit right atrium spontaneous contractile activity and tissue damage. Turkey Clinics Cardiology 1989; 2: 108-113.

[19] T. Ylikoski, J. Piirainen, O. Hanninen and J. Penttinen. Theeffect of coenzyme Q10 on the exercise performance of cross-country skiers. Molec Aspects Med. 1997; 18: 283-290.

[20] D.A. Porter, D.L. Costill, J.J. Zachwieja, K. Krzeminski W.J. Fink, E. Wagner and K. Folkers. Theeffect of oral coenzyme Q10 on the exercise tolerance of middle – aged untrained men. Clinical Neurop harmacology 1995; 27: 4, 187-191.

[21] S. Fujimoto, N. Kurihara, K. Hirata and T. Takeda. Effects of coenzyme Q10 administration on pulmonary function and exercise performance in patients with chronic lung diseases. Clin Investig 1993; 71:S 162 S 166.

[22] S.B. Weston, S. Zhou, Rp. Weatherby and SJ. Robson. Does exegenous coenzyme Q10 affect aerobic capacity in endurance athletes. Int J. Sport Nutr 1997; 7(3):197-206.

[23] A. Bonetti, F. Solito, G. Carmosino, A.M. Bargossi and PL. Fıorella. Effect of ubidecarenone oral treatment on aerobic power in middle-aged trained subject. Journal of Sports

[24] M. Cooke, M. Iosia, T. Buford, B. Shelmadine, G. Hudson, C. Kerksick, C. Rasmussen, M. Greenwood, B. Leutholtz and D. Willoughby. Effects of acuteand 14-day coenzyme Q1 supplementation on exercise performance in both trained and untrained individuals. Int Soc Sports Nutr 2008; March 4. doi: 10.1186/1550-2783-5-8.

Tripple-Ironman based on vegan raw vegetable/fruits diet: Physiological echocardiographic and blood analysis findings

Roman Leischik*, Norman Spelsberg, Birgit Dworrak, Melchior Seyfarth

Dept. Prevention and Sports Medicine, Chair Cardiology, University Witten-Herdecke, Hagen, Germany

Email address:
info@dr-leischik.de (R. Leischik)

Abstract: Endurance sport required healthy and balanced diet. This case report presents the findings of an ultra triathlete (three times Ironman with 11.4 km swimming, 540 km cycling and 126 km running in 41 hours 18 minutes) living and finished competitions based on vegan raw diet. To this end, the vegan ultra triathlete and a control group of 10 Ironman triathletes of similar age living on a mixed diet were investigated, using echocardiography and spiroergometry. In addition, blood samples were taken from the vegan athlete both in the sporting season and in the off-season. The vegan athlete showed no signs of dietary deficiencies or impaired health. In comparison with the control group, the vegan athlete showed a higher oxygen intake at the respiratory compensation point. This case demonstrates that even top-class sporting performance, like that of a three times Ironman, is possible on a vegan diet. Whether a vegan diet offers advantages or disadvantages for the performance of endurance athletes remains an open question.

Keywords: Vegetarian Diet, Vegan Diet, Endurance Sports, Triathlon

1. Case Report

A 48-years-old male finished Tripple-Ironman distance in 41 hours and 18 minutes (11.4 km swimming, 540 km cycling and 126 km running)at the time of the examinations, he had been practising his current diet of raw vegan diet for 6 years. Prior to this, the vegan athlete had been living as a vegan for 3 years and as a vegetarian for the previous 13.

All last competitions were performed only based on a raw diet. At the time of both examinations, the vegan athlete was 48 years of age and 1.80 metres in height. In the sporting season he was 79.7 kg in weight, with a body fat index of 12.9%; in the off-season he weighed 80.3 kg with a body fat index of 16.3%. Clinical examination showed a regular heart rhythm at 60 beats /min. Blood pressure was 115/70. The heart sounds were normal.

Previous the spiroergometry, echocardiography was performed based on ASA-Criteria (1).

For comparison purposes, we refer to the values for 10 Ironman triathletes of similar age living on a mixed diet.

The results of the spiroergometryare shown in tables 1, of echocardiography in table 2 and blood analysis findings are presented in table 3. The athletes of the control group were aged 47.4 ± 5.2, weighed 76.2 ± 8.9 kg (with 13.4 ± 2.0% body fat) and were 1.816 metres ± 6.6 cm in height. In the active phase the vegan athlete was training on average 18 hours per week, consisting of 2 hours of swimming, 11 hours of cycling and 5 hours running. This involved covering distances of 5 km (swimming), 330 km (cycling) and 50 km (running). The athletes of the control group were training for a total of 15.9 ± 2.1 hours weekly, involving 2.5 ± 0.7 hours and 5.6 ± 1.5 km swimming, 8.6 ± 1.5 hours and 215.5 ± 53.0 km cycling and 4.9 ± 0.7 hours and 55.2 ± 6.5 km running.

In terms of performance diagnostics, the vegan athlete showed comparable VO2max, VO2 at VAT and %VO2max at VAT values as compared with the control group. VO2 and %VO2max at RCP were somewhat higher for the vegan athlete. The maximum ergometric performance is higher for the vegan athlete in absolute terms, but not relative to the body weight. At RCP the ergometric performance of the vegan athlete is somewhat higher than that of the control group. The vegan athlete had lower pulse rates at rest, at VAT, RCP and at the endurance limit. In comparison with the off-season, in the active season the vegan athlete had a higher maximum ergometric performance, VO2 and %VO2max, as well as cardiac frequency at RCP.

In morphological terms, the vegan athlete showed a greater left ventricular end diastolic diameter, with consecutively higher end diastolic volume and stroke volume. The systolic and diastolic functions seem to be similar for the vegan athlete and the control group.

Apart from a mild thrombopenia, slight CK-NAC rise in the active season and (in both examinations) a slight drop in free testosterone, all the parameters registered fall within the reference zone.

2. Discussion

It is well known that a vegetarian or vegan diet, when sensibly managed, can make a contribution to the prevention and therapy of illnesses in all phases of life [1]. More and more people are thus adopting a vegetarian (2) or vegan (2) lifestyle. It is equally understandable that such people may want to take part in endurance sports. It follows that the effects of vegan diet on sporting performance are a matter of general interest.

This case report set out to investigate an ultraendurancetriathlete, who had been living on a vegetarian diet for 22 and a purely vegan diet for 9 years, with reference to his ability to perform, cardiac status and any symptoms of deficiency. It was also a matter of interest for the study to ascertain whether his performance parameters were different from those of mixed diet triathletes in any significant degree.

Even competitive athletes can adopt a diet of this kind with a view to the health benefits, without any risk of suffering from dietary deficiencies [2–4].

With its disciplines of swimming, cycling and running, the triathlon is a very popular type of endurance sport. As well as competitions involving classic sprint distances (0.5,20 and 5 km), short distances (1-1.5, 40 and 10 km) and medium distances (ca. 2, 80-90 and 21.2 km), it also offers competitions involving ultra distances: Ironman(3,8, 180 and 42.2 km) and multiple (2x until 10x) Ironman.

As is the case with other types of endurance sport, triathletes undergo various physical adaptations in the course of training. These include an increased cardiac output under stress and increased arteriovenous oxygen extraction with consecutive rises in the maximum oxygen intake (VO2max)[5]. In echocardiographic terms, triathletes show physical changes similar to those of cyclists, resembling a mixed state of static/dynamic stress and involving a significant increase in the left ventricular muscle mass and internal left ventricular diameter [6]. In terms of spiroergometry, successful triathletes not only show an increased oxygen intake – they also demonstrate a capacity for continuous high performance over long periods, as a result of effective internal economy, high fractional extraction of VO2max at the given stress level (%VO2max) and a high anaerobic threshold [7].Good indicators of the limit of endurance are the ventilatory anaerobic threshold (VAT) and the respiratory compensation point (RCP) [7,8].

The physiological profile of short distance and long distance triathletes has already been mapped out, based on the study of small groups. It is not known whether or to what extent triathletes living on a vegan or vegetarian diet differ from triathletes living on a mixed diet. It is known that non-sporting vegans show better metabolic parameters than mixed diet athletes (9).To the best of our knowledge, no data are to be found in the extant literature on the spiroergometric, echocardiographic or haematological parameters of ultra endurance athletes living on a vegan diet. As a result, this is a ground-breaking case-report – involving the first ever presentation of the characteristic parameters of a vegan ultra endurance athlete.

In view of the equivalence in terms of age and other similar anthropometric features, the data for the vegan athlete are well comparable with those of the control group. On the other hand, we are dealing here with an individual case, so the meaningfulness of the results, in the nature of the case, remains limited. Both the vegan athlete and the control group trained for a comparable number of hours. The vegan athlete's cycling training, on the other hand, was more intense and more prolonged. Comparison of the competition results would be a way of checking this, but in view of the fact that the athletes' preferred competition distances are vary from one another, this is not possible. Here, however, we should draw attention to the considerably higher age of the athletes under consideration. Millet et al[8] report on athletes of 24.8 ± 2.6 years of age. In comparison with the off-season, in the active season the RCP and themaximum ergometric performancerose moderately, whereas the VAT and VO2max remained at a constant level. This study demonstrated a significant rise in the RCP and maximum ergometric performance (with VAT and VO2max remaining constant), based on comparison between the pre-competitive and competitive seasons.

The echocardiographic parameters of the vegan athlete are hardly different from those of the control group. Essentially the vegan athletehas a greater LVEDD value, with higher EDV and SV, which however do not exceed standard and normal values [10]. Overall the echocardiographic values of the sporting season and the off-season do not differ in any significant degree.

Laboratory parameters showed no signicant pathology. A slight thrombopenia in the sporting season can be explained by the reduced thrombocyte activation and adhesion caused by training. In itself this is not necessarily a pathological manifestation. In conjunction with a threshold value for vitamin B12 and standard iron, ferritin and folic acid status, the standard haemoglobin, haematocrit, MCH, MCV and MCHC readings exclude the possibility of manifest or latent anaemia. Raised CK-NAC levels are not unusual with active athletes. Mougious et al. have therefore written about the necessity of separate CK reference values for active sportspersons. Reduced testosterone values in the blood have also been described. An influence on the bone density or the muscle mass, however, cannot be demonstrated. None of the usual laboratory parameters gives grounds for suspecting the presence of any detriment to health caused by sport or by diet. Quite on the contrary, the vegan athleteeven shows ideal cholesterol values.

3. Critical Remarks

The case report of a vegan triathlete can only provide indications that a vegan diet is at least not detrimental to health, even in connection with a long-distance triathlon, and that a vegan diet results in similar performance as compared with a mixed diet. These conclusions cannot be extrapolated to short distances and Olympic distances, where an explosive performance – above all, a performance in the lactic acid zone – is frequently necessary. Taking place for the most part in the aerobic range, long-distance races may work more in favour of vegan diet than races that approach the anaerobic threshold. In view of the shortage of suitable and willing test subjects, it will not be easy to arrange a group comparison of vegan and traditional triathletes for study purposes. A case study like the present one can supply indications, but the meaningfulness of its findings remains subject to limit.

This case report seems to suggest that an ultra triathlete living on a vegan diet has a similar profile, physiologically and in performance terms, to that of triathletes of similar age living on a conventional diet. The cardiac adaptations are likewise similar in both cases. The higher laboratory parameters do not permit conclusions with regard to dietary deficiency or any detriment to health. A well planned vegan diet can apparently also be adopted by ultra endurance athletes without any risk to health necessarily being incurred. To what extent a vegan diet offers benefits or disadvantages for the performance capacity / health of a triathlete would be a matter for investigation in a future study, though in view of the highly individual training regimes of triathletes, this would be difficult to arrange.

Data relating to financial interests and relationships (patents, fees, support by companies etc.): none.

Table 1.*Spiroergometric parameters of the vegan athlete and the control group (values given as a mean value ± standard deviation)*

		V OS	V S	CG (n=10)
VO2max	L/min	4.8	4.7	4.3 ± 0.6
	ml*min-1*kg-1	60.0	60.0	56.9 ± 7.5
VO2 VAT	L/min	3.4	3.3	3.3 ± 0.6
	ml*min-1*kg-1	43	42	43.7 ± 7.4
	% VO2max	71	70	76.1 ± 9.3
VO2 RCP	L/min	3.9	4.4	3.6 ± 0.6
	ml*min-1*kg-1	48	55	48.2 ± 8.3
	% VO2max	80.6	92	84.4 ± 6.9
HF	At rest	55	49	58.6 ± 2.9
	At VAT	127	123	147.7 ± 11.4
	At RCP	141	147	157.0 ± 13.1
	Maximal load	163	159	176.7 ± 11.0
W	At VAT	280	280	262 ± 42.9
	At RCP	340	370	286 ± 56.2
	Maximal load	370	400	337 ± 53.8
	Maximal load / kg body weight	4.61	5.02	4.46 ± 0.73

CG = control group, HF = heart frequency / min, OS = off-season, S = active season, V = vegan athlete, VO2max = maximum oxygen intake, VO2 VAT = oxygen intake at ventilatory anaerobic threshold, VO2 RCP = oxygen intake at respiratory compensation point, W = ergometric performance)

Table 2. *Echocardiographic parameters*

		Vegan athlete, off-season	Vegan athlete, active season	Control group (n=10)
Aortic root	cm	3.7	3.4	3.1 ± 0.4
Left atrium	cm	3.0	3.0	2.6 ± 0.3
Left atrium	ml	36	30	29.6 ± 8.6
LVEDD	cm	5.0	5.4	4.64 ± 0.4
IVSD	cm	1.2	1.1	1.2 ± 0.1
PWTD	cm	1.2	1.0	1.2 ± 0.1
LVMM	g	211.3	206.3	203.0 ± 35.3
LVMM	g/m²	105.68	103.67	103.1 ± 14.5
EDV	ml	119	140	100.2 ± 16.7
ESV	ml	48	58	39 ± 6.1
SV	ml	72	82	61.2 ± 11.2
EF	%	60	59	61.0 ± 2.1
SF	%	32	31	35.5 ± 9.4
MV E/A ratio		1.45	1.56	1.39 ± 0.20

EDV = end diastolic volume, EF = ejection fraction, ESV = end systolic volume, IVSD = intraventicular septum in diastole, LVEDD = left ventricular end diastolic diameter, LVMM = left ventricular muscle mass, MV E/A ratio = mitral valve E/A ratio, PWTD = posterior wall thickness in diastole, SF = shortening fraction, SV = stroke volume

Table 3.*Results of blood investigation of the vegan ultra triathlete*

Analysis	Off-season	Active season
Leukocytes (1000s/ul)	4.6	4.7
Erythrocytes (Mill.ul)	5.1	4.9
Haematocrit (%)	43	42
Haemoglobin (g/dl)	14.9	14.1
MCV (fl)	83	87
MCH (pg)	29.0	29.1
MCHC (g/dl)	35.1	33.3
Thrombocytes (1000s/ul)	171	138
Alkaline phosphatase (U/l)	68	70
Glutamyltranspeptidase	8	15
Glutamate oxalacetate transaminase (U/l)	36	40
Glutamate pyruvate transaminase (U/l)	32	42
Lactate dehydrogenase (U/l)	199	238
Amylase (U/l)	63	61
Lipase (U/l)	35	36
CK-NAC (U/l)	155	209
Protein (g/dl)	6.6	6.7
Cholesterol (mg/dl)	134	113
HDL (mg/dl)	47	51
LDL (mg/dl)	74	50
Triacylglyceride (mg/dl)	148	84
TSH basal (mU/l)	1.23	0.73
Iron (µg/dl)	95.0	82.0
Free testosterone (pg/ml)	5.5	5.7
Vitamin B12 (pg/ml)	329	347
Ferritin (ng/ml)	83.7	82.6
Folic acid (ng/ml)	16.8	14.3

References

[1] *Craig WJ, Mangels AR.* Position of the American Dietetic Association: vegetarian diets. J Am Diet Assoc 2009; 109: 1266 – 1282

[2] *Fuhrman J, Ferreri DM.* Fueling the vegetarian (vegan) athlete. Curr Sports Med Rep 2010; 9: 233 – 241

[3] *Barr SI, Rideout CA.* Nutritional considerations for vegetarian athletes. Nutrition 2004; 20: 696 – 703

[4] *Venderley AM, Campbell WW.* Vegetarian diets: Nutritional considerations for athletes. Sports Med 2006; 36: 293 – 305

[5] *O'Toole ML, Douglas PS.* Applied physiology of triathlon. Sports Med 1995; 19: 251 – 267

[6] *Hoogsteen J, Hoogeveen A, Schaffers H, Wijn PFF, van Hemel NM, van der Wall EE.* Myocardial adaptation in different endurance sports: an echocardiographic study. Int J Cardiovasc Imaging 2004; 20: 19 – 26

[7] *Sleivert GG, Rowlands DS.* Physical and physiological factors associated with success in the triathlon. Sports Med 1996; 22: 8 – 18

[8] *Millet GP, Dréano P, Bentley DJ.* Physiological characteristics of elite short- and long-distance triathletes. Eur. J. Appl. Physiol 2003; 88: 427 – 430

[9] Fontana L,MeyerTE,KleinS,Holloszy JO. Long-term low-protein vegan diet and endurance exercise are associated with low cardiometabolic risk. Rejuvenation Res. 2007;10(2):225-34.

[10] *Lang RM, Bierig M, Devereux RB et al.*Recommendations for chamber quantification. Eur J Echocardiogr 2006; 7: 79 – 108

The effect of vestibular stimulation on eye-hand coordination and postural control in elite basketball players

William W. N. Tsang[1,*], Shirley S. M. Fong[2], Yoyo T. Y. Cheng[1,3], Dinisha D. Daswani[1], Hiu Yan Lau[1], Carina K. Y. Lun[1], Shamay S. M. Ng[1]

[1]Department of Rehabilitation Sciences, The Hong Kong Polytechnic University, Hong Kong
[2]Institute of Human Performance, The University of Hong Kong, Hong Kong
[3]Institute of Child Health, University College London, UK

Email address:
William.Tsang@polyu.edu.hk (W. W. N. Tsang)

Abstract: The game of basketball requires complex eye-hand coordination and exceptional postural control ability. This study compared eye-hand coordination and postural control before and after vestibular stimulation in trained basketball players with healthy, age-matched controls. Fifteen trained basketball players and 17 healthy adults (all male, age range 19-25 years) were recruited. The participants were required to perform a fast finger-pointing task involving a moving visual target in a standing position, before and after whole head-and-body rotation at 150°s-1 for 30 s seated in a rotational chair. Results show that the trained basketball players had shorter reaction times in eye-hand coordination tasks (a decrease of 23.3% vs an increase of 8.1% of controls, p=0.008) and regained postural control more quickly (mediolateral direction: 0.4% vs 43.3%; p=0.009; anteroposterior direction: 3.9% vs 21.5%, p=0.038) after vestibular stimulation. These data suggest that vestibular stimulation could enhance balance and eye-hand coordination among young basketball players. The findings may provide information for sports training and further research work.

Keywords: Eye-Hand Coordination, Postural Control, Vestibular Stimulation, Basketball

1. Introduction

Good eye-hand coordination and postural control are essential for superior athletic performances [1-3]. Eye-hand coordination refers to the integrated use of vision, arms, hands and fingers to accomplish goal-directed hand movements [4]. Postural control is the ability to control the centre of mass in relation to the base of support. It depends on the integration of proprioception, vision and vestibular cues in the central nervous system. Among the three sensory cues, vestibular input is particularly important for postural control in sensory challenging environments (e.g. during dynamic sport activities) [5].

Basketball is a dynamic sport where athletes need extremely good eye-hand coordination and postural control for faultless catching, throwing, shooting, jumping, turning and pivoting movements in challenging environments [6]. The complex basketball tasks such as a turn and a jump shot, involve eye-hand coordination combined with excellent postural control. Vestibular input is particularly important for maintaining postural stability during the turning movements [5]. Therefore, it is logical to postulate that vestibular stimulation/strengthening might enhance balance performance and so eye-hand coordination in basketball players. However, to the best of our knowledge, no study has investigated the effect of vestibular stimulation on the aforementioned outcomes thus far.

Based on a study conducted by Tsang and Hui-Chan [7], the horizontal semi-circular canals of the vestibular apparatus can be stimulated by using a rotational chair. This swift rotational movement in the horizontal plane closely simulates the rotational basketball manoeuvres. Therefore, we hypothesize that basketball players might demonstrate better concurrent eye-hand coordination and balance performance after receiving the vestibular stimulation in a rotational chair.

This study was designed to compare eye-hand coordination and postural control before and after vestibular stimulation in elite basketball players and healthy adults.

2. Methods

2.1. Participants

Thirty-two males aged 19 to 25 years were recruited by convenience sampling. Fifteen of them were elite basketball players representing their university, and they participated in regular basketball training at least twice per week. The other 17 participants were healthy young active university students who had no regular sport-specific training. Participants who had musculoskeletal injuries such as ankle sprain injury in the previous 6 months or who had a history of vestibular problems or neurological diseases were excluded. All of the participants were screened using a general health questionnaire to ensure that they are healthy individuals. The study was approved by the Human Subjects Ethics Review Committee of the administering University. Written informed consent was obtained from all participants before data collection. All requirements stipulated in the Declaration of Helsinki were conformed.

2.2. Experimental Set-up

The equipment used in the experiment included a rotational chair (System 2000; Micromedical Technologies Inc, Chatham, IL, USA), a force platform (Model 9286AA; Kistler, Gommiswald, Switzerland), a visual display unit (VDU) (Clear Tek 3000 LCD screen; MicroTouch Systems Inc., Methuen, USA) and a mono-axial accelerometer (K-beam 8302B10; Kistler, Switzerland). The force platform was placed in front of the rotational chair. The VDU was set at arm's length of each individual standing on the force platform at 90° of shoulder flexion. The height of the VDU was adjusted to be at each participant's eye level, and the accelerometer was affixed with adhesive tape to the dorsal aspect of the dominant hand at the third meta-carpal phalangeal joint. The equipment was recalibrated before each trial. Each participant performed a standing balance test with concurrent fast finger pointing task toward a moving visual target for three times with the first one as familiarisation trial. The procedure was repeated after vestibular stimulation with a rotational chair. Two minute of rest were given in between each trial of vestibular stimulation.

2.2.1. Standing Balance with Fast Finger-Pointing

The participants stood on the force platform with their feet together, arms by their sides for 20 s. Three seconds after stepping onto the force plate, a moving visual target appeared on the VDU. The target was 3 cm in diameter, and moving at 10 mm s^{-1} from left to right across the screen. The participants were instructed to touch the target with the index finger of their dominant hand as fast and as accurately as possible, and return their hand to their side.

2.2.2. Vestibular Stimulation

To stimulate the vestibular system, particularly the horizontal semicircular canals [8], each participant sat in the rotational chair with their head fixed at 30° of flexion, eyes closed and hands on the armrests. A clockwise whole head-and-body rotation at 150° s^{-1} was applied for 30 s. The speed and duration were based on a similar study conducted by Goebel and Paige [9] with young healthy participants aged 20 to 35 years using a rotation speed of 180° s^{-1} for 30s. Here, 150° s^{-1} was used because 6 participants reported dizziness and unsteadiness after fast finger-pointing in a pilot study using 180° s^{-1}. Once the chair had stopped, the participants were instructed to open their eyes, get up as fast as possible, stand on the force platform with their feet together and arms by their sides and perform a finger-pointing task.

2.2.3. Data Recording

The age, height, weight, hand dominance and arm length of each participant were recorded. Eye-hand coordination was evaluated in terms of each participant's reaction times, movement times and touch accuracy. Reaction time was defined as the time between the appearance of the visual target on the VDU and the onset of acceleration in the hand movement. Movement time was defined as the time between the onset of acceleration and touching the screen. Touch accuracy was defined as the absolute deviation of the touched location from the centre of the circular target at that moment. The VDU being used in the present study was 34 cm wide and 27 cm tall, with resolution of 1024x1024 and accuracy of > 99% of true position. The test-retest reliability using such instrumentation has been found to be satisfactory with ICC values range from 0.68 to 0.97. The known groups validity has also been verified between young and older adults [10].

2.2.4. Data Reduction

Postural control was assessed in terms of the time to stabilisation (TTS) in both the mediolateral (ML) and anteroposterior (AP) directions. TTS was used because it can evaluate dynamic postural stability, which is more functional [11]. During the 20 s standing on the force platform, the trajectory of the centre of pressure (COP) was recorded continuously. The COP data from the force platform were sampled at 100 Hz and were smoothed using a second-order Butterworth low-pass filter with a cut-off frequency of 0.85 Hz. The sway signals in the ML and AP directions were rectified. The peak values in both the ML and AP directions from 10 to 15 s and from 15 to 20 s were detected. For each direction, the lower of the two peak amplitudes was selected for further analysis. The sway signal was then fitted into a polynomial curve with third order, and the amplitude of the curve was checked. The time to stabilisation was defined as the time after which the magnitude of the signal remained smaller than the peak value detected [12,13] (Figure 1).

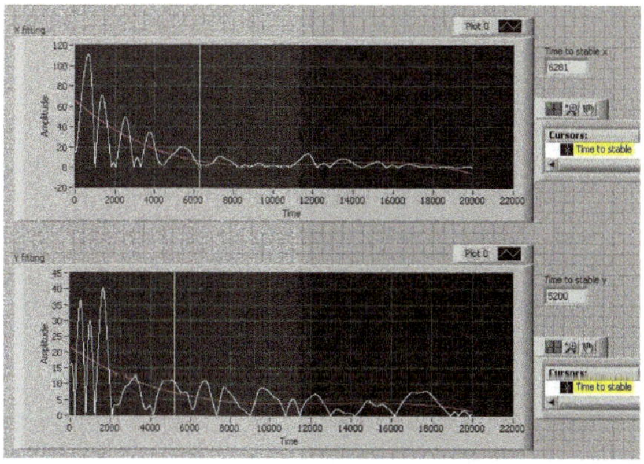

Figure 1. An illustration to demonstrate the determination of the time to stabilization.

2.2.5. Statistical Analysis

The average age, weight, height and arm-length of the two groups were compared using independent t-tests. Arm-length was used to normalise the movement time, since a longer arm should require more time to execute a given movement. Paired t-tests with Bonferroni adjustments were performed to compare the eye-hand coordination and time to stabilisation measures before and after vestibular stimulation within each group. Multivariate analysis of variance (MANOVA) was used to compare the eye-hand coordination measures, the times to stabilization, and the percentage changes after vestibular stimulation between the two groups. If statistically significant differences were found, univariate tests were conducted for each outcome measure. The time needed to get up from sitting and step onto the force platform after vestibular stimulation was compared between the two groups using independent t-tests. This was also used as a covariate in the statistical analysis because the effect of vestibular stimulation on balance control could be minimised if participants stayed in the chair too long. Any significant difference in this time interval would then be a confounding variable in between-group comparisons. A significance level (α) of 0.05 (two-tailed) was chosen for statistical comparisons.

All statistical analyses were performed using the SPSS software, version 17.0.

3. Results

3.1. Demographic Data

Table 1 presents the demographic profiles of the 15 basketball players and the 17 control participants. Independent t-tests showed no statistically significant difference in age between the two groups, but as might be expected, there were statistically significant differences in average height, body weight and arm length between the two groups. Basketball players are generally taller, heavier and have longer arms than other men of similar age.

Table 1. Demographic data of the controls and basketball players.

Characteristics	Health Adults (n=17)	Basketball players (n=15)	p-value
Age (year)	21.1 ± 0.6	21.3 ± 1.6	0.643
Height (cm)	171.2 ± 4.6	183.2 ± 7.6	0.003*
Body weight (kg)	63.8 ± 9.7	75.4 ± 10.2	<0.001*
Arm length (cm)	74.5 ± 3.6	82.1 ± 5.4	<0.001*

Note: Values are mean ± standard deviation for this and subsequent tables.
* Between-group difference significant at $p<0.05$ (using independent t-tests).

3.2. Effects of Vestibular Stimulation on Eye-Hand Coordination and Standing Balance Control

For the healthy young adults, after vestibular stimulation, the average reaction time of the control participants increased by 8.1%, movement time decreased by 2.4% and touch accuracy decreased by 0.8%. However, none of these changes were statistically (or indeed practically) significant (Table 2). The controls did, however, exhibit a highly significant increase in the average time to stabilisation—by 43.3% in the ML direction and by 21.5% in AP direction.

Table 2. Comparison of reaction time, movement time, touch accuracy, and time to stabilization before and after vestibular stimulation in healthy controls and basketball players.

Measures	Healthy Adults (n=17)			Basketball Players (n=15)		
	Pre-vestibular Stimulation	Post-vestibular Stimulation	p-value	Pre-vestibular Stimulation	Post-vestibular Stimulation	p-value
Reaction time (ms)	191.4 ± 49.0	200.8 ± 58.2	0.539	193.3 ± 66.4	154.5 ± 33.5	0.117
Movement time (ms)	770.7 ± 154.9	737.5 ± 136.7	0.422	706.6 ± 140.0	791.0 ± 204.4	0.141
Touch accuracy (mm)	11.2 ± 4.5	10.5 ± 3.9	0.489	9.7 ± 4.6	10.2 ± 5.2	0.467
Time to stabilization in:						
ML direction (ms)	6015.9 ± 1230.4	8266.1 ± 1113.1	0.000*	5702.0 ± 1961.1	6589.8 ± 1831.5	0.297
AP direction (ms)	6603.7 ± 1064.2	7850.0 ± 1237.1	0.004*	6193.5 ± 1229.1	6856.8 ± 1400.4	0.121

Notes: ML = Mediolateral; AP = Anteroposterior.
* Within-group difference significant at $p<0.025$ (using paired t-tests; with Bonferroni's adjustment).

For the basketball players, after vestibular stimulation, the average reaction time among the basketball players decreased by 23.3%, movement time increased by 8.8%, and touch accuracy increased by 14.8%. Time to stabilisation in

ML direction increased by 0.4%, while that in AP direction increased by 4.0%. Paired t-tests confirmed that none of these changes was statistically significant (Table 2).

3.3. Comparisons of Eye-Hand Coordination and Postural Control between Basketball Players and Healthy Young Adults

Before vestibular stimulation, the basketball players and the control participants performed similarly with regard to reaction time, movement time, touch accuracy and time to stabilisation in both the ML and AP directions. Multivariate tests of eye-hand coordination results and stabilisation times revealed no significant differences between the two groups.

After Vestibular Stimulation, the time taken to get up from the rotational chair onto the force platform was measured. Basketball players required 2.1 s on average and the controls required 1.7 s. An independent t-test showed this to be a statistically significant difference between the two groups. Therefore, it was used as a covariate in the multivariate and univariate tests for the analysis of time to stabilisation.

Percentage changes reflecting the differences before and after vestibular stimulation were significantly different between the basketball players and the controls in terms of both the eye-hand coordination measures (p=0.046) and the time to stabilisation (p=0.008). Univariate tests revealed a significantly shorter average reaction time among the basketball players than among the controls (Table 3). However, no significant differences were found in the percentage changes for touch accuracy or movement time. In terms of the time to stabilisation, the controls had a significantly greater percentage increase in both the ML and AP directions when compared with the basketball players.

Table 3. *Changes in reaction time, movement time, touch accuracy and time to stabilization for healthy controls and basketball players after vestibular stimulation.*

Measures	Healthy Adults (n=17) percentage change	Basketball Players (n=15) percentage change	p-value
Eye-hand coordination:			
Reaction time (ms)	8.1 ± 29.3	-23.3 ± 30.2	0.008*
Movement time (ms)	-2.4 ± 18.4	8.8 ± 22.6	0.137
Touch accuracy (mm)	-0.8 ± 38.3	14.8 ± 40.3	0.272
Time to stabilization in:			
ML direction (ms)	43.3 ± 38.3	0.4 ± 47.1	0.009*
AP direction (ms)	21.5 ± 25.6	3.9 ± 24.4	0.038*

Notes: ML = Mediolateral; AP = Anteroposterior.

* Between-group difference significant at p<0.05 using univariate tests, after MANOVA test p=0.046 and p=0.008 for eye-hand coordination measures and time to stabilization, respectively.

4. Discussion

The basketball players had a greater average decrease in reaction time after vestibular stimulation. This might be explained in the context of sports psychology by an inverted-U relationship between performance and arousal state. Arousal is a combination of psychological and physiological activity that can be controlled by an individual. A highly aroused person is activated both mentally and physically [14]. The inverted-U hypothesis states that arousal will increase together with performance to an optimal point of best performance. A further increase in arousal will lead to a decrease in performance. A group led by Collardeau [15] has shown that running can improve reaction time during the exercise due to an increase in arousal level. In our study, the vestibular stimulation may have mimicked the swift turning movements in a basketball game. The basketball players may have adapted to the effect of the stimulation and become aroused to their optimal levels for best performance, as in a basketball game. This might have led to the decrease in reaction time after the vestibular stimulation. The controls, on the other hand, may have been over-aroused, leading to slower reaction times. This suggests that basketball trainings may allow the élite basketball players to better regulate their arousal level and focus their attention in performing an eye-hand task in situations like that of a game [14].

A second possible mechanism which might cause shorter reaction times would be "learning effect" due to weekly basketball training. Libet and his co-workers [16] have shown that it takes almost half a second for the brain to be properly conscious of a fast-moving object in the surroundings. In another study, they also demonstrated that it takes 350 to 500 ms for the mind to complete all the recognition and filtering process to come to a settled field of awareness [17]. In addition, research by Haggard's group [18] suggests that when we anticipate an action to initiate an event, it will appear to happen earlier than if we did not anticipate it. This indicates that consciousness lags reality by approximately half a second, and any more rapid reaction presented by the athletes should have been achieved subconsciously. Basketball involves a lot of speed, turning and eye-hand coordination similar to that set up in these experiments. The elite basketball players may have been able to anticipate the fast-pointing task subconsciously much faster than the controls because they were better accustomed to the effect of vestibular stimulation subconsciously. This would in turn have increased the availability of neural resources for the basketball players to respond to the moving visual target, resulting in the faster reaction times observed.

Under normal circumstances, multisensory information from the vestibular, somatosensory and visual systems is essential to control postural stability. When the accuracy of vestibular input is affected by stimulation, a person uses "sensory channel reweighting" and relies on other sensory inputs, mainly proprioception, to keep the centre of mass (CoM) within his stability limit [19]. If the individual's proprioceptive system is not adapted to such demands, such alteration could lead to significant deterioration in postural control. Earlier studies have illustrated the decline in static bipedal standing balance after vestibular stimulation in healthy individuals [20,21].

Previous studies have found that young adults mostly employ ankle torque to minimise AP body sway during stable surface bipedal standing [22]. In such a strategy, synergistic muscle activation sequences are involved. To counteract an anterior sway, the gastrocnemius muscle would first be activated, followed by hamstring and paraspinal muscles. On the other hand, the tibialis anterior, quadriceps and abdominal muscles would be used to resist a posterior sway [5]. When the postural sway amplitude or velocity is too large to be overcome by ankle torque alone, hip torque might also be used in combination with the ankle strategy [23]. Allum and Pfaltz [24] have suggested that coordination of the anterior and posterior muscle systems is maintained through the vestibulo-spinal reflex system. Vestibular input is therefore important in controlling the timing and intensity of the muscle contractions to avoid unidirectional destabilisation. This could explain the delayed AP postural stabilisation observed after vestibular stimulation.

The standardised feet-together stance used in this experiment could have imposed a significant challenge for postural control in the ML direction, leading to the larger percentage change in ML time to stabilisation (43.3% versus 21.5% in AP direction) in the control group. With a normal wide stance, ML stability is usually maintained through sideways motion at the pelvis controlled by the hip adductors and abductors. Any stance width narrower than 8 cm can restrict movement at the hips and induce significant sideways motion at the ankle [25]. However the structural and biomechanical properties of the ankle limit its ML adjustment capacity. Thus, more effortful responses are needed to keep the CoM within the stability limits [26].

The basketball players' better postural control after vestibular stimulation, especially in the ML direction, could be related to their general fitness and sports specific training. Previous studies have shown that percentage lean body mass and muscle strength are positively correlated with postural control [24,27]. Basketball players' ability to generate forces sufficient for controlling their body position in space should also contribute to better postural control [5]. Daily activities such as walking and running involve mostly sagittal plane movement, but basketball training involves foot-work, balance and agility drills performed in multiple directions with lots of turning and pivoting [28]. Such training is designed to impose excessive demands on a player's somatosensory system, muscle recruitment and vestibular system. Adaptations to such training could have led to their superior performance in this experiment.

There are some limitations in this study. First, only male participants between 17 and 20 years old were recruited. Thus, the results may not be generalised to other age groups and to women. Second, the laboratory version of vestibular stimulation was generated by clockwise rotation at a fixed velocity, targeting only on the horizontal semicircular canal. This would certainly be different from the stimulation during dynamic head movement on-court. Postural strategies employed during sports might also be different from that used in bipedal standing. Third, since we used a non-randomized pre-test, post-test control group design in this study, cause-and-effect relationship between vestibular stimulation and balance/eye-hand coordination in basketball players cannot be well established. Further randomised trials are recommended.

Nevertheless, this study serves as a basis for future research into the causal relationship between vestibular stimulation and sports performance. The effect of basketball-related vestibular training for young athletes in general would also be worth exploring.

5. Conclusions

The basketball players showed better postural control and faster average reaction times in eye-hand coordination tasks following vestibular stimulation when compared to the control group. On the contrary, young control participants showed a significant increase in time to stabilisation after vestibular stimulation by whole head-and-body rotation. Vestibular stimulation could enhance balance performance and eye-hand coordination among young basketball players.

References

[1] A.S. Fu, and C.W. Hui-Chan. Ankle joint proprioception and postural control in basketball players with bilateral ankle sprains. Am J Sports Med. 2005, 33, 1174–82.

[2] J. Joyce, J. Graydon, T. McMorris, and K. Devranche. The time course effect of moderate intensity exercise on response execution and response inhibition. Brain Cogn. 2009, 71, 14-9.

[3] H. Nakamoto, and S. Mori. Sport-specific decision-making in a go/ no go reaction task: Difference among nonathletes and baseball and basketball players. Percept Mot Skill. 2008, 106, 163-71.

[4] H. Bekkering, and U. Sailer. Commentary: Coordination of eye and hand in time and space. Prog Brain Res. 2002, 140, 365-73.

[5] A. Shumway-Cook, and M. Woollacott. Motor control: Translating research into clinical practice (3rd ed.). Philadelphia: Lippincott Williams & Wilkins, 2007.

[6] J.V. Krause, D. Meyer, and J. Meyer. Basketball skills & drills (3rd ed.). Champaign, IL: Human Kinetics, 2008.

[7] W.W.N. Tsang, and C.W. Hui-Chan. Standing balance after vestibular stimulation in tai chi-practicing and nonpracticing healthy older adults. Arch Phys Med Rehabil. 2006, 87, 546-53.

[8] G.V. Bekesy. Subjective cupulometry: Threshold, adaptation, and sensation intensity of the vestibular organ for rotations in the horizontal plane. AMA Arch Otolaryngol. 1955, 61, 16-28.

[9] J.A. Goebel, and G.D. Paige. Posturography following rotation: A model of posture control during vestibular dysfunction. Otolaryngol Head Neck Surg. 1990, 102, 722-6.

[10] J.C. Kwok, C.W. Hui-Chan, and W.W. Tsang. Effects of aging and Tai Chi on finger-pointing toward stationary and moving visual targets. Arch Phys Med Rehabil. 2010, 91, 149-55.

[11] M.Y. Shaw, P.A. Gribble, and J.L. Frye. Ankle bracing, fatigue, and time to stabilisation in collegiate volleyball athletes. J Athl Train. 2008, 43, 164-71.

[12] P.A. Gribble, J. Hertel, C.R. Denegar, and W.E. Buckley. The effects of fatigue and chronic ankle instability on dynamic postural control. J Athl Train. 2004, 39, 321-9.

[13] S. Ross, and K. Guskiewicz. Examination of static and dynamic postural stability in individuals with functionally stable and unstable ankles. Clin J Sport Med. 2004, 14, 332-8.

[14] R.S. Weinberg, and D. Gould. Foundations of sport and exercise psychology. Champaign, IL: Human Kinetics, 2007.

[15] M. Collardeau, J. Brisswalter, and M. Audiffren. Effects of a prolonged run on simple reaction time of well-trained runners. Percept Mot Skill. 2001, 93, 679-89.

[16] B. Libet, E. Wright, B. Feinstein, and D. Pearl. Subjective referral of the timing for a conscious sensory experience. Brain. 1979, 102, 193-224.

[17] B. Libet, C. Gleason, E. Wright, and D. Pearl. Time of conscious intention to act in relation to onset of cerebral activity (readiness potential): The unconscious initiation of a freely voluntary act. Brain. 1983, 106, 623-42.

[18] P. Haggard, S. Clark, and J. Kalogeras. Voluntary action and conscious awareness. Nat Neurosci. 2002, 5, 382-5.

[19] R.J. Peterka. Sensorimotor integration in human postural control. J Neurophysiol. 2002, 88, 1097-118.

[20] B.L. Day, A. Severac Cauquil, L. Bartolomei, M.A. Pastor, and I.N. Lyon. Human body-segment tilts induced by galvanic stimulation: A vestibularly driven balance protection mechanism. J Physiol (Lond). 1997, 500, 661-72.

[21] A.E. Pavlik, J.T. Inglis, M. Lauk, L. Oddsson, and J.J. Collins. The effects of stochastic galvanic vestibular stimulation on human postural sway. Exp Brain Res. 1999, 24, 273-80.

[22] F. Horak, and L. Nashner. Central programming of postural movements: Adaptation to altered support surface configurations. J Neurophysiol. 1986, 55, 1369-81.

[23] P. Allard, M.L. Nault, S. Hinse, R. LeBlanc, and H. Labelle. Relationship between morphologic somatotypes and standing posture equilibrium. Ann Hum Bio. 2001, 28(6), 624-33.

[24] J.H.J. Allum, and C.R. Pfaltz. Visual and vestibular contributions to pitch sway stabilisation in the ankle muscles of normals and patients with bilateral peripheral vestibular deficits. Exp Brain Res. 1985, 58, 82-94.

[25] B.L. Day, M.J. Steiger, P.D. Thompson, and C.D. Marsden. Effect of vision and stance width on human body motion when standing: Implications for afferent control of lateral sway. J Physiol. 1993, 469, 479-99.

[26] D.A. Winter. Human balance and posture control during standing and walking. Gait Posture. 1995, 3, 193-214.

[27] L. Angyán, T. Téczely, and Z. Angyán. Factors affecting postural stability of healthy young adults. Acta Physiol Hung. 2007, 94(4), 289-99.

[28] H. Wissel. Basketball: Steps to success (2nd ed.). Champaign: Human Kinetics, 2004.

Effect of different practice schedules on learning and performance in handball task

Vahid Rouhollahi, Mansoorehossadat Rozan, Akhil Mehrotra

Department of Physical Education, Banaras Hindu University, Varanasi, India

Email address:
rouhollahi.vahid@gmail.com (V. Rouhollahi), rozan.mansoore@gmail.com (M. Rozan), drakhilhockey@yahoo.com(A. Mehrotra)

Abstract: The purpose of this study was to investigate different effects of various practice schedules in handball task. 30 participants have been divided into three equal practice groups randomly. Participants have performed a task under blocked, random and serial practice schedules and they were tested in acquisition phase conducted on five consecutive sessions with knowledge of results (KR). Delayed retention test and transfer test had been done on the next day without KR. On the basis of results of this study, there were not significant differences between various practice schedules in acquisition phase, retention and transfer tests. These findings were consistent with Magill and Hall (1990) hypothesis that the learning benefits of contextual interference are more likely to occur, when skill variations are from different classes of movement.

Keywords: Contextual Interference, Performance, Learning

1. Introduction

Motor learning has been described as a problem-solving process in which the goal of an action represents a problem and the development of an appropriate movement pattern represents the solution (Guadagnoli & Lee, 2004). Shea and Morgan (1979) are credited with being the first to demonstrate the contextual interference (CI) effect for motor skill learning (Heather Wilde et al., 2012). Contextual interference effect is "the effect on learning of the degree of functional interference found in a practice situation when several tasks must be learned and are practiced together (Magill et al., 1990). Skill acquisition researchers are interested in understanding which practice variables serve to optimize this process and consequently to understand the mechanisms that sub serve these variables. The scheduling of practice trials is one variable that has been shown to influence the efficacy of motor learning. Randomly sequencing practice trials throughout a training session (high contextual interference) has been shown to result in successful performance on tests of retention and transfer, despite poor performance during acquisition. The learner practices more than one skill is interspersed between the skills, i.e. one skill is practiced for a set number of trails, followed by practices on another skill, followed by practice on a third skill and back to beginning , then the cycle is repeated. In contrast, repeating all practice trials for one task before switching to another (low contextual interference or blocked practice) has been shown to result in impaired performance on tests of retention and transfer, despite superior performance during acquisition (Megan et al.,2011). In addition to blocked and random practice schedules, research has also been conducted on a type of serial schedule knows as moderate CI With a typical moderate schedule, a subject practices 2 or 3 trials of the same task and then is randomly switched to another task for 2 or 3 trials. However, there can be slight variations on a moderate schedule that affect acquisition and learning. A type of variation is a transitional schedule where subjects start off practicing under blocked schedules but are "transitioned" throughout acquisition into a more randomized schedule until they are practicing under a fully randomized schedule in their final trials (Gregory C. Snider,2009).Pigott & Shapiro (1984) and Al-Ameer and Toole (1993) supported this "middle of the round" type contextual interference because they argued that performance during acquisition wasn't nearly as degraded as it was during randomization and the moderate schedule was just as beneficial to learning as was the randomized schedule. Landin and Herbert (1997) would later confirm these conclusions in an applied setting with a study on basketball shooting where the group that performed under a moderate CI schedule actually performed best during both the acquisition stage as well as during retention. The researchers argued that moderate levels of contextual interference may be superior because it combines the best features of both high CI and low CI. Moderate CI allows the learner to make adjustments on the task because of the 3 trials in a row but also still offers the benefits of high CI by requiring each subject to perform several different tasks per practice session. There are various viewpoints on the contextual interference and its processes. Shea and Morgan (1979) and Shea and Zimny (1983 & 1988) proposed that when practice is performed in a random order, it has some advantages to learn via interaction between the working memories of two or more similar tasks. An increase in the interference in working memory during practice results in an increase in a distinctive and vast processing and ultimately facilitates retention (Al-Ameer, H. et al.1993).

During the last three decades, many motor learning studies have focused on dissociating between temporary performance effects and relatively permanent learning effects. These studies have demonstrated some paradoxical phenomena whereby practice schedules that hinder acquisition performance actually facilitate as assessed by retention and transfer test.

Since Shea & Morgan's (1979) study, many studies have found and explain the CI effect in motor learning. Some of these studies directly focus on investigating why the CI effect occurs; for example Shea and Morgan (1979) explained the CI effect from a viewpoint of level of elaboration imposed on learners. This explanation has some empirical support (e.g. Limon & Shea, 1998; Shea & Zimny, 1983; Wright, 1991; Wright, Li, &Whitacre, 1992). The Elaboration hypothesis has explained that when individuals shift from one skill to another during a random practice session, they are forced to become aware of the distinctiveness among the skills, making each one more meaningful in their long-term memory. More meaningful or distinctive memories are presumably more durable and therefore, more easily retrieved for use at a later time, resulting in more effective performance in retention tests (Richard A. Schmidt et al., 1999).

Lee and Magill (1985) from a view point of reconstruction of action plans explained that under high level of CI, an action plan for a particular task needs to be reconstructed every time that task is performed because the action plan is completely or partially forgotten from the working memory by intervening other tasks. Although this reconstruction process hinders acquisition performance, retention and transfer are enhanced because the reconstruction process is required during retention and transfer tests.

Other groups of studies investigated the generalizability of the effect in variety of setting. One of these groups included studies that investigated the influence of task characteristics on the CI effect. The CI effect was found with real world motor skill such as volleyball (Bortoli, Robazza Durigon & Carra, 1992), badminton serves (Goode&Magil, 1986; Wrisberg, 1991) and baseball batting (Hall, Dominguez & Cavazos, 1994).These studies provided evidence that the CI effect can occurred outside a laboratory.

Carnahan, Van Eerd, and Allard (1990) proposed that the CI effects occurs only when tasks require generation of overt movement, suggesting that different levels of CI are attributed to the process of learning motor components of a task, Similarity of task variation is another task characteristics that has recently intrigued many researchers following the Magill and Hall (1990) hypothesis. Similarity has been defined in terms of characteristics of generalized motor program (GMP) in their hypothesis and controversial finding have been reported by (Hall & Magill,1995; Lee, Wulf, & Schmidt,1992; Sekiya, Magill, & Anderson,1996; Sekiya, Magill, Sidaway, & Anderson, 1994; Wood and Ging,1991;Wulf ,1992;Lee,1993;& etc.).

Magill and Hall hypothesis proposed a limitation to the generalizability of the CI effect with respect to underlying GMP structures of task variation to be learned.

Magill and Hall (1990) hypothesis indicating that the CI effect would be found when task variations to be learned are governed by different Generalized Motor Programs(GMPs), but should not be found when task variation are governed by the same GMP. The GMP is a hypothetical notion for a memory representation that governs a class of movements (Schmidt, 1988).The GMP has invariant features such as relative timing and relative force and variant features such as overall duration and overall force. The variant features are parameters added to the fundamental GMP. Under this conceptualization, task variation with different invariant and variant feature belong to different movement classes and are controlled by different GMPs. On the other hand, when task variation share the same invariant features but differ along in variant features, the task variation belong to the same movement class and are controlled by the same GMPs. According to this hypothesis, the CI effect is unlikely to occur when task variations from the same GMP are learned. Some investigations that support the Magill and Hall (1990) hypothesis implies to this point that no CI effect with task variation controlled by the same GMP (Heitman & Gilley, 1989; Whitehurst & Del Rey, 1983; Wulf, 1992; Wulf & Lee,1993 and etc.), but some recent studies found the CI effect with task variations that are considered to be controlled by the same GMP (Carnahan et al.1990; Shea et al.1990; Young chon & Husak,1993;Hall et al.1994; Sekiya et al.,1994; etc.).

Based on Magill and Hall (1990) hypothesis, present study was designed to investigate effects of CI on performance and learning of handball center shot in novice participants because any movement has specific nature in learning process and there has been no investigation of CI effect in regards to the learning of a skill in Handball sport. This research will help to formulate, evaluate and refine techniques developed to teach and cultivate motor skill performance as effectively and efficiently as possible.

2. Method

2.1. Participants

Thirty male Physical Education students (Mage = 22.6 years, SD = 1.3 years) from Banaras Hindu University which divided into three equal blocked, random and serial practice groups has been selected randomly (see table 1). The participants had no prior experience with the task (Handball Center Shot) and were not aware of the specific purpose of the study. All participants were right-hand dominant as determined by self-report prior to the experiment. The participants read and signed an informed consent prior to participation.

***Table 1.** Participant Characteristics*

Variable	Blocked Group	Random Group	Serial Group
Age (years)	23.06±1.69	22.21±0.90	23.10±1.45
Height (cm)	169±4.64	168.90±9.25	170±6.61
Weight (kg)	61.9±3.80	64.5±7.13	63.4±2.32

2.2. Materials and Procedure

Cornish Handball Test has been constructed with an objective to measure the power of handball drive and is frequently used for testing handball skill (Devinder k.Kansal, 2008).The field was marked with a restraining line at a distance of 18 feet from a 22feet wide hard wall. This line at a distance of a 5feet behind it, made the service zone. Four additional horizontal lines at a distance of 5.75 feet were drawn behind the service zone. The subject was required to throw the ball against the front wall on which a horizontal line was marked at the height of 6 feet. Each subject was informed that he has to hit the ball up to the height marked by the horizontal line on the wall and also he was instructed clearly that he has to stroke the ball from behind the front service line. In case, the ball hits the front wall above the 6 feet line or the subject makes the foot fault that is he hits the ball in front of the service line, he was asked to restart the test. For scoring, service zone is marked as one score zone and each of 5.75 feet board zone behind the service zone was labeled as zone scoring 5, 10, 15, 20&25 respectively.

In first session, explanation and illustration of the Handball Center Shot skill was taught by coach; then subjects continued to their training with the use of Cornish test with consideration of their practice schedule. The study consisted of pre-test, acquisition phase, delayed retention test and delayed transfer test which will be explained as follows:

Pre-test: After viewing the skill, the participants performed a blocked schedule pre-test of the task that included 15 trials from 34.5 feet distance.

Acquisition phase: Prior to the first acquisition session, participants were assigned to one of three groups, which differed in the practice schedule used: blocked (n = 10), random (n = 10) and serial (n=10). The acquisition phase consisted of 225 practice trials of task for per participant in total. Participants had been trained for 5 sessions (consecutive days), in every session participants completed 45 trails according to Cornish test, and subjects have been received knowledge of their result after each block. Within each session, the blocked learners practiced all trials in blocked order. For the random group, participants practiced each task in a random order during each session and the random schedule was different for each practice session, but the same for each participant and serial schedules performed in a serial order. The task order was counterbalanced across participants.

Delayed retention test: The delayed retention test was conducted 24 hours after the last Acquisition phase session in one day. All participants completing 15 trails from 34.5 feet distance, same as pre-test performance.

Delayed transfer test: After 5min rest, each subject performed transfer test which include 15 trails on one new task, which was Handball Center Shot with 45° from center point of target with 34.5 feet distance. During delayed retention test and delayed transfer test, trials were done without KR.

3. Results

Pre-test: The pre-test confirm that there were no significant performance differences between the groups for task, $F (2, 27) = 1.11$, $p = .345$, (see figure1).

Acquisition phase results: During the acquisition period, we were evaluated with separate Learning Group × Acquisition Session (3 × 5) analyses of variance (ANOVAs) with repeated measures on the acquisition session factor. There was a significant improvement in performance across the acquisition sessions ($F (4, 135) =14.50$, $p < .05$, partial $\eta2 = .300$) .However, there was no significant main effect for learning group $F (2, 54) = 1.094$, $p = .338$. There were also no significant learning group by acquisition session interaction effects, $F (4, 135) = .219$, $p = .987$(see figure 1).

Delayed retention test results: We expected that relative to blocked practice and serial practice, random practice would result in superior performance on tests of delayed retention, to test this hypothesis, performance during the pretest and the delayed retention test were analyzed with three separate Learning Group × Test Occasion (3 × 2) ANOVAs with repeated measures on the test occasion factor. There was a significant main effect for test occasion ($F (2, 54) = 6.68$, $p < .001$, partial $\eta2 = .012$), such that the level of performance for all groups improved from the pre-test to the retention test (see Figure1). There was neither a significant main effect for learning group ($F (2, 54) = 1.90$, $p = 159$), nor a significant interaction effect ($F (2, 54) 1.17$, $p = .316$).

Paired sample t tests confirmed the impression given in Figure 1 that there were no significant differences from pretest to retention for the blocked group ($t (9) = -1.63$, $p = .138$), and also for serial group ($t (9) = -2.71$, $p = .024$), whereas the random group showed a significant improvement in performance from the pre-test to the retention test (t (9) = – 6.16, p < .001).

Delayed transfer test results: The results of transfer test showed that, there were no difference in performance between groups in this period (F (2, 27) = .809, p = .456), it means that effect of CI was not apparent in delayed transfer test (see Figure 1).

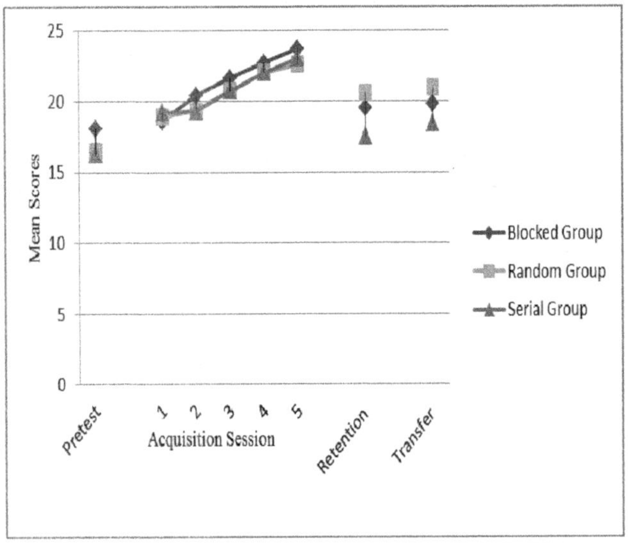

Figure 1. *Mean scores for the blocked, random and serial groups during pre-test, acquisition phase, delayed retention and delayed transfer tests*

4. Discussion

The purpose of present experiment was to investigate the effect of various practice schedules on performance and learning of a task with different distance parameters. In line with previous researches showing that random learners experience high levels of cognitive effort (e.g. Brady, 1998; Lee et al., 1994; Li & Wright, 2000; Young et al., 1993), we expected that, relative to blocked practice, random practice and serial practice would result in poor performance during acquisition phase. The results delivered mixed findings regarding this hypothesis. We found that there were no differences between the level of performance of the blocked, random and serial learners during acquisition phase. These findings contradict the traditional contextual interference effect; but support research suggesting that high contextual interference schedules are less likely to adversely affect performance during acquisition of applied tasks than laboratory based tasks. For example, Goode and Magill (1986) did not observe CI between different groups during acquisition in their applied study of blocked, random and serial practice of badminton serves (despite finding significant differences between the learning groups on both the retention and transfer tests).

With reference to retention, in the retention test, which was the critical test of learning, there were no retention benefits for the random and serial practice schedule compared to the blocked schedule, it means that effect of CI no appear in delayed retention test.

Magill and Hall (1990) suggested that including skills from different motor programs is likely to increase the amount of interference caused during the learning process (this is based on Schmidt's [1975, 1988] view of a motor program). Magill and Hall suggested that when tasks were consistent on aspects such as relative timing, sequence of events, and spatial configurations, then the tasks were unlikely to introduce a sufficient level of interference to produce the traditional interaction effect. Also according to Lee (1990) and Herbert (1996), due to the inherent attractiveness of applied task, to appear the effect of CI in this type of task, we need a lot of practice compared to laboratory tasks; thus, the significant difference between the fifth session scores with scores of previous sessions implies that further efforts are needed.

In the transfer test, there were no difference in performance between groups; it means that effect of CI was not apparent in transfer test. Our results in transfer test was consistent with the some applied studies like Chamberlin et al. (1990) in basketball jump shot but it was inconsistent with such studies Piggott & Shapiro(1984), Hall & Boyle(1993), Guadagnoli et al.(1996) and Pollock et al.(1997). Therefore, considering to lack of effect of CI in acquisition, delayed retention and transfer tests, by supporting Magill and Hall hypothesis (1990), we conclude that for the appearance of CI effect, variability of motor program parameters is not enough. Also, its seem that results of this study should await for applied investigations about effect of CI with other variables such as number of sessions and efforts, subject s experience and reliability of scoring system.

Reference

[1] Al-Ameer, H. and T. Toole, (1993). Combinations of blocked and random practice orders: Benefits to acquisition and retention. J. Human Movement

[2] Bortoli, Robazza Durigon & Carra. (1992). Effects of contextual interference on learning technical sports skills. Perceptual and Motor Skills, 75,552-56.

[3] Brady, F. (1998). A theoretical and empirical review of the contextual interference effect and the learning of motor skills. Journal of Research Quarterly for Exercise and Sports, 50, 266–293.

[4] Brady, F. (2008). The contextual interference effect and sport skills. Perceptual and Motor Skills, 106, 461–472.

[5] Carnahan, H.,Van Eerd, D.l., & Allard, F. (1990). A note on the relationship between task requirement and contextual interference. Journal of Motor Behavior, 22, 159-169.

[6] Chamberlin, C.J. et al. (1990). The ecological validity of contextual interference effect: A practical application to learning the jump shot in basketball. Paper presented at the annual meeting of North American Society for the Psychology of Sport and Physical Activity, Houston, T X.

[7] Devinder k.Kansal(2008).Applied measurement, evaluation & sports selection, Sport &spiritual science.

[8] Gregory C. Snider (2009).The effect of random, blocked, and transition practice schedules on children's performance of a barrier knockdown test,p.g.6-7

[9] Goode, S., & Magill, R. A. (1986). Investigation of the contextual interference effect in the manipulation of the motor parameter of over-all force. Perceptual and Motor Skills, 83, 735–743.

[10] Guadagnoli,M.A & Holcomb,W.R. (1996). The effect of variable and constant practice on the skill of putting. Science of Golf ш. Human Kinetics, campaign, IL.

[11] Hall, K.G. & Boyle, M. (1993). The effects of contextual interference on shuffleboard skill in children. Research Quarterly for Exercise and Sports, 64, 74-78.

[12] Hall, K.G., Dominquez, D.A., & Cavazos, R. (1994). Contextual interference effects with skilled baseball players. Perceptual and Motor Skills, 78, 835- 841.

[13] Hall, K.G., & Magill, R.A. (1995).Variability of practice and contextual interference in motor skill learning. Journal of Motor Behavior, 27,299-309.

[14] Heather Wilde, Curt Magnuson, & Charles H. Shea (2012). Random and Blocked Practice of Movement Sequences: Differential Effects on Response Structure and Movement Speed. Research Quarterly for Exercise and Sports,76,416-425.

[15] Heitman, R.J., & Gilley, W.F. (1989). Effects of blocked versus random practice by mentally retarded subjects on learning a novel skill. Perceptual and Motor Skills, 69, 443-447.

[16] Herbert, E.P. et al. (1996). Practice schedules effects on the performance and learning of low and high skilled studies: An applied study. Research Quarterly for Exercise and Sports, 67, 52-58.

[17] Landin, D., & Hebert, E.P. (1997). A comparison of three practice schedule along the contextual interference continuum. Research Quarterly for Exercise and Sport,68, 357-361.

[18] Lee,T.D., & CARNAHAM,H.(1990). When to provide knowledge of results during motor learning: Scheduling effects. Human performance, 3, 87-105.

[19] Lee, T.D. & Magill, R.A. (1985). Can forgetting facilitate skill actuation? In D. Goodman, R.B. Wilberg, & I.M. Frank (Eds), Differing perspectives in motor learning memory, and control (pp.3-22). Amsterdam: North-Holland.

[20] Lee, T. D., Swinnen, S. P., & Serrien, D. J. (1994). Cognitive effort and motor learning. Research Quarterly for Exercise and Sport, 46, 328–344.

[21] Lee, T. D., & Simon, D. A. (2004). Contextual interference. In A.M. Williams & N. J. Hodges (Eds.), Skill Acquisition in sport: Research, theory, and practice (pp. 29–44). London, England: Routledge.

[22] Lee, T.D. & Weeks, D.J. (1987).The beneficial influence of forgetting on short-term retention of movement information. Human movement science, 6,233-245.

[23] Li, Y., & Wright, D. L. (2000). An assessment of the attention demands during random- and blocked-practice schedules. Quarterly Journal of Experimental Psychology, 53A, 591–606.

[24] Limons, E., & Shea , J.B. (1988). Deficient processing in learning and performance. In A.M. Colley & J.R.Beech (Eds.), Cognition and action in skilled behavior, (pp.333-347).

[25] Magill, R. A., & Hall, K. G. (1990). A review of the contextual interference effect in motor skill acquisition. Journal of Human Movement Science, 9, 241–289.

[26] Megan A. Rendell1, Rich S. W. Masters, Damian Farrow & Tony Morris, (2011). An Implicit Basis for the Retention Benefits of Random Practice. Journal of Motor Behavior, Vol. 43, No. 1.

[27] Pigott, R.E. & Shapiro,D.C (1984). Motor schema: The structure of the variability session. Research Quarterly for Exercise and Sports, 55, 41-45.

[28] Keating, D.P. (1980). Four faces of creativity: The continuing plight of the intellectually under served. Gifted Child Quarterly, 24: 56-61.

[29] Pigott, R.E., & Shapiro, D.C. (1984). Motor Schema: The structure of the variability session. Research Quarterly for Exercise and Sport, 55, 41-45.

[30] Pollock, B.J. & Lee, T.D. (1997). Dissociate contextual interference in children and adults. Perceptual and Motor Skills, 84,851-858.

[31] Richard A. Schmidt, Craig A. Wrisberg (1999). A situation based learning approach, p.g.259.

[32] Schmidt, R. A. (1975). A schema theory of discrete motor skill learning. Psychological Review, 82, 225–260.

[33] Schmidt, R. A. (1988). Motor control and learning: A behavioral emphasis (2nd Ed.). Champaign, IL: Human Kinetics.

[34] Sekiya,H.(1997). Interactive influence of task characteristics and amount of practice on the contextual interference effect in motor learning. Mem,Fac.Integrad Arts and Sci., Hiroshima Uni.,23,87-105.

[35] Sekiya, H., Magill R.A. & Anderson, D.I. (1996). The contextual interference effect in parameter modifications of the same generalized motor program. Research Quarterly for Exercise and Sport, 67, 59-68.

[36] Sekiya, H., Magill, R.A., Sidaway, B., & Anderson, D.I. (1994). The contextual interference effects for skill variations from the same and different generalized motor programs. Research Quarterly for Exercise and Sports, 65, 330-338.

[37] Shea, C. H., Kohl, R., & Indermill, C. (1990). Contextual interference: Contributions of practice. Acta Psychological, 73, 145-157.

[38] Shea, J. B., & Morgan, R. L. (1979). Contextual interference effects on the acquisition, retention and transfer of a motor skill. Journal of Experimental Psychology, Human Learning and Memory, 5, 179–187.

[39] Shea,J.B., & Zimny, S.T. (1983). Context effects in memory and learning movement information. In R.K. Magill (Ed.), Memory and control of action, (pp.345-366).

[40] Whitehurst, M. & Del Ray, P. (1983). Effects of contextual interference, task difficulty, and levels of processing on pursuit tracking. Perceptual and Motor Skills, 57, 619–628.

[41] Wood, C.A., & Ging, C.A. (1991). The role of interference and task similarity on the acquisition, retention and transfer of simple motor skill. Research Quarterly for Exercise and Sport, 62, 18-26.

[42] Wright, D. L. (1991). The role of inter task and intra task processing in acquisition and retention of motor skills. Journal of Motor Behavior, 23, 139–145.

[43] Wright, D. L., Li, Y., & Whitacre, C. (1992). The contribution of elaborative processing to the contextual interference effect. Research Quarterly for Exercise and Sport, 58, 369–374.

[44] Wrisberg, C.A. (1991). A field test of effect of contextual variety during skill acquisition. Journal of Teaching in Physical Education, 11, 21-33.

[45] Wulf, G. (1992). Reducing knowledge of results can produce context effects in movements of the same class. Journal of Human Movement Studies, 22, 71-84.

[46] Wulf, G. & Lee,T.D. (1993). Contextual interference effects in movements of the same class: Differential effects on program and parameter learning. Journal of Motor Behavior, 25,263.

[47] Young, D. E., Cohen, M. J., & Husak, W. S. (1993). Contextual interference and motor skill acquisition: On the processes that influence retention. Human Movement Science, 12, 577–600.

Permissions

All chapters in this book were first published in AJSS, by Science Publishing Group; hereby published with permission under the Creative Commons Attribution License or equivalent. Every chapter published in this book has been scrutinized by our experts. Their significance has been extensively debated. The topics covered herein carry significant findings which will fuel the growth of the discipline. They may even be implemented as practical applications or may be referred to as a beginning point for another development.

The contributors of this book come from diverse backgrounds, making this book a truly international effort. This book will bring forth new frontiers with its revolutionizing research information and detailed analysis of the nascent developments around the world.

We would like to thank all the contributing authors for lending their expertise to make the book truly unique. They have played a crucial role in the development of this book. Without their invaluable contributions this book wouldn't have been possible. They have made vital efforts to compile up to date information on the varied aspects of this subject to make this book a valuable addition to the collection of many professionals and students.

This book was conceptualized with the vision of imparting up-to-date information and advanced data in this field. To ensure the same, a matchless editorial board was set up. Every individual on the board went through rigorous rounds of assessment to prove their worth. After which they invested a large part of their time researching and compiling the most relevant data for our readers.

The editorial board has been involved in producing this book since its inception. They have spent rigorous hours researching and exploring the diverse topics which have resulted in the successful publishing of this book. They have passed on their knowledge of decades through this book. To expedite this challenging task, the publisher supported the team at every step. A small team of assistant editors was also appointed to further simplify the editing procedure and attain best results for the readers.

Apart from the editorial board, the designing team has also invested a significant amount of their time in understanding the subject and creating the most relevant covers. They scrutinized every image to scout for the most suitable representation of the subject and create an appropriate cover for the book.

The publishing team has been an ardent support to the editorial, designing and production team. Their endless efforts to recruit the best for this project, has resulted in the accomplishment of this book. They are a veteran in the field of academics and their pool of knowledge is as vast as their experience in printing. Their expertise and guidance has proved useful at every step. Their uncompromising quality standards have made this book an exceptional effort. Their encouragement from time to time has been an inspiration for everyone.

The publisher and the editorial board hope that this book will prove to be a valuable piece of knowledge for researchers, students, practitioners and scholars across the globe.

List of Contributors

Francesco Feletti
U.O.Radiologia, Presidio Ospedaliero di Ravenna, Viale Randi 5, Ravenna, Italia.

Raja Ben Sassi
Hôpital militaire de Tunis, centre d'oxygénothérapie hyperbare, 1008, Tunis, Tunisie.

Karima Taamallah
Université de Tunis El Manar, Faculté de Médecine de Tunis, 1007, Tunis, Tunisie
Hôpital militaire de Tunis, service de chirurgie cardiaque, 1008, Tunis, Tunisie.

Imen Mezoughi
Hôpital militaire de Tunis, centre d'oxygénothérapie hyperbare, 1008, Tunis, Tunisie.

Walid Belhaj Brahim
Hôpital militaire de Tunis, centre d'oxygénothérapie hyperbare, 1008, Tunis, Tunisie.

Zied Hajjej
Université de Tunis El Manar, Faculté de Médecine de Tunis, 1007, Tunis, Tunisie
Hôpital militaire de Tunis, service d'anesthésie réanimation, 1008, Tunis, Tunisie.

Hedi Gharsallah
Université de Tunis El Manar, Faculté de Médecine de Tunis, 1007, Tunis, Tunisie
Hôpital militaire de Tunis, centre d'oxygénothérapie hyperbare, 1008, Tunis, Tunisie.

Hugo Machado Sanchez
Master Physical Therapy, Teacher of Physical Therapy in UniRV (University of Green River), Rio Verde-GO, Brazil.

Eliane Gouveia de Morais Sanchez
Master in Education (UFU), Rio Verde-GO, Brazil.

Mario Antonio Baraúna
PhD. in Motricity Human for University of Lisboa (POR), Uberlândia-MG, Brazil.

Roberto Sérgio de Tavares Canto
Post-doctoral in Traumatology for University of Liverpool (ING), Uberlândia-MG, Brazil.

Pouya Jalilian, Patrick K. Kreun, MohammadHady M. Makhmalbaf and William W. Liou
Department of Mechanical and Aerospace Engineering, Western Michigan University, Kalamazoo, MI 49008, USA.

Sridip Chatterjee
Department of Physical Education, Jadavpur University, Kolkata - 700032, West Bengal, India.

Aloke Sen Borman
Seva Bharati Mahavidyalaya, Department of Physical Education, Kapgari - 721505, Paschim Midnapore, West Bengal, India.

Aparup Konar
Director of Physical Instruction, Office of the Sports Board, Jadavpur University, Kolkata - 700032, West Bengal, India.

Samiran Mondal
Department of Physical Education, Vinaya Bhavana, Visva Bharati, Santiniketan - 731235, West Bengal, India.

Makram Zghibi
LASELDI, University of Franche-Comté, Besançon, France.

Nabila Bennour
UMR EFTS, Le Mirail University, Toulouse II, France.

Mohamed Jabri and Hajer Sahli
Higher Institute of Sports and Physical Education, Kef, Tunisia, Tunisia .

Index